Practical Techniques in Periodontics and Implant Dentistry

Practical Techniques in Periodontics and Implant Dentistry

Edited by

Edgard El Chaar, DDS, MS
Department of Periodontics
University of Pennsylvania, Dental Medicine
Philadelphia, PA, USA

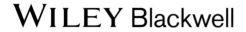

Registered Office
John Wiley & Sons, Inc., 111 River Street, Hoboken, NJ 07030, USA

Editorial Office
111 River Street, Hoboken, NJ 07030, USA

For details of our global editorial offices, customer services, and more information about Wiley products visit us at www.wiley.com.

Wiley also publishes its books in a variety of electronic formats and by print-on-demand. Some content that appears in standard print versions of this book may not be available in other formats.

Library of Congress Cataloging-in-Publication Data applied for

ISBN: 9781119793557 (hardback)

Cover Design: Wiley
Cover Images: Courtesy of Edgard El Chaar

Set in 9.5/12.5pt STIXTwoText by Straive, Chennai, India

Printed in Singapore
M115720_270922

Contents

List of Contributors

Thierry Abitbol
Arthur Ashman Department of Periodontics and Implant Dentistry
New York University
New York, NY
USA

Roya Afshar-Mohajer
Ashman Department of Periodontology and Implant Dentistry
New York University College of Dentistry
New York, NY
USA

Zahra Bagheri
Ashman Department of Periodontology and Implant Dentistry
New York University College of Dentistry
New York, NY
USA

Michael Bral
Department of Periodontics and Implant Dentistry
New York University College of Dentistry
New York, NY
USA

Edgard El Chaar
Department of Periodontics
University of Pennsylvania
Dental Medicine
Philadelphia, PA
USA

Steven Engebretson
Department of Periodontology and Implant Dentistry
New York University College of Dentistry
New York, NY
USA

Aikaterini Georgantza
Ashman Department of Periodontology and Implant Dentistry
New York University College of Dentistry
New York, NY
USA

Babak Hamidi
Ashman Department of Periodontology and Implant Dentistry
New York University College of Dentistry
New York, NY
USA

Arthi M. Kumar
Department of Oral and Maxillofacial Pathology
Radiology & Medicine
New York University College of Dentistry
New York, NY
USA

Wayne Kye
Ashman Department of Periodontology and Implant Dentistry
New York University College of Dentistry
New York, NY
USA

Claire Mc carthy
King's College
London
UK

Dena M. Sapanaro
Department of Pediatric Dentistry
New York University
New York, NY
USA

Stuart L. Segelnick
Arthur Ashman Department of Periodontics and
Implant Dentistry
New York University
New York, NY
USA

Mea A. Weinberg
Arthur Ashman Department of Periodontics and
Implant Dentistry
New York University
New York, NY
USA

Cecilia White
Private practice
Princeton, NJ
USA

Introduction

In the past 28 years, from being a resident to academician and clinical practitioner in the science of Periodontics and Implant Dentistry, I have witnessed an exponential evolution in the possibilities of treatments. Consequently, that comes with a wealth of information to the practitioners making the discernment between validity of treatment choices difficult. I worked throughout the years on basing my treatments and my teaching around solid biological foundation because I always believed that fundamentals never change. With that in mind, the practitioner has to always set the goal of treatment and then work his/her way back to evaluate the steps it takes to execute it. These steps have to be based on, as stated before, solid biological foundations.

In order to understand these solid foundations, we built this manuscript in a way to start with a review of fundamentals, mainly the wound healing, preparing a more in depth focused vented information that the practitioner can review. These will be done in a facilitated manner without compromising on the needed fundamentals. This manuscript will help either a practitioner in preparing a surgical decision, a resident preparing for his/her boards, or a dental student/surgical resident learning the science of Periodontics and Implant Dentistry.

I am grateful for my colleagues that contributed to this manuscript, without their invaluable participation this manuscript would have not become a reality, thus benefiting the user of this work. I would like to specifically thank my oldest daughter, Lauren, for encouraging me and helping me in the writing of the proposal to the publisher during the lockdown for the Covid-19 pandemic. I hope that she, or one of my other children, one day use it for their studies if they decide to take dentistry as their vocational professional career. Finally, for you the reader, I am honored and humbled that you chose this book in your endeavor. Periodontology-Implant Dentistry has been a great journey for me and I hope it will be the same for you. Keep learning and always remember three things: biology always wins, fundamentals never change, set your goal, and work your way back.

Sincerely,
Edgard El Chaar

Part I

Fundamentals

1

Anatomy and Physiology

Edgard El Chaar[1] and Thierry Abitbol[2]

[1] *Department of Periodontics, University of Pennsylvania, Dental Medicine, Philadelphia, PA, USA*
[2] *Arthur Ashman Department of Periodontics and Implant Dentistry, New York University, NY, USA*

Overview of Gingival Tissue and Periodontium

Macroscopically, the dental organ appears to be limited to the dental crown surrounded by soft tissue, which is scalloped around a well delineated circular line called the cementoenamel junction (CEJ).

The morphology of the dental crowns change shape from the midline to the posterior dentition and with it, the function and dimension change. The soft tissue changes as well to accommodate these differences. That soft tissue will comprise two distinct parts, the mucosa and the keratinized tissue separated by the mucogingival line (MGL). In the keratinized zone, we have the attached gingiva and the marginal gingiva. The latter is a non-attached tissue that extends few millimeters from the margin to the junctional epithelium (JE), delineating the sulcus that is a gap on the inner side of the non-attached gingiva around the CEJ. JE is non-keratinized epithelium as it is on the border of the attached and non-attached gingiva.

In a microscopic cross-sectional view, we can appreciate the different parts of hard and soft tissue interacting together making the periodontium of the dental organ from its incisal tip apically (Figure 1.1). This figure shows the intricate components of the dental organ and the harmony needed to make this interaction work reminding us of a well-tuned opera. All of this hard and soft tissue requires irrigation from perfectly lined up blood circulation, which originates from an alveolar artery dividing itself in a periodontal ligament (PDL) branch, dental branch, and an intra-marrow branch. Inside the mucosa, an intricate circular system leads to a supra-periosteal artery crossing into the keratinized gingiva in a linear manner up to the gingival collar in which the three arteries,

PDL, intra-marrow, and supra-periosteal form the gingival crevicular plexus (Figure 1.2).

Radiographically, the PDL space can be observed and its width ranges between 0.1 and 0.25 mm (Figure 1.3). Any widening beyond these margins is considered a "widening of the periodontal ligament," which can be a sign of inflammation either from an early periodontal disease at the coronal level or excessive occlusal trauma.

This harmonious intricate system called the dental periodontium will be reviewed in this manual, wishing you great reading and enjoyment.

Embryonic Development

At approximately four to five weeks into embryonic development, there is downgrowth of the ectoderm of the primitive oral stomatodeum into the underlying ectomesenchyme. At the terminal end of this downgrowth, the cells form a knoblike structure or bud. Cells in the surrounding ectomesenchyme begin to concentrate around this bud.

Several weeks later, this ectodermal bud has developed into a cuplike structure with four distinct layers: an outer enamel epithelium (OEE), an inner enamel epithelium (IEE), a stellate reticulum (SR), and a stratum intermedium (SI). Directly beneath the IEE, cells of the underlying ectomesenchyme have condensed into a dental papilla (DP). Surrounding these two structures is a third condensation, the dental follicle (DF), which will give rise to most of the cementum, periodontal ligament, and alveolar bone.

At the apical extent of the root, the IEE and OEE have fused to form Hertwig's epithelial root sheath (HES). More coronally, this root sheath breaks down to form islands of

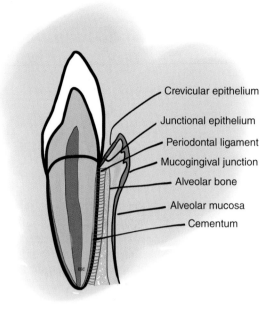

Figure 1.1 Different components of the periodontium in a cross section.

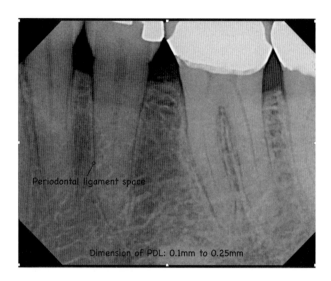

Figure 1.3 Dimension of periodontal ligament.

epithelial cells in the developing PDL space, the epithelial rests of Malassez (ERM). The breakdown of the root sheath and subsequent exposure of the dentin (D) to the DF allows cells in the DF nearest the developing root surface to differentiate into cementoblasts (CB) and lay down the first cementum matrix (CM). Further away from the tooth follicle, cells differentiate into fibroblasts and lay down the first bundles of collagen in the PDL (Figures 1.3–1.6).

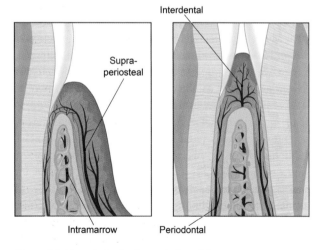

Figure 1.2 Vascularity in the periodontal ligament.

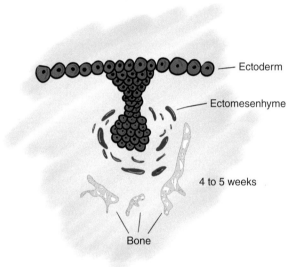

Figure 1.4 Bud stage in embryologic formation of the dental organ.

to CEJ. During eruption, the tip of the tooth approaches the oral mucosa leading to a fusion of the RED with oral epithelium (OE). Once the tip emerges, the RED is termed Epithelial Attachment. As the tooth erupts, the attached epithelium gradually separates from its surface creating a groove called the Gingival Sulcus.

Formation of the Epithelial Attachment

After formed, the enamel is covered by an epithelium called the reduced dental epithelium (RED) extending

Formation of the Cementum, Periodontal Ligament, and Alveolar Bone

The deposition of cementum on the root surface that gradually thickens toward the PDL space is somewhat similar

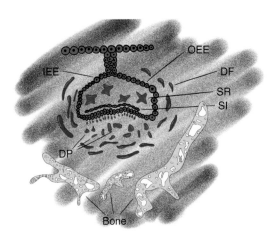

Figure 1.5 Bell stage in embryologic formation. (OEE: outer enamel epithelium; IEE: inner enamel epithelium; SR: stellate reticulum; SI: stratum intermedium; DF: dental follicle; DP: dental papilla).

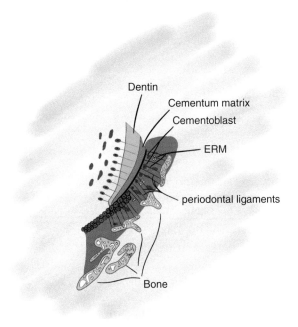

Figure 1.6 Apical formation of the different periodontal ligament. ERM, epithelial rest of malassez; HES, Hertwig's epithelial root sheath.

to the deposition of alveolar bone that thickens the alveolar bone support from the opposite side of the ligament space. As a result, the cementum does have some structural and biochemical similarities (as well as some critical differences) with alveolar bone.

As with the development of the alveolar bone proper, an organic matrix of cementum composed primarily of type I and type III collagen is secreted by a layer of formative cells (the cementoblasts) over the thin hyaline-like

layer secreted by HES covering the root dentin. This fine fibrillar matrix calcifies to form a relatively uniform and well-organized layer of cementum free of cellular elements called primary acellular cementum. This first thin layer of mineralized cementum contains only the fibrillar matrix from the cementoblasts themselves. These fibers are therefore called intrinsic fibers of cementum.

As the cementum continues to thicken by apposition of cementum by the cementoblast layers, this thickening cementum will encounter and incorporate bundles of the forming periodontal ligament. These ligament bundles incorporated into the cementum surface will calcify along with the surrounding intrinsic fibers to form a significant portion of the more superficial layers of the cementum. These insertions of calcified ligament fibers are termed extrinsic fibers of the cementum. A similar entrapment and calcification process occurs on the forming alveolar bone side. The general term for these calcified insertions of bundles of ligament fibers into the cementum and bone are Sharpey's fibers. On the cementum side, these Sharpey's fibers are much thinner in diameter and insert at closer intervals when compared with the alveolar bone side.

These differences in the pattern of insertion have clinical importance in the distribution of forces that are generated within the PDL during occlusion, tooth movement, and traumatic forces. Specifically, these forces are more evenly distributed along the cementum surface and are more concentrated along the more widely spaced insertions on the alveolar bone side. As a result, in response to mechanical forces, there is generally a remodeling of the periodontal housing on the alveolar bone side and not on the cementum side. This prevents the possibility of significant cementum and root resorption. In addition, the root cementum is protected from this relatively extensive remodeling because it is avascular, and therefore not as exposed to osteoclast-like precursor cells in the circulation. Although small areas of microscopic cementum resorption and repair have been frequently observed in histologic sections, more extensive resorption of cementum is usually not seen unless there is a force on the tooth of a high enough magnitude, or duration, or both, that cannot be accommodated by the remodeling of the alveolar bone.

As the tooth completes actively erupting into the oral cavity and meets its opposing tooth in the other arch, the formation of cementum becomes somewhat less regular and organized. This type of cementum formation that occurs over the more organized primary cementum is called secondary cementum. It occurs mainly along the apical one third of the root. During the formation of secondary cementum, cells in the layer of secreting cementoblasts will often become entrapped within the CM. These entrapped cementoblasts become cementocytes similar in appearance to the entrapped osteoblasts that become osteocytes on the alveolar bone side. These areas of cementum that contain cementocytes are called cellular cementum. Layers of cellular cementum are generally seen in the apical one third of the root surface. In secondary cementum, these layers of cellular cementum often alternate with layers of acellular cementum.

Soft Tissue Physiology

Gingiva

The gingiva consists of free and attached tissue. The attached gingiva is the portion of the gingiva that is firm, dense, stippled, and tightly bound to the underlying periodontium, tooth, and bone. The free gingival margin is defined as the coronal border of the free gingiva that surrounds the tooth and is not directly attached to the tooth surface. The free gingival margin generally corresponds to the base of the gingival sulcus. It is present in 30–40% of adults and most frequently occurs in the mandibular premolar and incisor regions. The mucogingival junction (MGJ) represents the junction between the gingiva (keratinized) and alveolar mucosa (non-keratinized) (Lindhe 1983).

Width and Thickness of the Gingiva
Bowers (1963) measured the widths of the facial attached gingiva in the primary and permanent dentitions of 240 subjects. The width of attached gingiva ranged from 1 to 9 mm. Values were greatest in the incisor regions (especially the lateral incisor) and the least in the canine and first premolar sites. The maxilla usually exhibited a broader zone of the attached gingiva than the mandible. Clinically healthy gingiva was noted in subjects with less than 1 mm of the attached gingiva, but the tissue was usually inflamed in areas of no attached gingiva. Buccal–lingual tooth position affected the amount of the attached gingiva present, and high frenum and muscle attachments were generally associated with narrow zones of attached gingiva. Facially positioned teeth had narrower zones of attached and keratinized tissue than well-aligned or lingually positioned teeth. As teeth moved lingually, an increase in the width of attached and keratinized tissue and a slight decrease in clinical crown height were observed. Teeth moving facially had a decrease in the width of the attached and keratinized tissue.

Voigt et al. (1978) measured the width of lingual attached gingiva in the mandible. The keratinized tissue ranged from 1 to 8 mm. Greatest widths were recorded on the first and second molars (4.7 mm), decreasing at premolar and third molar sites. The smallest widths were observed on the incisors and canines (1.9 mm).

Goaslind et al. (1977) measured the thickness of the free and attached facial gingiva in a population consisting of 10 males (ages 25–36). Results demonstrated considerable variation of gingival thickness among subjects and among areas within individual subjects. Free gingival thickness averaged 1.56–0.39 mm, increased from anterior to posterior and was directly proportional to sulcus depth. Thickness of the attached gingiva averaged 1.25–0.42 mm, increased from anterior to posterior in the mandibular arch, remained relatively constant in the maxillary anterior, and was inversely proportional to attached gingival width. The overall mean thickness for all areas was 1.41 mm.

Histological Composition
As discussed in the tooth development section, while tooth emerges and eruption continues, three distinct zones of epithelium form: outer epithelium, crevicular epithelium, and the JE. Each is different in stratification, organization, and function.

Like the epidermis, the OE has multiple layers:

1. **Stratum basale**: one to two layer of cuboidal-shaped cells that divide and migrate to the superficial layers
2. **Stratum spinosum or prickle cell layer**: spinous-shaped cells with large intercellular spaces
3. **Stratum granulosum**: flattened granular cells with flattened and condensed nuclei, increased accumulation of keratohyalin granules, and intracellular and extracellular membrane-coated granules
4. **Stratum corneum**: flattened cells packed with keratin; nuclei may be undiscernible known as orthokeratinized or may have visible dense nuclei called parakeratinized; cells shed and are replaced by cells from the deeper layers migrating upward.

In both the basal and prickle cell layers connect to each other via desmosomes, which appear microscopically as a thickening. Each half is made of a hemi-desmosome that attach to underlying cell through intermediate filaments. Within the oral gingival epithelium, there are several other cells not derived from keratinocytes. These include melanocytes that transfer melanin pigment granules to the surrounding basal layer of keratinocytes, Langerhans cells that are part of the reticulo-endothelium system and are responsible for processing and presenting foreign antigens to the immune system, and Merkel cells that may be responsible for perception of sensation in the gingiva.

On the outer layer, in 45% of the patient, stippling is noticed. It used to be thought that its presence is a sign of health but later it was refuted. Based on Karring and Loe (1970), the stippling coincides with the intersection with epithelial ridges. Epithelial (rete) ridges represent areas of epithelial proliferation into the underlying connective tissue (CT). These are believed to promote anchoring of epithelium to the CT by increasing the surface area of attachment. They are more pronounced in the gingiva than in the alveolar mucosa.

The CT of the gingiva consists of cells, fibers, and ground substance (proteoglycans [PGs] and glycoproteins [GPs]). Cells constitute about 5% of the CT and include fibroblasts (65%), mast cells, PMNs, macrophages, lymphocytes, and plasma cells. Fibers account for approximately 60–65% of the CT, with collagen predominating reticulin and elastic fibers. Ground substance comprises 35% of the CT and consists of protein-polysaccharide macro-molecules made up of PGs and GPs. The PGs contain glycosaminoglycans (GAGs) as the polysaccharide units that are covalently bonded to one or more protein chains. PGs are usually large molecules in the ground substance that function to regulate diffusion and fluid flow through the matrix, acting as molecular filters. GPs function in cell-to-cell and cell-to-matrix interactions. Fibronectin (FN) is the principal GP in CT, serving to orient fibroblasts to collagen and provide protein attachment for cell–matrix adhesions. FN may influence the migration of fibroblasts and play a crucial role in maintaining structural integrity of CT. Laminin (LN) is the attachment GP for epithelial cells, which mediates attachment of these cells to the basement membrane and preferentially binds type IV collagen.

Epithelial–Connective Tissue Interaction

Karring et al. (1975) examined the role of CT in determining differentiation of the epithelium by implanting CT from the palates of monkeys (with the epithelium removed) into pouches created in the buccal alveolar mucosa. Three to four weeks later, the grafts were exposed and allowed to re-epithelialize from surrounding non-keratinized alveolar mucosa. The sites with CT transplants from the palate healed with a keratinized surface displaying the same characteristics as normal gingival epithelium. The results of this study demonstrated conclusively that the determinant for epithelial differentiation (keratinization or non-keratinization) is the underlying CT and is not the functional stimuli as previously thought.

Gingival Fiber Groups

Hassell (2000), described the gingival collagen fibers and divided them into five principal and six minor groupings.

The principal groupings:

a. Dentogingival
b. Alveolo-gingival
c. Dento-periosteal
d. Circular
e. Transseptal

The secondary grouping:

a. Periosteogingival
b. Interpapillary
c. Transgingival
d. Intercircular
e. Intergingival
f. Semicircular

The dentogingival fibers extend from the cementum into the lamina propria laterally. Alveolo-gingival fibers "fan" coronally into the lamina propria from the periosteum at the alveolar crest. The dento-periosteal fibers extend from the cementum (close to CEJ) into the periosteum at the alveolar crest. Circular fibers circumscribe the tooth and are present in the attached gingival coronal to the alveolar crest and in the free marginal gingiva. The transseptal fibers extend mesially and distally, inserting into the cementum of the adjacent teeth coronal to the alveolar crest.

Alveolar Mucosa

The alveolar mucosa covers the basal part of the alveolar process and continues without demarcation into the vestibular fornix and the floor of the mouth. It is movable and loosely attached to the periosteum.

The main difference with the gingiva is the vascular network distributed within the periosteum of the alveolar mucosa. It is densely arranged, consisting of arterioles, venules, and a large number of capillaries. This difference in distribution of vessels is considered to reflect the histological difference. In the attached gingiva, the CT is firmly attached to the alveolar process and that is mainly due to its function which is to resist the compression and friction of mastication (Squier and Hill 1985). In contrast, the lamina propria and submucosal tissue beneath the alveolar mucosa have a fibrous structure consisting of many elastic fibers that are loosely attached to the periosteum to handle the vascular meshwork that is mainly circular and stacked. According to Lozdan and Squier (1969), the marked difference in elastic tissue content between the gingiva and alveolar mucosa was used as a reference to define this transition and the position of the MGJ.

Junctional Epithelium

As discussed earlier in the tooth development, with the tooth eruption, the OE and the reduced enamel epithelium (REE) fuse and the JE is formed. In periodontal health the JE consists of a single or multiple layers of non-keratinizing cells adhering to the tooth surface and functions as a security seal-barrier at the base of the sulcus.

Sabag and Saglie (1981) described the attachment of epithelium to the cementum root surface to be mediated by four to eight hemidesmosomes per micron at the coronal zone of epithelial attachment and two hemidesmosomes per micron in the apical zone. Because of this arrangement, the authors suggested that the coronal zone of the cemental surface may exhibit enhanced adhesion of epithelial attachment when compared with the apical zone Gargiulo et al. (1961) studied the dimensions and relations of the dento-gingival junction in man. The mean average length of the epithelial attachment (phases I–IV) was 0.97 mm with a range of 0.71–1.35 mm mean average.

Histologically, Ten Cate (1989) found that the immature character of the JE was characterized by the presence of hemidesmosomes that are necessary for epithelial attachment but are not seen in gingival and sulcular epithelium.

Biotype

The periodontal biotype and its clinical significance have fascinated clinicians and researchers since the early twentieth century. As early as 1923, Hirschfeld conducted an anthropometric study on human skulls, in which he noted the existence of a thin alveolar contour. He postulated that such a thin bony contour was likely accompanied by a thin gingival form. Later on, in 1969, Oschenbein and Ross classified the gingival anatomy as either flat or pronounced scalloped. They suggested that flat gingiva was related to square tooth forms and pronounced scalloped gingiva was related to tapered tooth forms. In 1977, Weisgold asserted that a thin, scalloped gingival architecture has an increased susceptibility to recession.

Later in 2009, De Rouck et al. illustrated the presence of two distinct gingival biotypes. The first type was thin-scalloped, making up one-third of the study population. These subjects typically had a slender tooth form, a narrow zone of keratinized tissue, and tended to be females. The second type was described as thick-flat, occurring in two-thirds of the study population. These cases were comprised of a more square tooth form, a broad zone of keratinized tissue, and were typically found in males.

In a 2010 systematic review, Fu et al. detailed the different clinical methods of diagnosing biotype and the differences noted between the two, as illustrated in the following table:

Characteristics	Thin	Thick
Profile	Highly scalloped soft tissue and bone contours	Relatively flat soft tissue and bone contours
Soft tissue texture	Delicate, friable	Dense, fibrotic
Width of keratinized and attached gingiva	Narrow	Wide
Bone thickness	Thin; presence of bony dehiscences and fenestrations	Thick; presence of ledges
Reaction to insults	Reacts readily with recession	Relatively resistant to gingival recessions; reacts with pocket formation or intrabony defects

Periodontal Biotype

One way to describe individual differences as they relate to the focus of this review is the periodontal "biotype." The biotype has been labeled by different authors as gingival or periodontal biotype, morphotype, or phenotype. In this review, it will be referred to as periodontal biotype. The assessment of periodontal biotype is considered relevant for outcome assessment of therapy in several dental disciplines, including periodontal and implant therapy, prosthodontics, and orthodontics. Overall, the distinction among different biotypes is based upon a multitude of anatomic characteristics of the components of the masticatory complex, including:

1. Gingival biotype, which includes in its definition gingival thickness (GT) and keratinized tissue width (KTW)
2. Bone morphotype (BM)
3. Tooth dimension

A recent systematic review Zweers et al. (2014), using the parameters reported previously, classified the biotypes in three categories:

Biotype	Crown form	Cervical convexities	Location of contacts	Zone of KT	Tissue quality	Alveolar bone quality
Thin scalloped	Slender, Triangular	Subtle	Incisal	Narrow	Clear, thin	Thin
Thick flat	Square	Pronounced	Cervical	Broad	Thick, fibrotic	Thick
Thick Scalloped	Slender	Variable	Variable	Narrow	Thick, fibrotic	Variable

The strongest association within the different parameters used to identify the different biotypes is found among GT, KTW, and BM. These parameters have been reported to be frequently associated with the development or progression of mucogingival defects, gingival recession in particular. Keratinized tissue width ranges in a thin biotype from 2.75 (0.48) mm to 5.44 (0.88) mm and in a thick biotype from 5.09 (1.00) mm to 6.65 (1.00) mm. The calculated weighted mean for the thick biotype was 5.72 (0.95) mm (95% CI 5.20; 6.24) and 4.15 (0.74) mm (95% CI 3.75; 4.55) for the thin biotype. Gingival thickness ranges from 0.63 (0.11) mm to 1.79 (0.31) mm. An overall thinner GT was observed with canine teeth and ranged from 0.63 (0.11) mm to 1.24 (0.35) mm, with a weighted mean (thin) of 0.80 mm (0.19).

When discriminating between either a thin or thick periodontal biotype, in general, a thinner GT can be found in a thin biotype population regardless of the selected study. Bone morphotype (BM) resulted in a mean buccal bone thickness of 0.343 (0.135) mm for thin biotype and 0.754 (0.128) mm for thick/average biotype. BMs have been radiographically measured with cone-beam computed tomography (CBCT).

Anatomy Is Destiny

Anatomy

A healthy periodontium is largely derived from a physiologic equilibrium among essential elements conducive to a stable environment against chronic deterioration. As a therapeutic objective it is in fact these components that, once identified, are recreated surgically or non-surgically.

To that end osseous surgery, for example, results ideally in the artificial recreation of a physiologic architecture of bone and its relation to the overlying soft tissue. A surgically recreated periodontal environment is where presumably health may be maintained with a reasonable regimen of home care and office hygiene visits.

Of the components that must be given due attention in the understanding of periodontal health disease and subsequent treatment, the anatomy of the natural dentition is a key.

A thorough student of the fundamentals of periodontics cannot escape the uncanny near mathematical system, which exists and binds basic dental anatomy as its most recurrent variations articulate and coexist with the elements of the periodontium, namely, soft tissue and bone. To that end we will concentrate primarily on the radicular anatomy of the permanent human dentition and some relevant aspects of coronal anatomy as well.

Understanding "the system" is one way to see clearly through the maze that represents periodontal health and resting equilibrium, disease, and the recreation of a remissive state through treatment. This chapter is an attempt to review some of the more salient features of dental anatomy as they relate to periodontal parameters.

Root Surface Anatomy

Facial and palatal or lingual root surfaces are for the most part convex to flat. The relative position of these root surfaces as well as their inherent geometry make these surfaces more accessible and less prone to the accumulation of biofilm, presumably with adequate home care and hygiene. Interproximal and interradicular root surfaces are primarily concave to flat; these surfaces on the other hand, because of their relative position in the arch and because of their shape are more likely to be susceptible to periodontal breakdown.

Proximal and interradicular surfaces however because of their outline, which is generally concave, and their inter proximal or interradicular position are in fact less amenable to maintenance and more prone to periodontal breakdown than facial or lingual surfaces.

This pattern tends to worsen anteroposterior for at least two reasons:

Anterior teeth are inherently accessible for hygiene, whereas posterior teeth would be more problematic in that respect. Inter proximal contacts and corresponding septa are also generally broader from the anterior part of the arch back. This particular anatomy makes the posterior contact area, the area initially susceptible to an etiological insult and lesion more difficult to access.

Also as periodontal disease progresses, the formation of osseous craters or for that matter any type of intrabony lesion is now more likely to form where broad posterior septa are initially present. This adds to the overall inaccessibility of these areas. Again the reasons why crater formation is more probable with broader septa is the purpose of a subsequent part of the book where the biologic fundamentals of disease progression and healing will be entertained.

Anterior Teeth

We know anterior teeth for the most part to be single rooted with a mostly conical radicular shape apico-coronally. They are relatively accessible for debridement because of their forward position in the arch. From the point of view of a periodontist the fact that anterior teeth have conical roots implies the following:

Vertical loss of attachment becomes exponentially more severe as it progresses apically on an increasingly fluted radicular area. Also, as periodontal disease increases in severity, these may become more difficult to restore and recreate an esthetic outcome, particularly in the maxillary anterior segment where fluted divergent roots lead to black inter proximal triangles with a receded periodontium. Anterior teeth with an accentuated facial or buccal parabolic contours are more difficult to restore as opposed to teeth with a flatter profile. Coronal anatomy of anterior teeth is usually described as square, ovoid, or tapered/triangle. Square crowns are usually associated with relatively broad inter proximal contact areas in all three dimensions. For this particular anterior tooth morphology the soft tissue biotype is usually thick.

Square crowns are more often short apico-coronally. These may be indicative of altered passive eruption, a condition where adult teeth that are fully erupted have a soft tissue margin positioned more coronal than the norm. These square shaped teeth tend to be associated with broad interproximal septae where interproximal craters are more likely to form. Esthetics are a consideration when periodontal disease is present and resective periodontal surgical treatment is not planned unless a prosthetic commitment is secured to address contingent issue, usually of anesthetic nature.

Ovoid or triangular shaped anterior teeth coronally present with a contact that is more point than area. These are associated with corresponding thinner interproximal septae.

As a result interproximal craters are not as probable as with square shaped crowns. Also with more ovoid shaped teeth, the tissue biotype and the alveolus tend to be thinner; soft tissue recessions are therefore likely with either periodontal disease or treatment.

Mandibular anterior teeth have relatively small contact points. These teeth, which are typically short and squarish have a thinner osseous septum and thin alveolar bone as well as a thin soft tissue biotype; as a result, these teeth are prone to recessions. Mandibular anterior teeth however are

not in the esthetic zone and thus marginal soft tissue recessions may not be critical (Glickman 1953).

Developmental Anterior Grooves

Maxillary incisors will sometimes present with a facio-gingival developmental groove.

Although this condition is more frequently found on the palatal surface of maxillary incisors, it has sometimes been observed on the facial aspect of these teeth. These usually present as a narrow developmental groove that courses over the cingulum area from a point coronally.

The groove itself is anatomically prone to localized periodontal breakdown. Prognosis and treatment alternatives depend largely on the severity and the geometry, the number of bony walls for example, of the lesion associated with the anatomical groove.

Canines have bulbous prominent roots both mandibular and maxillary. As a result the alveolar bone is thin and the biotype associated with these is relatively thin alveolus and soft tissue biotype. These facts have an impact of treatment approach and should be addressed with caution as tissue manipulation may result in recessions from fenestrations and dehiscence likely to be present with a thin buccal wall. Cone beam imagery may be useful in arriving at the correct diagnosis (Lee and Lee 1968; Everett and Kramer 1972; Kogon 1986; Avital et al. 1988).

Premolars

Premolars are relatively small teeth coronally and may deceivingly appear, perhaps as a result of their relative size coronally to be single rooted.

The maxillary first premolar is the classic example as to why that is not the case. In the majority of cases, the first premolar is bifurcated, has two roots associated with a short root trunk or, in the least, a deep mesial groove. With that in mind, assumptions should not be made regarding the anatomy of premolars rather they should be looked at individually with no pre conceived notion (Dababneh and Rodan 2013).

For the purpose of diagnosis, prognosis, and treatment, furcation involvements have been classified and categorized according their degree of severity itself a measure of the clinical penetrability of a calibrated periodontal probe.

For the most part it is the horizontal involvement that has been used as a measure of prognosis and treatment potential. In one particular publication however the vertical component of the furcation involvement was addressed in terms of severity and potential for treatment. Again in subsequent chapters, the issue of furcation involvement will be revisited as it is related to periodontal disease, prognosis, and treatment alternatives (Hamp et al. 1975; Tarnow and Fletcher 1984).

The Root Trunk

The root trunk is essentially a measure of the distance between the CEJ to the anatomical roof of a furcation area. It is also an estimate of the anatomical potential of a furcated multirooted tooth to periodontal breakdown. A short root trunk is more susceptible to a furcation involvement than a long root trunk; in effect, the latter provides more leeway in the face of periodontal breakdown. When a tooth with a long root trunk is affected with a furcation involvement, that is indicative of a severe periodontal condition and an unfavorable prognosis. Once an anatomical furcation becomes clinically detectable, this represents a significant prognosis downturn for the given tooth. Treatment options and treatment outcomes are, as we will see inn subsequent chapters of this book, severely compromised and will depend as the literature supports it, on the severity of the lesion Gargulio (1961).

Maxillary First Molars

As is the case in general for molar teeth, their anatomy has been reported and is described in terms of the first molar. This includes the first maxillary molar.

The first maxillary molar typically has three roots, a mesiobuccal, a distobuccal, and a palatal.

As such, three anatomical furcations are present: a buccal, a mesial, and a distal.

If the root trunk of the maxillary first molar is measured from the CEJ to the roof of each anatomical furcation, the literature indicates that the buccal root trunk is the shortest followed by the mesial and the distal, respectively. One should note however that the furcation on the buccal is midway from mesial to distal; the distal furcation is directly below the contact area so midway bucco-palatally, whereas the mesial furcation is slightly off center. These all have significant implications with respect the susceptibility to periodontal disease as well as treatment implications.

The surface area of each of the three maxillary first molar roots has been reported with the mesiobuccal, the palatal, and the distobuccal roots usually in that order of decreasing size.

As with any furcated or multirooted teeth intraradicular root concavities are present with maxillary molars. Because of the three roots here as opposed to the two roots for mandibular molars, furcation involvements tend to be unidirectional for mandibular molars. For maxillary molars however, the presence of three furcations means that these can be affected internally rather than simply

from the furcation entrance. This adds to the potential on prognosis and the ability to treat or maintain these areas.

One should note that root anatomy should be seen not only as it relates to each individual tooth in isolation but also with respect to their relative position in the arch. For example, the maxillary first molar often presents with a distobuccal root that angles distally and buccally. That may lead to a thin alveolar buccal housing where a fenestration or dehiscence are to be considered. Also the distal divergence of the distobuccal root often results in a thin interdental septum with the adjacent second molar. This has significant implications in terms of disease progression and treatment alternatives. Such anatomical relationships may potentially found anywhere in the arch (Herman et al. 1983; Gher and Dunlap 1985; Roussa 1998).

Mandibular First Molars

First molars represent the classic anatomy for mandibular molars with variations expected for second molars and particularly third molars.

The mandibular first molar typically has two roots, a mesial and a buccal, with two corresponding anatomical furcations, a buccal and a lingual. The root trunk, measured from the CEJ to the roof of the furcation, is shorter on the buccal then on the lingual then on the buccal. Root trunk length has implications both in terms of prognosis and treatment. When furcation involvements are diagnosed as opposed to shorter root trunk, that is indicative of more loss of attachment and therefore a more unfavorable prognosis in terms of treatment. A shorter furcation however can be more of a potential challenge with respective to any type of resective osseous surgery where the anatomical furcal entrance is closer to the CEJ apicoronally. This constitutes a physical limit to the apical positioning of the alveolar margin. This would include a crown lengthening for example where the establishment of the biologic width may be the intended objective but where the length of the root trunk may represent a limiting factor.

The furcal entrance is usually wider on the buccal than on the lingual although the literature indicates that in most instances the furcal entrance is narrower in diameter then instruments used for debridement. Both roots of the mandibular molar are usually kidney shaped in a horizontal cross with the interproximal and intraradicular root surfaces being more concave on the mesial then the distal root. Because both roots are concave on the furcal aspect, this access for debridement is challenging endeavor. Also the fact the mesial root is more kidney shaped has often led clinicians to favor the distal root over the mesial root in root resection procedures because it is comprehensively more treatable periodontally and restoratively. In some instances and with good judgement, root surfaces may be reshaped with fine diamonds to modify their anatomy to a more treatable or maintainable one.

One additional important aspect of intra furcal root anatomy is the intermediate bifurcational ridge, which runs in a mesio distal direction. Its position within the furcation can potentially interfere with an accurate clinical estimate of a given furcation involvement (Everett et al. 1958; Bower 1979a,b; Gher and Vernino 1980).

Cervical Enamel Projections (CEPs)

CEPs may be described as fingerlike extensions of enamel from the coronal portion of the tooth at various depths beyond the CEJ. Because they are enamel in their composition their soft tissue interface is not a CT attachment but a long JE. As such they are often the focus of localized periodontal breakdown. CEPs are classified according their proximity to the furcation area, the most severe being one that is actually within a furcation.

Intermediate CEPs are found most commonly on the buccal aspect of mandibular second molars mostly as class II projections.

Cementicles and enamel pearls are usually small isolated globules made of cementum or enamel respectively. They can be detected usually within the body of the PDL and are of little known significance. Accessory canals have been described coursing laterally to the periodontal ligament. The potential for these as pathways for cross contamination is not clear from the available literature (Swan and Hurt 1976; Masters and Hoskins 1984; You and Tsai 1987; Moskow and Canut 1990).

It may be important to note the following as far the enamel relates to the cementum at the CEJ: sixty percent of the cementum and enamel overlap; thirty percent form a butt joint; ten percent are separated by a gap (Gutman 1978).

References

Avital, K., Tal, H., Yechenskhy, N., and Mazei, O. (1988). Facial lingual grooves. *J. Periodontol.* 59: 615–617.

Bower, R.C. (1979a). Furcation morphology relative to periodontal treatment. Furcation root surface anatomy. *J. Periodontol.* 50: 366–374.

Bower, R.C. (1979b). Furcation morphology relative to periodontal treatment furcation entrance architecture. *J. Periodontol.* 50: 23–27.

Bowers, G.M. (1963). A study of the width of the attached gingiva. *J. Periodontol.* 34: 201–209.

Dababneh, R. and Rodan, R. (2013). Anatomical landmarks of maxillary bifurcated first pre molar and their influence on periodontal disease and treatment. *J. Int. Acad. Periodontol.* 15: 8–15.

De Rouck, T., Eghbali, R., Collys, K. et al. (2009). The gingival biotype revisited: transparency of the periodontal probe through the gingival margin as a method to discriminate thin from thick gingiva. *J. Clin. Periodontol.* 36 (5): 428–433.

Everett, F.G. and Kramer, G.M. (1972). The Disto Lingala Groove in the maxillary lateral incisors. a periodontal hazard. *J. Periodontol.* 43: 352–361.

Everett, F.G., Jump, E.B., Holder, T.D., and Williams, G.C. (1958). The intermediate bifurcational ridge: a study of the morphology of the bifurcation of the lower first molars. *J. Dent. Res.* 37: 162–169.

Fu, Jia-Hui, Chu-Yuan Yeh, Hsun-Liang Chan, et al. Tissue biotype and its relation to the underlying bone morphology. *J. Periodontol.* 2010; 81(4): 569–574.

Gargiulo, A.W., Wentz, F.M., and Orban, B. (1961). Dimensions and relations of the dentogingival junction in humans. *J. Periodontol.* 32: 261–267.

Gargulio, A.W. (1961). Dimensions and relations of the dentogingival junction in humans. *J. Periodontol.* 32: 261–267.

Gher, M.E. and Dunlap, R.M. (1985). Linear variations of the root surface of the maxillary first molar. *J. Periodontol.* 56: 39–43.

Gher, M.E. and Vernino, A.R. (1980). Clinical significance in the pathogenesis and treatment of periodontal disease. *J. Am. Dent. Assoc.* 101 (4): 6227–6263.

Glickman, I. (1953). *Clinical Periodontology: The Periodontum in Health and Disease: Diagnosis and Treatment of Periodontal Disease in the Practice of General Dentistry.* Philadelphia: Saunders.

Goaslind, G.D., Robertson, P.B., Mahan, C.J. et al. (1977). Thickness of facial gingiva. *J. Periodontol.* 48: 768–771.

Gutman, J.L. (1978). Prevalence, location, and patency of accessory canals in the furcation region off the permanent molars. *J. Periodontol.* 49: 21–26.

Hamp, S.E., Nyman, S., and Lindhe, J. (1975). Periodontal treatment of the multirooted teeth. Results after five years. *J. Clin. Periodontol.* 2: 126–135.

Hassell, T. (2000). Tissues and cells of the periodontium. *Periodontology* 1993 (3): 9–38.

Herman, D.W., Gher, M.E., Dunlap, R.M., and Pelieu, G.B. Jr., (1983). The potential attachment area of the maxillary first molar. *J. Periodontol.* 54: 431–434.

Hirschfeld, I. (1923). A study of skulls in the American Museum of Natural History in relation to periodontal disease. *J. Dent. Res.* 5 (4): 241–265.

Karring, T. and Loe, H.B. (1970). The three-dimensional concept of the epithelium connective tissue boundary of gingiva. *Acta Odontol. Scand.* 28: 917–933.

Karring, T., Lang, N.P., and Loe, H.B. (1975). The role of gingival connective tissue in determining epithelial differentiation. *J. Periodontol. Res.* 10: 1–11.

Kogon, S.L. (1986). The prevalence location and conformation of palate radicular grooves. *J. Periodontol.* 57: 231–234.

Lee, K.W., Lee, E.C., and Poo, K.Y. (1968). Palatal gingival grooves in maxillary incisors and localized periodontal disease. *Br. Dent. J.* 124: 114–111.

Lindhe, J. (ed.) (1983). *Textbook of Clinical Periodontology*, 19–66. Copenhagen: Munksgaard.

Lozdan, J. and Squier, C.A. (1969). The histology of the muco-gingival junction. *J. Periodontol.* 4: 83–93.

Masters, D.H. and Hoskins, S.W. (1984). Projections of cervical enamel into molar furcation. *J. Periodontol.* 35: 49–53.

Moskow, B.S. and Canut, P.M. (1990). Studies on root enamel (2). Enamel pearls. A review of their morphology, localization, nomenclature, classification, histogenesis, and incidence. *J. Clin. Periodontol.* 17: 275–281.

Ochsenbein, C. and Ross, S. (1969). A reevaluation of osseous surgery. *Dent. Clin. N. Am.* 13 (1): 87.

Roussa, E. (1998). Anatomic characteristics of the furcation and root surface of molar teeth and their significance in the clinical management of marginal periodontitis. *Clin. Anat.* 11: 177–186.

Sabag, N. and Saglie, R. (1981). Ultrastructure of the normal human epithelial attachment to the cementum root surface. *J. Periodontol.* 52: 94–95.

Squier, C.A. and Hill, M.W. (1985). *Oral Histology, Development, Structure, and Function*, 2e, 372. St. Louis: The C.V. Mosby Co.

Swan, R.H. and Hurt, W.C. (1976). Cervical enamel projection as an etiologic factor in furcation involvement. *J. Am. Dent. Assoc.* 93: 342–345.

Tarnow, D. and Fletcher, P. (1984). Classification of the vertical component of the furcation involvement. *J. Periodontol.* 55: 283–284.

Ten Cate, A. (1989). Connective tissue influence on junctional epithelium. In: *Oral Histology, Development, Structure, and Function*, 3e (ed. A. Ten Cate), 264–267. St. Louis: CV Mosby.

Voigt, J.P., Goran, M.L., and Fleisher, R.M. (1978). The width of lingual mandibular attached gingiva. *J. Periodontol.* 49: 77–80.

Weisgold, A.S. (1977). Contours of the full crown restoration. *Alpha Omegan* 70: 77–89.

You, G.I. and Tsai, L. (1987). Relationship between periodontal furcation involvements molar cervical enamel projections. *J. Periodontol.* 58: 715–722.

Zweers, J., Thomas, R.Z., Slot, D.E. et al. (2014). Characteristics of periodontal biotype, its dimensions, associations and prevalence: a systematic review. *J. Clin. Periodontol.* 41: 958–971.

Further Reading

Cortellini, P. et al. (2018). Mucogingival conditions in the natural dentition: narrative review, case definitions, and diagnostic considerations. *J. Periodontol.* 89 (Suppl 1): S204–S213.

Nobuto, T., Yanagihara, K., Teranishi, Y. et al. (1989). Periostea! microvasculature in the dog alveolar process. *J. Periodontol.* 60: 709–715.

Termeie, D.A. (2013). *Periodontal Review*. Hanover Park: Quintessence.

2

Wound Healing

Steven Engebretson

Department of Periodontology and Implant Dentistry, New York University College of Dentistry, New York, NY, USA

Definitions and Terms for Clinical Outcomes

Repair is defined as healing of a wound by tissue that does not fully restore the architecture or the function of the part. *Reattachment* means to attach again such as the reunion of epithelial and connective tissues (CT) with root surfaces and bone such as occurs after an incision or injury. *New attachment* is the union of CT or epithelium with a root surface that has been deprived of its original attachment apparatus. This new attachment may be epithelial adhesion and/or CT adaptation or attachment and may include new cementum. *Regeneration* is the reproduction or reconstitution of a lost or injured part. *Guided tissue regeneration* refers to procedures aimed at regeneration of lost periodontal structures by guiding differential tissue responses using barrier materials such as expanded-polytetrafluoroethylene, polyglactin, polylactic acid, titanium mesh, or collagen to exclude epithelium from the root surface.

Inflammatory Phase

When a surgical wound is created bleeding occurs, the cascade of events leading to hemostasis is initiated and a clot is formed. Collagen attracts platelets to the wound site and a platelet plug is formed, creating a fibrin matrix, providing the basis for tissue repair. Neutrophils are the first immune cells recruited to the wound in response to the activation of complement, the degranulation of platelets and the products of bacterial degradation. Polymorphonuclear leukocyte (PMN) or the "poly band" reaches peak activity 24–48 hours followed by the influx of monocytes, which act to debride the site of bacteria and necrotic tissue. Platelets release growth factors and cytokines and regulate subsequent healing. Platelet-derived growth factor (PDGF)

stimulates chemotaxis of neutrophils and macrophages in the wound site as well as chemotaxis and mitogenesis of fibroblasts and stimulates collagen synthesis. Transforming growth factor beta (TGF-β) is a key modulator of wound healing and is chemotactic for macrophages, fibroblasts, and smooth muscle cells and stimulate collagen synthesis, while modulating collagenase and tissue inhibitor of metalloproteinases (TIMPS). After two to three days monocytes differentiate into macrophage and secrete factors that stimulate angiogenesis and fibroblast proliferation that promotes the proliferative phase.

During the inflammatory stage flap tensile strength is still weak, as fibrin holds the flap in place (Hiatt et al. 1968). Following hemostasis, vasodilation of tissues adjacent to the wound, mediated by histamine, prostaglandins, kinins, and leukotrienes result in vascular permeability allowing blood plasma and white blood cells to permeate via diapedesis to the extravascular space. The classical signs of inflammation are thus observed: swelling (tumor), redness (rubor), heat (calor), and pain (dolor).

Proliferative Phase

The cytokines and growth factors secreted during the inflammatory phase stimulate the succeeding proliferative phase. The proliferation of fibroblasts from the surrounding tissue induces production of collagen and proteoglycans. Collagen production restores tissue stability and serves to support the newly formed blood vessels supplying the wound. Proteoglycans function as a reservoir of moisture essential for early wound hydration. Angiogenesis is essential for the transport of nutrients and oxygen and begins post injury and lasts up to three weeks. The proliferative phase is distinguished by the formation of granulation tissue containing macrophages, fibroblasts, and budding vasculature in a loose collagen matrix. Angiogenesis induced by vascular endothelial growth factor (VEGF) and fibroblast growth factor 2 (FGF-2). Epithelialization is facilitated by underlying CT, which draws the wound margins together and contraction begins leading to the remodeling phase.

Remodeling Phase

During the remodeling stage the collagenous matrix is synthesized continually and broken down in an effort to achieve tissue homeostasis. Cross-links are formed between collagen molecules and tensile strength of the wound increases. Osteoclasts ruffled borders act to resorb the bone, while osteoblasts form new bone tissue in response to mechanical stress. New haversian systems are developed as concentric layers of cortical bone are deposited along blood vessels. The bone has the capacity to undergo regeneration as part of a repair process and can heal without scarring.

Epithelium and Connective Tissue Healing

Following a procedure such as gingivectomy or gingivoplasty, an incision to the gingiva results in a clot formation followed by an infiltrate of PMN, which forms a band around the wound. The acute inflammatory response ensues (Ramfjord et al. 1966). Blockage and withdrawal of cut capillary ends occur during the first day, and by day 2 new sprouts are observed, capillary loops form by day 3–5, and anastomoses and normal vasculature are restore by day 11 (Cutright 1969). The fate of the root surface is determined by the cells present. Epithelial attachment, CT attachment, bone, cementum, or periodontal ligament (PDL) cells may repopulate the root. Healing by long junctional epithelium following root planing occurs in the absence viable PDL cells, while in the presence of viable PDL cells CT attachment may occur (Waerhaug 1955; Caton et al. 1980). Teeth denuded of cementum by scaling showed no CT attachment (Karring et al. 1980). Epithelium originates from the basal and deep spinous layers of the adjacent epithelial tissues (Engler et al. 1966). Migration begins within 12–24 hours and continues at a rate of approximately 0.5 mm per day, resulting in a complete reformation of the gingival sulcus in three to five weeks (Engler et al. 1966). Epithelial attachment to the tooth occurs at seven to eight days (Sabag et al. 1984) by long junctional epithelium (Karring et al. 1984), that may aid resistance to plaque induced inflammation (Magnusson

et al. 1983). Cementum growth can be observed after three weeks (Hiatt et al. 1968) and is key to CT attachment and PDL regeneration. PDL cells form the basis of granulation tissue at adjacent sites (Karring et al. 1975). CT matrix formation begins one to two days after surgery and peak activity is observed at three to four days. Collagenous maturation and functional orientation of collagen fibrils that results in a restored gingiva requires four to six weeks (Ramfjord et al. 1966; Novaes et al. 1969).

Flap Surgery

Following elevation of a periosteal flap, and suturing, the immediate events include blood clot formation and a fibrin adhesion of the flap to bone, infiltration with PMN, and epithelial cell migration. During the period of one to three days, post-operation epithelial migration continues. Vascular sprouts begin to form and fibroblasts begin to migrate into the fibrin clot. By seven days epithelium has begun to attach to the root surface via hemidesmosomes and basal lamina. Capillary loops reform at the edges of the wound. After 14 days collagen fibers have begun to orient parallel to the tooth surface and the flap tensile strength has increased, while maturation of capillary loops and return of normal vasculature occurs. After 28 days the gingival unit has been reformed with collagen fibrils in their preoperative state.

Free Graft

Following free soft tissue allograft procedures, the initial healing events are observed, with the graft being maintained through plasma diffusion and hydration from the adjacent tissue bed. CT grafts become edematous and undergo degeneration. By day 2, granulation tissue begins to form and capillary buds from the recipient site can already be observed. During day 3–14, capillaries anastomose and infiltrate the graft. Epithelial grafts will necrose and slough with new epithelium appearing by day 4 and rete pegs by day 7. After 14 days the overlying epithelium of a CT graft begins to differentiate into stratified squamous keratinized epithelium. By four to six weeks remodeling occurs. Free allografts maintain their histological character. Keratinized tissue grafts remain keratinized (Karring et al. 1975). CT grafts may form new keratinized tissue at recipient sites previously devoid of keratinized tissue.

Bone Healing

The events that occur during normal wound healing of soft tissue injuries (e.g. inflammation, proliferation, and remodeling) also take place during the repair of injured bone. Osteogenic cells (osteoblasts and osteoclasts) derived from periosteum, endosteum, and circulating pluripotential mesenchymal cells reconstitute and remodel bone. Osteoblasts produce osteoid, which later calcifies. Osteoclasts, derived from monocyte precursor cells, function to resorb necrotic bone and bone to be remodeled.

Following flap elevation, bone undergoes a period of superficial necrosis lasting one to three days that peaks at four to six days. By day seven days osteoblastic activity begins and peaks at three to four weeks. A net loss of approximately 0.8 mm of bone can occur as a net result of the resorption and osteoblastic activity (Wilderman et al. 1970). Activated macrophage and PMN produce cytokines that directly or indirectly stimulate osteoclast formation and activation. IL-6, TNF-alpha, IL-1-beta, prostaglandins matrix metalloproteases, and chemokines such as IL-8 are released by activated PMN and macrophage and influence osteoclastic and osteoblastic activity. As with oral mucosa and gingiva, bone healing undergoes an inflammatory phase, a proliferative phase, and a remodeling phase. In the initial days following flap elevation, following clot formation and PMN infiltrate, macrophage functions to debride the wound of debris and release cytokines while PMNs phagocytose bacteria. PDGF, VEGF, and TGF beta recruit bone cells and stimulate proliferation. Fibroblasts infiltrate the granulation tissue and convert the fibrin clot to granulation tissue while osteoclastic activity is already present during the first week. Osteoblastic activity begins after seven days and continues for weeks to months and gradually infiltrates the granulation tissue to form new bone. The remodeling phase continues for weeks to years through osteoclastic resorption, osteoblastic bone apposition, and maintenance by osteocytes. Woven bone is gradually remodeled and becomes lamellar (or cortical) bone.

Healing of Extraction Sockets

The removal of a tooth initiates the same sequence of inflammation, proliferation, and remodeling seen in mucosal wounds. The inflammatory stage occurs during the first days of healing. White blood cells enter the socket to remove contaminating bacteria from the area and phagocytose debris. Fibroblasts and capillaries begin to infiltrate during the first week. The epithelium migrates into the socket wall until it reaches a level at which it contacts epithelium from the other side of the socket or it encounters the bed of granulation tissue over which the epithelium can migrate. Finally, during the first week of healing, osteoclasts accumulate along the crestal bone. Within five days of extraction, early granulation tissue

composed of immature capillaries and fibroblasts appears at the bottom of the socket and spreads upward along the socket walls. The second week is marked by continued formation of granulation tissue that fills the socket. Osteoid deposition has begun along the alveolar bone lining the socket.

These processes continue during the third and fourth weeks of healing, with epithelialization of most sockets complete at this time. The cortical bone continues to be resorbed from the crest and walls of the socket, and new trabecular bone permeates the socket. At three weeks new bone formation begins. Bone growth continues at four to five weeks and new trabeculae forms on socket walls and apical regions and fills two-thirds of the socket. At six weeks bone formation may be seen radiographically. However, bone fill in the alveolus takes up to four months. At four to six months after extraction the cortical bone lining a socket is fully resorbed; this is recognized radiographically by a loss of a distinct lamina dura. At one year the only visible remnant of the socket is the rim of fibrous (scar) tissue that remains on the edentulous alveolar ridge.

Osseointegration

A surgically created osteotomy for a dental implant is accomplished by drilling into the bone with sharp burs and copious sterile saline irrigation, resulting in a bleeding wound. Upon placement of a dental implant consisting of an osteoconductive and biocompatible surface such as a sandblasted and acid etched titanium or titanium zirconium alloy, and where primary stability has been achieved, wound healing events are similar to those described earlier: hemostasis and coagulum in the form of a fibrin clot at day 1, followed by granulation tissue formation at day 1–3. Bone resorption of the osteotomy occurs through day 7, while new bone apposition consisting of woven bone takes place from one to six weeks with increasing trabeculae and direct bone to implant contact leading to osseointegration. After 6 weeks, increases in bone density occur and remodeling then continues throughout the life of the patient (implant) (Bosshardt et al. 2017).

Modifiers of Wound Healing

Systemic illnesses such as alcoholism, diabetes mellitus, and habits such as smoking may impede the wound healing process. The use of certain medications such as bisphosphonates may interfere with bone remodeling and result in adverse healing events such as osteonecrosis.

References

Bosshardt, D.D., Chappuis, V., and Buser, D. (2017). Osseointegration of titanium, titanium alloy and zirconia dental implants: current knowledge and open questions. *Periodontology* 2000 (73): 22–40. https://doi.org/10.1111/prd.12179.

Caton, J., Nyman, S., and Zander, H. (1980). Histometric evaluation of periodontal surgery. II. Connective tissue attachment levels after four regenerative procedures. *J. Clin. Periodontol.* 7: 224–231.

Cutright, D.E. (1969). The proliferation of blood vessels in gingival wounds. *J. Periodontol.* 40 (3): –137, 41.

Engler, W.O., Ramfjord, S.P., and Hiniker, J.J. (1966). Healing following simple gingivectomy. A tritiated thymidine radioautographic study. I Epithelialization. *J. Periodontol.* 37: 298–308.

Hiatt, W.H., Stallard, R.E., and Butler, E.D. (1968). B Badgett Repair following mucoperiosteal flap surgery with full gingival retention. *J. Periodontol.* 39 (1): 11–16.

Karring, T., Lang, N.P., and Loe, H. (1975). The role of gingival connective tissue in determining epithelial differentiation. *J. Periodontol. Res.* 10: 1–11.

Karring, T., Nyman, S., and Lindhe, J. (1980). Healing following implantation of periodontitis affected roots into bone tissue. *J. Clin. Periodontol.* 7: 96–105.

Karring, T., Nyman, S., Lindhe, J., and Sirirat, M. (1984). Potentials for root resorption during periodontal wound healing. *J. Clin. Periodontol.* 11: 41–52.

Magnusson, I., Runstad, L., Nyman, S., and Lindhe, J. (1983). A long junctional epithelium – a locus minoris resistentiae in plaque infection? *J. Clin. Periodontol.* 10: 333–340.

Novaes, A.B., Kon, S., Ruben, M.P., and Goldman, H.M. (1969). Visualization of the microvascularization of the healing periodontal wound. 3. Gingivectomy. *J. Periodontol.* 40: 359–371. https://doi.org/10.1902/jop.1969.40.6.359.

Ramfjord, S.P., Engler, W.O., and Hiniker, J.J. (1966). A radioautographic study of healing following simple gingivectomy. II The connective tissue. *J. Periodontol.* 37: 179–189.

Sabag, N., Mery, C., Garcia, M. et al. (1984). Epithelial reattachment after gingivectomy in the rat. *J. Periodontol.* 55: 135–141. https://doi.org/10.1902/jop.1984.55.3.135.

Waerhaug, J. (1955). Depth of incision of gingivectomy. *Oral Surg. Oral Med. Oral Pathol.* 8: 707–718.

Wilderman, M.N., Pennel, B.M., King, K., and Barron, J.M. (1970). Histogenesis of repair following osseous surgery. *J. Periodontol.* 41: 551–565. https://doi.org/10.1902/jop.1970.41.10.551.

3

Diagnosis and Pathology of Periodontal Diseases
Cecilia White

Private practice, Princeton, NJ, USA

Formulating a Periodontal Diagnosis

An accurate periodontal diagnosis involves the merging of our current understanding of disease with patient-specific information.

Historically, the American Academy of Periodontology together with the European Federation of Periodontology have worked to provide updated guidelines for diagnosis based on current scientific understanding. In 2017, a series of papers were published as the *Classification of Periodontal and Peri-Implant Diseases and Conditions*. The workshop aimed to clarify previously unclear nomenclature and provided a completely restructured method of periodontal diagnoses.

In this format, a branch of peri-implant diseases and conditions was created to address implant-related issues and standardize specific diagnoses. This reflects the growing importance of implant therapy in the field of periodontics.

Data collection in the form of a systematic approach to patient examination is essential in the process of determining an accurate diagnosis. Complete records should be gathered including relevant systemic and local factors, history of condition, and thorough examination of the patient. There are factors to consider in the process of data collection can be informed by our current understanding of periodontal disease activity. For example, certain infections periodontal conditions have been attributed to the presence bacterial biofilm and the host response process. Thus, the presence or absence of certain bacteria can be used to inform a diagnosis.

Periodontal Health and Gingival Health

Defining and recognizing periodontal health are important in order to recognize standards in which disease can be compared. *Periodontal health* can be defined as the state in which tissues are free from periodontal inflammation.

There is a difference between histological and clinical periodontal health: Histologic features of health include a low bacterial load with bacterial species mostly gram-positive and nonmotile such as *Streptococcus* and *Actinomyces* species. The confirmation of this status may not be practical for all patients in a clinical setting. Instead, clinical indicators of health include information, which can be gathered chairside during a thorough examination including bleeding upon probing (BOP), probing depth, radiographic bone levels, and tooth mobility.

Host determinants in clinical health include microbiological, host, and environmental categories. Each of these may be considered a predisposing factor, which contributes to the accumulation of dental plaque or a modifying factor or one which alters the way in which an individual responds to subgingival plaque accumulation. Some of these factors may be controllable while others are not.

- **Local predisposing factors:** periodontal pockets, dental restorations, root anatomy, tooth position, and crowding
- **Systemic modifying factors**: host immune function, systemic health, and genetics

While the determinants of health are important in understanding the disease process, the indicators of clinical health are essential for the practitioner to recognize and accurately diagnose a periodontally healthy patient. The best method for monitoring the health or inflammation of gingival tissues is through bleeding on probing (Lang et al. 1986), usually measured as bleeding provoked by applying a probe to the bottom of a gingival sulcus or pocket.

Other factors such as periodontal probing depth, radiographic bone loss, and tooth mobility have been used in the past; however, these are not always useful in assessing patients who have experienced periodontal disease in the past.

Practical Techniques in Periodontics and Implant Dentistry, First Edition. Edited by Edgard El Chaar.
© 2023 John Wiley & Sons, Inc. Published 2023 by John Wiley & Sons, Inc.

Diagnoses of periodontal health can include clinical health on an intact periodontium or clinical health on a reduced periodontium. Patients with a history of disease can further be identified as stable periodontitis patients or non-periodontitis patients.

Gingivitis: Dental Plaque-Induced

Gingivitis is defined as inflammation of the gingival tissues. The most common form of which involves a plaque-induced host response. Studies on the natural history of gingivitis in man have found that there are a greater number of bacteria in gingivitis sites compared with healthy sites. Additionally, there is a shift from Gram positive, non-motile species to a more Gram negative, motile species.

Gingival inflammation can be categorized according to its extent and severity. Gingivitis is considered localized when <30% of teeth are affected and generalized when ≥30% of teeth are affected. Additionally, mild gingivitis occurs in an area with minor change in color and little change of texture; moderate in areas with glazing, redness, edema, enlargement, and BOP; severe in areas of overt redness and edema with bleeding occurring with slight touch.

Modifying factors in the process of gingivitis include sex steroid hormones (puberty, menstrual cycle, pregnancy, oral contraceptives), hyperglycemia, leukemia, smoking, malnutrition local factors affecting plaque accumulation: prominent subgingival restorative margins, hyposalivation, and drug-induced gingival enlargement.

Necrotizing Periodontal Diseases

Necrotizing conditions of the periodontium involve ulceration of the epithelial barrier, allowing for microflora to invade the underlying connective tissue. These conditions clinically manifest as painful lesions presenting in patients with specific underlying risk factors, such as poor oral hygiene smoking, stress, poor nutrition, or compromised immune status.

The microflora is considered widely varied and many species are difficult to identify as they are unculvable; however the most frequent bacteria associated with these conditions are gram-negative, anaerobic spirochetes. *Prevotella intermedia, Fusobacterium,* and *Selenomas* species are frequently associated with necrotizing conditions (Horning and Cohen 1995).

Necrotizing periodontal diseases include necrotizing gingivitis, necrotizing periodontitis, and necrotizing stomatitis. While microbiological testing may be recommended in certain cases, most often a diagnosis can be determined based on clinical signs. Necrotizing gingivitis is recognized as necrosis and ulceration of the gingival papilla, gingival bleeding, pain, pseudomembrane formation, and halitosis. In addition to these, the presence of periodontal attachment loss and bone destruction indicates a diagnosis of necrotizing periodontitis. In a diagnosis of necrotizing stomatitis, bone denudation through the alveolar mucosa with larger areas of bony sequestrum, often in immunocompromised patients, may be typical (Herrera et al. 2018).

Periodontitis

The primary goals in the staging of a periodontitis patient include classifying the severity and extent of the condition as well as assessing the complexity of controlling current disease and managing the condition long-term. The primary goals of the grading process include estimating future risk of disease progression and responsiveness to therapy as well as estimating the potential influence of periodontitis on systemic health and vice versa.

The staging process represents factors that indicate severity of disease (interdental CAL, radiographic bone loss, and tooth loss attributable to loss of bony support), complexity (local factors such as vertical defects, furcation involvement, ridge defects and need for complex rehabilitation), and extent and distribution.

Extent and distribution are added as descriptors and may include localized, generalized, or molar/incisor pattern.

Stage I periodontitis represents those cases at the early stages of attachment loss. At this stage, a diagnosis of gingivitis will switch to periodontitis resulting from persistent gingival inflammation and biofilm dysbiosis.
Stage II periodontitis is diagnosed when inflammation has caused identifiable damage to the tooth support; however management remains straightforward.
Stage III periodontitis occurs when there is significant damage to the attachment apparatus and, in the absence of advanced treatment, tooth loss may occur. In this stage,
Stage IV periodontitis is the most advanced diagnosis in which there has been considerable damage to the periodontal support, which can lead to significant tooth loss and thus, loss of masticatory function. At this phase, in the absence of adequate control and rehabilitation, the patient is at risk for losing the entire dentition.

A practical guide to beginning the staging process may be to consider whether the patient should fall into Stages I/II category of mild to moderate or III/IV category of moderate to severe. From here, individual patient data can be used to identify the appropriate stage of disease.

Grade of periodontitis allows rate of progression to be considered and designation is based on either direct or indirect evidence of progression. Direct evidence is based on longitudinal observation of criteria such as previous radiographs and indirect evidence is based on assessment of bone loss as a function of age.

In 2019, Kornman and Papapanou attempted to clarify certain aspects of the new classification system. They addressed issues with implementation of the classification system in a practical manner for example, the importance of distinguishing between a Stage I or II patient versus a Stage III or IV patient and important factors to consider when identifying specific diagnoses. Additionally, a series of "gray zones" were recognized and clarified based on the author's interpretation of the classification criteria.

Other Conditions Affecting the Periodontium

Periodontal Abscesses

The clinical presentation of abscess in the periodontal tissues may be a result of a number of etiologies, such as pulp necrosis, periodontal infection, pericoronitis, trauma, surgery, or foreign body reaction. A periodontal abscess is defined as a localized accumulation of pus located within the gingival wall of the periodontal pocket, with an expressed periodontal breakdown occurring during a limited period of time, and with easily detectable clinical symptoms (Herrera et al. 2000). Periodontal abscesses most often occur in periodontitis patients, however, can occur in non-periodontitis patients due to impaction of foreign bodies, gingival enlargement, or alterations of the root surface.

Diagnosis of such a condition should include patient symptoms such as pain and swelling, clinical features described as a round or ovoid elevation in the gingiva, and patient history including previous treatment or exposure to possible foreign body.

Endodontic–Periodontal Lesions

Endo–perio lesions are microbial contamination, which simultaneously affects the pulp and periodontal tissues. Etiology may be associated with primary endodontic–periodontal infections or by trauma or iatrogenic factors. A "true combined" lesion is a condition in which the etiology of infection can be attributed to both dental caries and periodontal breakdown. Lesions associated with trauma or iatrogenic factors may include perforation of the root during endodontic procedures, root fracture, external root resorption, or pulp necrosis due to trauma

and drainage through periodontium. The etiology of the condition corresponds to the case's prognosis and ultimate treatment plan.

Mucogingival Deformities and Conditions Around the Teeth

The 2017 Consensus focused primarily on dental recession, defined as the apical shift of the marginal gingiva caused by different conditions or pathologies and is associated with clinical attachment loss (Jepsen et al. 2018). Importantly, thin gingival phenotype has been shown to increase risk for gingival recession. Mucogingival conditions associated with gingival recession should be described via the extent of the apical shift of the gingival margin, or *recession depth*, as well as interdental CAL, gingival phenotype, keratinized tissue width, root surface condition (i.e. presence or absence of non-carious cervical lesions), detection of the cementoenamel junction (CEJ), tooth position, aberrant frenum, and number of adjacent recessions. Mucogingival conditions without gingival recessions may be described as the gingival phenotype of a dentition or particular site. Features of these conditions may include tooth position, aberrant frenum, or vestibular depth.

Traumatic Occlusal Forces

Traumatic occlusal forces are defined as any occlusal force resulting in injury of the teeth and/or periodontal attachment apparatus (Jepsen et al. 2018). Occlusal trauma is a lesion in the periodontal ligament (PDL), cementum, and adjacent bone caused by traumatic occlusal forces. This condition can be diagnosed clinically by the presence of: progressive tooth mobility, adaptive tooth mobility, radiographically widened PDL, tooth migration, discomfort on chewing, or root resorption. Further, occlusal trauma can be classified as either primary (increased occlusal forces on a healthy periodontium), secondary (increased or normal occlusal forces on a reduced periodontium), or orthodontic forces.

Prosthesis and Tooth-Related Factors

Several factors involved in the fabrication and presence of dental and tooth-related factors have on the periodontium have been described (Ercoli and Caton 2018; Jepsen et al. 2018). Certain factors such as tooth anatomic factors, root fractures, cervical root resorption, cemental tears, root proximity, or altered passive eruption can lead to increased plaque retention and thereby should be considered in diagnostic criteria associated with a periodontitis or gingivitis diagnosis. Other factors associated with dental prosthesis can directly impact the periodontium. For example, restorative margins placed within the junctional epithelium and supracrestal attached tissue may lead to inflammation and recession. Tissue trauma may occur during the process of fabrication of direct restorations and hypersensitivity or toxicity reactions may occur in response to dental materials used.

References

Ercoli, C. and Caton, J.G. (2018). Dental prostheses and tooth-related factors. *J. Periodontol.* 89 (Suppl 1): S024–S213.

Herrera, D., Alonso, B., de Arriba, L. et al. (2000). Acute periodontal lesions. *Periodontology* 2014 (65): 149–177.

Herrera, D., Retamal-Valdes, B., Alonso, B., and Feres, M. (2018). Acute periodontal lesions (periodontal abscesses and necrotizing periodontal diseases) and endo-periodontal lesions. *J. Periodontol.* 89 (Suppl 1): S85–S102.

Horning, G.M. and Cohen, M.E. (1995). Necrotizing ulcerative gingivitis, periodontitis, and stomatitis: clinical staging and predisposing factors. *J. Periodontol.* 66: 990–998.

Jepsen, S., Caton, J.G., Albandar, J.M. et al. (2018). Periodontal manifestations of systemic diseases and development and acquired conditions: consensus report of workgroup 3 of the 2017 World Workshop on the Classification of Periodontal and Peri-Implant Diseases and Conditions. *J. Periodontol.* 89 (Suppl 1): S237–S248.

Lang, N.P., Joss, A., Orsanic, T. et al. (1986). Bleeding on probing. A predictor for the progression of periodontal disease? *J. Clin. Periodontol.* 13 (6): 590–596.

4

Oral Pathology and Oral Medicine

Edgard El Chaar[2] and Arthi M. Kumar[1]

[1]*Department of Oral and Maxillofacial Pathology, Radiology & Medicine, New York University College of Dentistry, New York, NY, USA*
[2]*Department of Periodontics, University of Pennsylvania, Dental Medicine, Philadelphia, PA, USA*

Introduction

In this chapter, a description of a broad spectrum of oral lesions is listed with a focus on lesions related to the periodontium. The format of the chapter takes into consideration the recently revised classification by Holmstrup and Albandar. The aim is to create an easy reference of pathologic entities tailored to the periodontist. The periodontal pathology encountered, which is by far most common, encompasses the inflammatory processes of gingivitis or periodontitis. However, numerous other lesions exist, which require recognition and subsequent management. Moreover, oral pathology lesions may present anywhere in the oral cavity and gnathic bones. Therefore, periodontists need to be aware of the key characteristics of abnormal presentations regardless of the site. This compilation aids in the creation of a differential diagnosis (Ddx), which is essential in guiding management decisions to arrive at a definitive diagnosis.

Non-Dental-Biofilm Induced Gingival Diseases

Genetic/Developmental Disorders

Hereditary Gingival Fibromatosis (HGF)

Hereditary Gingival Fibromatosis (HGF)

- **Clinical presentation**: Slow, progressive gingival overgrowth with varying degrees of manifestation. May present in an isolated fashion or part of a syndrome. Gingival enlargement is typically of normal coloration and non-ulcerated.
- **Cause**: Association with mutation of the Son of Sevenless gene SOS1 and SOS2 (however not in all cases). Gingival expansion as a result of accumulation of extracellular matrix protein.
- **Diagnosis**: Clinical examination, biopsy, medical history, family history and laboratory tests.
- **Ddx**: Drug induced gingival hyperplasia and leukemia.
- **Histopathology**: Epithelial hyperplasia with elongated thin rete pegs extending into hypo-vascular fibrous connective tissue containing numerous collagen fibers, oriented in variable directions.
- **Management**: Non-surgical management entails scaling, root planing, and oral hygiene instruction. Surgical management involves gingivectomy.

Specific Infections

Infections of Bacterial Origin

Necrotizing Periodontal Diseases

- **Clinical**: Patient presents with painful and erythematous gingiva and "crater-like" necrosis in interdental papillae with ulceration. The lesions may be hemorrhagic and disseminate a strong foul odor. Consider the spectrum of lesions which vary depending on both localization of lesion and predisposing factors i.e. necrotizing-gingivitis, -periodontitis, -stomatitis, and noma.
- **Cause**: Due to bacterial infection by species that include *Treponema*, *Selenomonas*, *Fusobacterium*, and *Prevotella intermedia*. Immunosuppression, poor oral hygiene, smoking, stress, and poor nutrition are strongly associated with infection.
- **Diagnosis**: Clinical features and bacterial culture.
- **Ddx**: Primary herpetic gingivostomatitis, vesiculobullous diseases, and gonorrhea.
- **Histopathology**: Ulceration with necrotic tissue and prominent acute and chronic inflammatory cells in connective tissue stroma. Bacterial colonies are also noted.

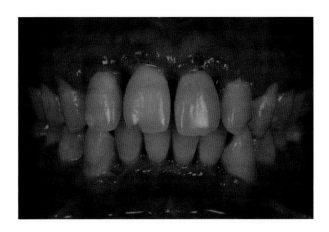

Figure 4.1 Crater-like necrosis of interdental papillae in necrotizing periodontitis. Source: EEC Institute, Inc.

- **Management**: Supportive care and pain control with debridement to remove debris and plaque. Consider antibiotics (Figure 4.1).

Gonorrhea

- **Clinical**: Rare oral manifestation of sexually transmitted disease with areas of erythema and ulceration of gingiva with a pseudomembranous coating. Oropharyngeal lesions appear markedly erythematous with scattered pustules. Lesions develop within one week of contact with infectious individual. This infection is associated with pelvic inflammatory disease and gonococcal ophthalmia neonatorum.
- **Cause**: Sexually transmitted infection caused by the bacterial organism Neisseria gonorrhea.
- **Diagnosis**: Culture of organism, gram stain of purulent material demonstrates gram negative diplococcic, and nucleic acid amplification tests (NAATs).
- **Ddx**: Necrotizing periodontitis (typical odor is not present in gonorrhea).
- **Management**: Symptomatic treatment of oral lesions after confirming patient is receiving care from physician with appropriate antibiotics.

Syphilis

- Clinical: Sexually transmitted disease with possible oral manifestations which vary in presentation depending upon stage.
  - **Primary**: Presents with the highly infectious usually painless chancre that may occur at any oral mucosal site including the gingiva (resolves in approximately two to eight weeks).
  - **Secondary**: Diffuse skin eruptions are the hallmark of this stage. Orally presents with elevated mucous patches and condylomata lata (2–12 weeks after primary lesion).
  - **Tertiary**: This stage may occur as many as 30 years after the secondary stage. Oral lesions include areas of granulomatous inflammation termed gumma, which results in significant ulceration (more common on palate and tongue).
  - Also consider congenital syphilis infection and oral manifestation of Hutchinson incisors and mulberry molars.
- **Cause**: Infection with spirochete bacterium *Treponema pallidum.*
- **Diagnosis**: Clinical features, histopathology, dark field microscopy of a smear and lab tests (i.e. venereal disease research lab (VDRL) test, rapid plasma reagin [RPR] test).
- **Ddx**: Depending upon stage the lesions may resemble various other oral pathologic processes.
  - **Primary**: The lesion may resemble the non-healing ulceration differential (traumatic ulcer, squamous cell carcinoma, tuberculosis ulcer, deep fungal ulcer).
  - **Secondary**: Mucous patches may resemble leukoplakic patches.
  - **Tertiary**: Palatal gumma may mimic sequelae from cocaine use, malignancy, or mucormycosis infection.
- **Histopathology**: In primary and secondary syphilis the oral lesions show ulceration with exocytosis of neutrophils with a dense chronic inflammatory infiltrate in the connective tissue stroma. Of note is the perivascular lymphoplasmacytic infiltrate. With special stain (Warthin Starry, silver stain) or immunohistochemistry, the spirochete organisms can be seen in surface epithelium. In tertiary lesions the organisms are difficult to ascertain however ulceration and granulomatous inflammation is noted.
- **Management**: Intramuscular Penicillin G.

Tuberculosis

- **Clinical**: Chronic granulomatous infectious disease, which usually affects the lungs. Secondary hematogenous spread from the lungs or rarely primary infection may lead to non-specific oral lesions. The most common manifestation however is a painful non-healing ulcer on the lateral tongue.
- **Cause**: Infection with Mycobacterium tuberculosis.
- **Diagnosis**: Biopsy, sputum culture, chest X-ray, Mantoux test, and systemic signs.
- **Ddx**: Traumatic ulcer, major aphthous ulcer, squamous cell carcinoma, deep fungal ulcer, syphilitic ulcer.
- **Histopathology**: Epithelioid histiocytes surrounding a central necrotic zone accompanied by multinucleated giant cells and lymphocytes. Special stain with Ziehl–Neelsen to demonstrate acid-fast bacilli.

- **Management**: Six month course of antibiotics (isoniazid, rifampin, pyrazinamide, and either ethambutol or streptomycin).

Streptococcal Gingivitis

- **Clinical**: Diffuse gingival inflammation and bone loss considered unassociated with plaque formation.
- **Cause**: Infection with streptococcal strains.
- **Diagnosis**: Culture of organism if regular phases of periodontal treatment are not providing resolution.
- **Ddx**: Other forms of periodontal disease.
- **Management**: Antibiotics with mechanical debridement.

Infections of Viral Origin

Hand, Foot, and Mouth Disease

- **Clinical**: Viral illness which usually presents in young children. The patient may display signs of fever, malaise, lack of appetite, and sore throat. Painful oral ulcers start to develop in the back of the mouth along with a rash/vesicles on the palms and soles.
- **Cause**: Most commonly Coxsackie virus A16, which is a type of Enterovirus.
- **Diagnosis**: Clinical presentation.
- **Ddx**: Herpetic gingivostomatitis, herpangina.
- **Histopathology**: Epidermal necrosis, infiltrate of lymphocytes along epithelial interface with connective tissue and extensive edema.
- **Management**: Self-limiting condition which lasts 7–10 days in most cases therefore supportive treatment to alleviate pain and prevent dehydration.

Primary Herpetic Gingivostomatitis

- **Clinical**: Initial herpes simplex virus infection which results in shallow ulcers on both keratinized and non-keratinized mucosa with systemic signs and symptoms (fever, lymphadenopathy, myalgia). More common in children.
- **Cause**: Herpes simplex virus type 1 (or type 2).
- **Diagnosis**: Cytologic smear, tissue biopsy, antibody studies, viral culture.
- **Ddx**: Other viral infections, necrotizing ulcerative periodontitis and erythema multiforme in some cases.
- **Histopathology**: Infected keratinocyte cells display balloon degeneration and nuclear changes consisting of margination of chromatin, multinucleation, and nuclear molding. The ulcer is composed of a fibrin membrane with viable and necrotic neutrophils.
- **Management**: Self-limited condition which resolves in approximately 10 days without scarring. Palliative treatment with adequate hydration, nutrition, and consideration given to pain relief.

Recurrent Herpes Simplex

- **Clinical**: Recurrent unilateral ulcers which occur on the skin of the lip (termed herpes labialis) and intraorally on the keratinized mucosa. Extraorally, the ulcerations initially appear as a cluster of vesicles which eventually open and finally crust over. Intraorally, crops of coalescing ulcers are seen. Prodromal symptoms may be present before clinical evidence of lesions. Atypical presentation of lesions may occur in HIV infected individuals.
- **Cause**: Reactivation of herpes simplex virus infection which is latent in the trigeminal ganglion. Triggers include exposure to sunlight, trauma, fever, and stress.
- **Diagnosis**: Clinical diagnosis if features are classic or cytologic smear/tissue biopsy.
- **Ddx**: Extraorally, may resemble impetigo (not unilateral). Intraoral recurrent herpes is usually distinct but may resemble localized necrotizing ulcerative gingivitis or traumatic ulcers.
- **Histopathology**: Infected keratinocyte cells display acantholysis, balloon degeneration, and nuclear changes consisting of margination of chromatin, multinucleation, and nuclear molding. The ulcer is composed of a fibrin membrane with viable and necrotic neutrophils.
- **Management**: Self-limited condition which heals without scarring. 1% penciclovir cream may be useful for extraoral lesions if applied during prodrome and for intraoral lesions consider systemic antivirals such as valacyclovir.

Oral Hairy Leukoplakia

- **Clinical**: Opportunistic infection by Epstein Barr virus (EBV) which results in a non-wipeable white lesion with corrugated vertical folds on lateral tongue.
- **Cause**: Immunosuppression (HIV infection or organ transplant patients) leading to EBV infection.
- **Diagnosis**: Biopsy and microscopic evaluation.
- **Ddx**: Frictional keratosis, tongue chewing, leukoplakia.
- **Histopathology**: Thickened parakeratin with surface projections overlying a "balloon cell" layer containing cells with excess cytoplasm. These cells display nuclear clearing and margination of chromatin in the pattern of a circular string of beads.
- **Management**: Treatment is usually not needed however lesions may be removed for esthetic reasons.

Human Papilloma Virus Infection

- **Clinical**: The squamous papilloma is an asymptomatic oral lesion caused by low risk human papilloma virus (HPV). This exophytic growth presents with papillary projections and either a pedunculated or sessile base. The common locations are the tongue and soft palate.
- **Cause**: Low risk human papilloma virus (types 6 or 11) causing a benign neoplasm of squamous cells.

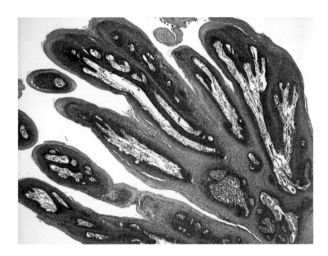

Figure 4.2 Papillary epithelium and fibrovascular cores in a squamous papilloma.

- **Diagnosis**: Microscopic examination.
- **Ddx**: Verruca vulgaris (cutaneous wart), condyloma acuminatum (genital wart), and occasionally a giant cell fibroma that has a similar bosselated surface.
- **Histopathology**: Proliferation of squamous epithelial cells in a papillary manner with fibrovascular cores (Figure 4.2). Other features include evidence of a viral cytopathic effect consisting of koilocytes and binucleated cells.
- **Management**: Surgical excision.

Chicken Pox (Varicella) and Zoster

- **Clinical**: Chicken pox or varicella is a viral infection that usually affects children and results in a pruritic maculopapular skin rash with associated systemic symptoms (headache, fever, malaise). In later stages, the lesions become vesicles and pustules which rupture and become crusted. The oral manifestation includes intraoral vesicles. In zoster or "shingles" there is a reactivation of the latent virus present in the dorsal root ganglion or trigeminal ganglion. The rash is distributed in a unilateral manner and presents with pain. In zoster, oral manifestations are rare however vesicles, bone necrosis, and tooth loss may occur in the affected area.
- **Cause**: Varicella zoster virus.
- **Diagnosis**: Clinical features, cytology, PCR, culture, antibody titers.
- **Ddx**: Rare oral gingival lesions resemble primary HSV infection.
- **Histopathology**: Cytology displays identical viral cytopathic effect as seen in HSV (i.e. nuclear margination of chromatin, molding of cells and multinucleation).
- **Management**: Supportive treatment (may consider antivirals in certain cases).

Molluscum

- **Clinical**: Commonly presents as pruritic, umbilicated papules on the skin of the face and trunk, rarely intraorally. More frequent in children and immunocompromised individuals. Sexually transmitted in adults.
- **Cause**: Poxvirus.
- **Diagnosis**: Clinical features, biopsy with microscopic examination.
- **Ddx**: Cryptococcus, verruca vulgaris, condyloma acuminatum.
- **Histopathology**: Viral cytopathic effect in epithelial cells leads to intracytoplasmic eosinophilic inclusions (Henderson-Paterson bodies or molluscum bodies).
- **Management**: May regress within 6-9 months or may be removed surgically.

Infections of Fungal Origin

Candidiasis

- **Clinical**: Opportunistic oral infection by the commensal fungal organism *Candida albicans* that results in five main presentations.
  1. **Pseudomembranous candidiasis**: White, wipeable curd-like plaques that occur most commonly on the buccal mucosa, palate, and tongue in immunosuppressed or individuals taking broad-spectrum antibiotics. Symptoms may include a burning sensation.
  2. **Erythematous candidiasis**: Red areas that may be a result of antibiotic use, xerostomia, or steroid inhalers (palate). The tongue may display patchy depapillation of the filiform papillae. The lesions may include symptoms of a burning sensation. This category also includes median rhomboid glossitis that presents as a well-defined central area of atrophy on the dorsal tongue infected with candida which is asymptomatic.
  3. **Denture stomatitis**: Erythematous lesion localized to denture-bearing areas due to continuous wear of denture. May present with petechiae to diffuse redness (Figure 4.3).
  4. **Chronic hyperplastic**: Uncommon form of candidiasis which presents as a non-wipeable white lesion. The hyperplastic response of the mucosa is a result of the presence of candida organisms. Common on the anterior buccal mucosa.
  5. **Angular cheilitis**: Candida infection presents with cracking and erythema at the commissures that are usually bilateral. The loss of vertical dimension may predispose the area to constant moisture which leads to the infected fissured lesions.
- **Diagnosis**: Clinical features and cytologic smear (Figure 4.4) or biopsy with microscopic evaluation after PAS stain (Figure 4.5)

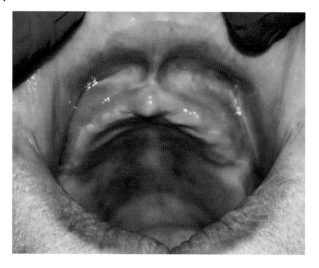

Figure 4.3 Erythematous palate in a case of denture stomatitis.

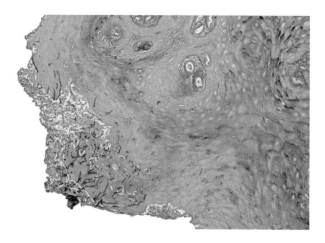

Figure 4.5 PAS stain to show presence of Candida organisms in the surface parakeratin layer.

Histoplasmosis

- **Clinical**: Rare intraoral presentation of solitary ulceration with firm borders due to extrapulmonary disseminated infection.
- **Cause**: Histoplasma capsulatum.
- **Diagnosis**: Biopsy and microscopic examination, culture, serology.
- **Ddx**: Squamous cell carcinoma.
- **Histopathology**: Granulomatous inflammation comprised of epithelioid histiocytes containing fungal organisms (Figure 4.6). GMS special stain used to highlight presence of fungal organisms.
- **Management**: Amphotericin B or itraconazole antifungal medications.

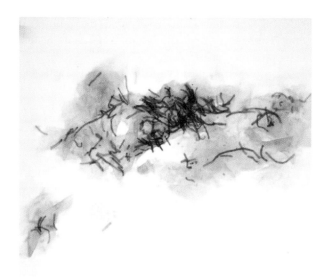

Figure 4.4 Candida organisms stained with PAS stain on a cytologic smear.

- **Ddx (number corresponds with type of candidiasis)**: 1. Materia alba, 2. & 3. Erythroplakia, localized inflammatory response, 4. Frictional keratosis, leukoplakia (dysplasia/squamous cell carcinoma), 5. Nutritional deficiencies (iron, B12, folic acid).
- **Histopathology**: Increased thickness of parakeratin layer containing neutrophilic microabscesses and candida hyphae. There is also elongation of epithelial rete ridges and a chronic inflammatory cell infiltrate in the connective tissue.
- **Management**: Antifungal medication (nystatin or clotrimazole).

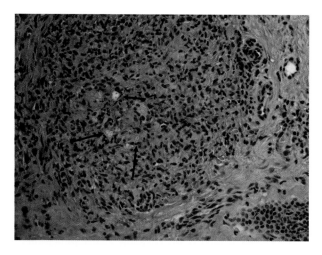

Figure 4.6 Granulomatous inflammation composed of epithelioid histiocytes. Fungal organisms observed within granuloma (black arrows).

Aspergillosis

- **Clinical**: Inhaled spores lead to various clinical presentations. Noninvasive form presents as an allergic fungal sinusitis or fungal ball (aspergilloma). Invasive form may present as disseminated disease or a localized intraoral lesion with a diffuse gray or violaceous hue.
- **Cause**: Aspergillus flavus and Aspergillus fumigatus.
- **Diagnosis**: Biopsy and microscopic examination or culture.
- **Ddx**: Other fungal infection, malignancy.
- **Histopathology**: Branching (acute angle) septate hyphae with fruiting bodies.
- **Management**: Debridement for non-invasive disease (corticosteroids are also added for allergic fungal sinusitis). Debridement, voriconazole, and amphotericin B for invasive aspergillosis.

Inflammatory and Immune Conditions

Hypersensitivity Reactions

Contact Allergy/Allergic Contact Mucositis

- **Clinical**: Erythematous and edematous lesions that may form vesicles and ulcers or appear lichenoid as a result of direct contact with allergens such as dental materials, toothpaste, chewing gum, food additives, and cinnamon. Symptoms include burning, itching, and stinging.
- **Cause**: Direct contact with allergen.
- **Diagnosis**: Consider history and perform allergy testing or possible biopsy in certain clinical situations.
- **Ddx**: Lichen planus, epithelial dysplasia.
- **Histopathology**: Lesions may present with interface mucositis and deeper perivascular inflammatory infiltrate with occasional eosinophils. Lichenoid type lesions display areas of hydropic degeneration of the basal cell layer and a dense band like infiltrate of lymphocytes and plasma cells subjacent to the basal cells. A deeper perivascular lymphoid infiltrate may also be seen.
- **Management**: Removal of allergen, antihistamines, or topical corticosteroids.

Plasma Cell Gingivitis

- **Clinical**: The gingival epithelium takes on a bright red hue and displays generalized involvement. Pain is associated with the condition especially if hot, spicy, and acidic foods are contacted.
- **Cause**: Allergy or idiopathic.
- **Diagnosis**: Histopathology combined with clinical features.
- **Ddx**: Desquamative gingivitis lesions.
- **Histopathology**: Hyperplasia of the mucosa in a psoriasiform manner with an intense plasma cell infiltrate in connective tissue stroma.

- **Management**: Allergy testing or dietary history to rule out offending agent. May consider topical steroids.

Erythema Multiforme

- **Clinical**: Acute self-limiting condition with abrupt onset that presents with oral mucosal and/or skin lesions. The diffuse oral lesions are usually large ulcerations on the buccal/labial mucosa and lateral tongue. A characteristic hemorrhagic crusting of the vermilion of the lip and "target lesions" (concentric erythematous rings) on the skin may also be seen. This condition is most commonly seen in young adults.
- **Cause**: Uncertain but most likely hypersensitivity reaction to preceding herpes simplex or Mycoplasma pneumonia infection, drugs, or idiopathic.
- **Diagnosis**: Clinical features and history. May consider biopsy to rule out other conditions since histopathology is not pathognomonic.
- **Ddx**: Paraneoplastic pemphigus and other vesiculobullous disorders may present similarly. Stevens Johnson syndrome and toxic epidermal necrolysis are similar however more severe in presentation and most likely due to drug exposure.
- **Histopathology**: The epithelium displays necrosis of basal cells and the presence of intercellular and intracellular edema. There is also intraepithelial and subepithelial vesicle formation with exocytosis of inflammatory cells. A mixed infiltrate of lymphocytes, neutrophils, and occasional eosinophils is seen in the submucosa. A perivascular inflammatory infiltrate is also noted in the connective tissue.
- **Immunofluorescence**: Non-specific.
- **Management**: Try to identify and avoid the probable etiologic agent. Usually self-limiting (lasts two to four weeks), however, may consider steroid or antiviral for recurrent cases. Maintain hydration and use topical anesthetic for pain during eating.

Autoimmune Diseases of Skin and Mucous Membranes

Pemphigus Vulgaris

- **Clinical**: Autoimmune vesiculobullous condition more common in adults 50–60 years old. Autoantibodies develop toward epithelial intercellular bridges and results in loss of cell to cell adhesion. This condition manifests clinically as painful skin and oral vesicles and bullae which quickly rupture to form ulcers. Clinical manifestation on the gingiva is called desquamative gingivitis.
- **Cause**: Binding of autoantibodies (IgG) to desmoglein-3 which is a component of desmosomes.
- **Diagnosis**: Biopsy (including intact epithelium) and consider a positive Nikolsky sign (formation of a bulla

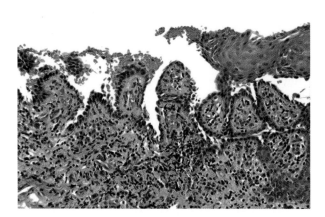

Figure 4.7 Histopathology of pemphigus vulgaris showing continued attachment of basal cells to connective tissue in "tombstone" arrangement.

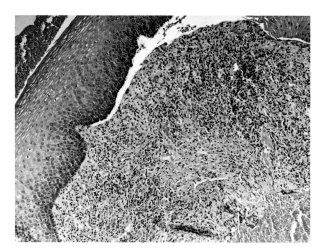

Figure 4.8 Subepithelial separation between epithelium and inflamed connective tissue in mucous membrane pemphigoid.

on normal mucosa with gentle lateral pressure) may also be noted.

- **Ddx**: Mucous membrane pemphigoid, erythema multiforme, erosive lichen planus, and paraneoplastic pemphigus.
- **Histopathology**: Acantholysis of the epithelium with an intact basal cell layer attached to the underlying connective tissue. Only the basal layer cells are attached to the basement membrane zone by hemidesmosomes and appear as a "row of tombstones." Loose rounded acantholytic cells are noted in the intraepithelial clefts which are termed Tzanck cells (Figure 4.7).
- **Direct immunofluorescence**: IgG, IgM, and C3 are demonstrated in the intercellular spaces ("fishnet pattern").
- **Indirect immunofluorescence**: Positive.
- **Management**: High dose steroids and immunosuppressives.

Mucous Membrane Pemphigoid

- **Clinical**: Autoimmune vesiculobullous condition more common in adults 50–60 years old. Autoantibodies develop toward a component of the basement membrane. This results in painful vesicles and bullae that rupture to leave large ulcerations that heal with scarring. Gingival lesions are clinically termed desquamative gingivitis. Ocular involvement may cause significant complications.
- **Cause**: Binding of autoantibodies (IgG, C3) to a component of the basement membrane (epiligrin) or a component of hemidesmosomes (alpha-6 integrin).
- **Diagnosis**: Biopsy (including intact epithelium), a positive Nikolsky sign may also be noted.

- **Ddx**: Pemphigus vulgaris, erosive lichen planus, bullous pemphigoid (skin usually, BP180 and BP230 are antigens), linear IgA bullous dermatosis (deposition of IgA along basement membrane, mostly in skin), angina bullosa hemorrhagica (rare with blood filled vesicles), and epidermolysis bullosa acquisita (mostly skin, type 7 collagen is antigen).
- **Histopathology**: The epithelium separates from the connective tissue at the basement membrane (subepithelial cleft) (Figure 4.8). The superficial connective tissue displays a chronic inflammatory infiltrate.
- **Direct immunofluorescence**: Linear pattern of deposition of IgG and C3 at basement membrane.
- **Treatment**: Topical steroids, immunosuppressives, referral to ophthalmologist.

Lichen Planus

- **Clinical**: Chronic T-cell mediated autoimmune disease which affects both the skin and oral mucosa. The condition is more commonly seen on the buccal mucosa, tongue, and gingiva in people older than age 40. The buccal lesions are usually bilateral in presentation. Two main forms exist: reticular and erosive. The reticular form presents with lace-like white lesions (Wickham striae) (Figure 4.9). On the dorsal of the tongue the white lesions are plaque like in appearance. The erosive form presents with pain, atrophy, and ulceration. Radiating white striae tend to rim the ulcerations. The erosive form is clinically termed desquamative gingivitis (Figure 4.10) when present on the attached gingiva. The skin lesions are described as purple, pruritic papules.
- **Cause**: T-cell mediated disease.

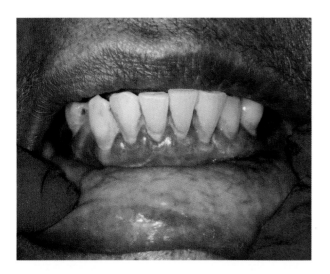

Figure 4.9 Faint white striae on mandibular gingiva in a patient with lichen planus.

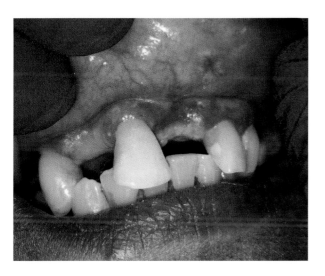

Figure 4.10 Desquamative gingivitis in a patient with erosive lichen planus.

- **Diagnosis**: Clinical features may be distinct in the reticular form however biopsy (including intact epithelium) is usually indicated for erosive form.
- **Ddx**: Clinical ddx: Lichenoid drug reaction (similar reaction as a result of systemic medication), graft versus host disease, epithelial dysplasia, mucous membrane pemphigoid, lupus erythematosus. Histopathologic ddx: Lichenoid drug reaction, graft versus host disease, lupus erythematosus, chronic ulcerative stomatitis, oral mucosal cinnamon reaction.
- **Histopathology**: The epithelium may show varying levels of parakeratosis and appear hyperplastic or atrophic depending on the form. Sub-epithelial separation may be noted in the erosive type. Hydropic degeneration of

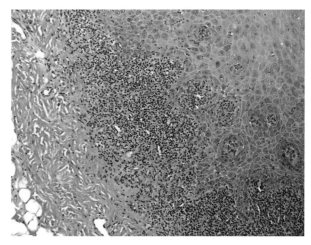

Figure 4.11 Dense band-like infiltrate of lymphocytes and "saw-tooth" rete ridges.

the basal cell layer of the epithelium associated with a dense band-like infiltrate of T-lymphocytes is seen (Figure 4.11). "Saw-tooth" rete ridges (Figure 4.11), colloid bodies (eosinophilic degenerating keratinocytes), and melanin incontinence may also be present.
- **Direct immunofluorescence**: Non-specific with shaggy band of fibrinogen at basement membrane zone. **Management**: No treatment is needed for the reticular form. Topical corticosteroids may be used for the symptomatic erosive form. Warn patient of waxing and waning nature of disease.

Chronic Ulcerative Stomatitis

- **Clinical**: Immune mediated condition affecting older women with ulcerations on tongue or buccal mucosa in a manner similar to erosive lichen planus. Desquamative gingivitis may also be a feature.
- **Cause**: Studies suggest autoantibodies to the nuclear protein deltaNp63alpha cause a disruption in the attachment of epithelium to connective tissue.
- **Diagnosis**: Biopsy with direct immunofluorescence.
- **Ddx**: Erosive lichen planus (chronic ulcerative stomatitis does not respond well to steroid treatment).
- **Histopathology**: Similar to lichen planus.
- **Direct immunofluorescence**: Autoantibodies (IgG) to the nuclei of stratified squamous epithelial cells in basal and parabasal regions.
- **Management**: Hydroxychloroquine if lesions do not respond to steroid treatment.

Paraneoplastic Pemphigus

- **Clinical**: Vesiculobullous disorder that affects patients with a neoplasm such as lymphoma or leukemia.

Clinically appears similar to pemphigus vulgaris however there is a diverse presentation.

- **Cause**: Precise mechanism is unknown; however antibodies to plakin family of desmosomal components have been identified in cases.
- **Diagnosis**: Tissue biopsy.
- **Ddx**: Pemphigus vulgaris, erythema multiforme (crusting of lips is similar), mucous membrane pemphigoid (eye scarring is similar), lichen planus (skin lesions are similar)
- **Histopathology**: A combination of features seen in pemphigus vulgaris and lichen planus (suprabasilar separation with acantholysis and vacuolization of basal cells with a lymphoid infiltrate).
- **Direct immunofluorescence**: Intercellular deposition of IgG and complement, with a granular deposition of complement at basement membrane.
- **Indirect immunofluorescence**: Positive.
- **Treatment**: Systemic steroids and immunosuppressive therapy are attempted however the morbidity and mortality rate is high.

Recurrent Aphthous Ulcers

- **Clinical**: Most common type of oral ulceration which appears on the movable non-keratinized mucosa. Young adults are affected most frequently. The three types include: (i) Minor, (ii) Major, and (iii) Herpetiform
  1. Minor aphthous presents as a circular ulcer less than 1.0 cm with a white fibrin pseudomembrane and an erythematous halo. Commonly presents on buccal and labial mucosa. There may be a prodrome and healing occurs in one to two weeks without scarring.
  2. Major aphthous ulcers are larger than 1.0 cm and extend deeper into the submucosa. These ulcers require more time to heal and heal with scarring.
  3. Herpetiform aphthous ulcers are the rarest type and appear as crops of coalescing ulcers similar to recurrent herpetic ulcers (on fixed mucosa). Healing occurs in one to two weeks.
- **Cause**: Possible T-cell mediated immune reaction causing epithelium to ulcerate.
- **Diagnosis**: Clinical features and exclusion of other diseases, biopsy is non-specific.
- **Ddx**: (i) Minor aphthous-Ulcers in systemic disorders, (ii) Major aphthous-Squamous cell carcinoma, traumatic ulcer, deep fungal and tuberculosis ulcer, (iii) Herpetiform aphthous-Herpetic ulceration (consider location).
- **Histopathology**: Ulcerated mucosa consisting of a fibrin membrane entrapping viable and necrotic neutrophils. Increased vascularity and an infiltrate of acute and chronic inflammatory cells are noted.

- **Management**: No treatment usually. May consider topical anesthetics or steroids. Systemic steroids may be used in major aphthous cases.

Graft versus Host Disease

- **Clinical**: Adverse reaction after allogeneic bone marrow transplantation to treat conditions such as leukemia, lymphoma, and multiple myeloma. Clinically oral lesions affect the tongue, labial mucosa, and buccal mucosa and may appear similar to lichen planus. Ulcerations and atrophy of the mucosa are noted.
- **Cause**: Engrafted cells start attacking cells in donor environment.
- **Diagnosis**: Consider clinical history and histopathology.
- **Ddx**: Lichen planus and potentially malignant lesions.
- **Histopathology**: Similar to lichen planus with less inflammation.
- **Management**: Topical corticosteroids, topical anesthetics (for comfort).

Granulomatous Inflammatory Conditions

Crohn's Disease

- **Clinical**: Type of inflammatory bowel disease with immune mediation affecting any part of the gastrointestinal tract. Oral manifestations include "cobblestone" appearance to mucosa and linear ulcers in buccal vestibule. Erythematous macules and plaques may be seen on the gingiva. May see pyostomatitis vegetans or yellow-white pustules on mucosa. Also noted is an increased frequency of periodontal disease.
- **Cause**: Unknown.
- **Diagnosis**: Based on clinical features and histopathology.
- **Ddx**: Histopathology resembles orofacial granulomatosis and Melkersson–Rosenthal syndrome.
- **Histopathology**: Non-necrotizing granulomatous inflammation.
- **Management**: Oral lesions are treated with topical or intralesional steroids however usually resolve with overall treatment of condition.

Sarcoidosis

- **Clinical**: Granulomatous disorder that affects multiple organ systems. Uncommon oral manifestations include swelling, areas of granularity, and ulcerations. Most commonly affected intraoral soft tissue sites include buccal mucosa and gingiva.
- **Cause**: Unknown.
- **Diagnosis**: Clinical features, histopathology, lab analysis, and radiographic evaluation (intraosseous lesions also possible).

- **Ddx**: Perform special stains to rule out fungal and bacterial infections.
- **Histopathology**: Granulomas composed of epithelioid histiocytes with a rim of lymphocytes.
- **Management**: Corticosteroids and chemotherapeutics (in resistant cases).

Reactive Processes

Epulides

Irritation Fibroma/Fibrous Epulis
- **Clinical**: Smooth surfaced nodular lesion composed of connective tissue with overlying normal mucosal coloration (Figure 4.12). Irritation fibromas may be sessile or pedunculated and may occur anywhere in the oral cavity. The most common location is the buccal mucosa. A variation includes the epulis fissuratum that occurs in association with a denture flange.
- **Cause**: Reactive proliferation after traumatic injury or irritation. Some possible etiologies include calculus, ill-fitting denture, overhanging restoration, or tissue injury from biting.
- **Diagnosis**: Consider clinical location and antecedent trauma. Biopsy is performed to obtain definitive diagnosis and rule out soft tissue tumor.
- **Ddx**: Other mesenchymal derived soft tissue tumor.
- **Histopathology**: Surface epithelium overlying a mass of dense fibrous connective tissue composed of collagen bundles.
- **Management**: Conservative surgical excision.

Peripheral Ossifying Fibroma
- **Clinical**: Exophytic pink to erythematous firm mass which presents exclusively on the gingiva. The lesion may be ulcerated.

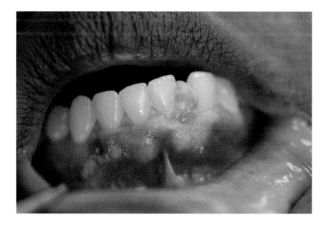

Figure 4.12 Fibrous proliferation in interdental papilla between teeth #23 and #24 diagnosed as an irritation fibroma.

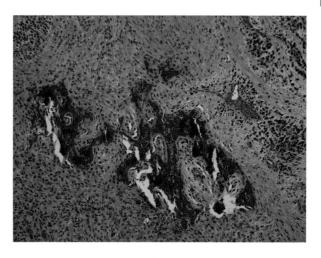

Figure 4.13 Cellular fibroblastic stroma containing irregular ossifications in a peripheral ossifying fibroma.

- **Cause**: Most likely a reactive proliferation of periodontal ligament derived tissue in response to local irritation.
- **Diagnosis**: Biopsy and microscopic evaluation.
- **Ddx**: Peripheral giant cell granuloma, pyogenic granuloma, irritation fibroma, and peripheral odontogenic fibroma.
- **Histopathology**: Cellular fibrous proliferation with scattered bone and cementum-like calcifications (Figure 4.13).
- **Management**: Local surgical excision down to periosteum and thorough scaling of adjacent teeth to prevent possible recurrence.

Pyogenic Granuloma
- **Clinical**: Erythematous nodule with frequent ulceration which may present anywhere in the oral cavity. Lesion tends to bleed easily due to vascular proliferation. May be sessile or pedunculated. Also called a "pregnancy tumor" when the lesion occurs during pregnancy.
- **Cause**: Possibly develops in response to trauma or irritants such as calculus.
- **Diagnosis**: Biopsy and microscopic evaluation.
- **Ddx**: Peripheral ossifying fibroma, peripheral giant cell granuloma, irritation fibroma, peripheral odontogenic fibroma, and malignant tumors in some cases.
- **Histopathology**: Vascular proliferation that resembles granulation tissue with an abundance of endothelial lined channels (Figure 4.14). The overlying epithelium may be ulcerated with a fibrin membrane entrapping viable and necrotic neutrophils. A mixed infiltrate of acute and chronic inflammatory cells is noted in the edematous stroma. When the vessels appear to be organized into lobules the term "lobular capillary hemangioma" is used.

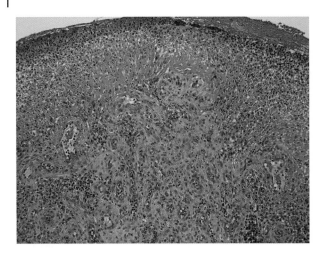

Figure 4.14 Ulcerated surface epithelium overlying an abundance of endothelial lined capillaries and an infiltrate of acute and chronic inflammatory cells.

Figure 4.15 Dense collection of mononuclear cells with scattered multinucleated giant cells and numerous red blood cells.

- **Management**: Local surgical excision down to periosteum and thorough scaling of adjacent teeth to prevent possible recurrence.

Peripheral Giant Cell Granuloma
- **Clinical**: Exophytic red to blue firm mass which presents exclusively on the gingiva with a tendency to bleed easily. The lesion is more common in adults between 30 and 45 with a female predilection. These lesions may be ulcerated and may cause superficial resorption of the underlying bone.
- **Cause**: Most likely a reactive proliferation in response to local irritants.
- **Diagnosis**: Biopsy and microscopic evaluation.
- **Ddx**: Peripheral ossifying fibroma, pyogenic granuloma, irritation fibroma, and peripheral odontogenic fibroma.
- **Histopathology**: Proliferation of mononuclear spindle cells with numerous multinucleated giant cells set in abundant hemorrhage (Figure 4.15).
- **Management**: Local surgical excision down to periosteum and thorough scaling of adjacent teeth to prevent possible recurrence.

Pre-Malignant Lesions and Malignant Neoplasms

Oral Potentially Malignant Disorders: Leukoplakia/ Erythroplakia
- **Clinical**: Clinical terms for white or red lesions of the oral mucosa which cannot be attributed to any other cause and carry an increased risk of progression to cancer (Figure 4.12). Leukoplakic lesions may display dysplasia or squamous cell carcinoma in 20% of cases. Erythroplakia, while rare on the gingiva have a

much higher potential for dysplasia or squamous cell carcinoma at 85%.
- **Risk factors**: Tobacco, alcohol, radiation, areca nut, and HPV (oropharyngeal squamous cell carcinoma).
- **Diagnosis**: Biopsy and microscopic evaluation.
- **Ddx**: Frictional keratosis, hyperplastic candidiasis.
- **Histopathology**: Dysplastic epithelium displays architectural and cytologic alterations in the surface epithelium. These features consist of irregular epithelial stratification, loss of basal cell polarity, tear-drop shaped rete ridges, dyskeratosis, nuclear/cellular pleomorphism, nuclear hyperchromatism, increased nuclear-to-cytoplasmic ratio, prominent nucleoli and increased mitotic activity with irregular mitoses (Figure 4.16). Dysplasia is characterized into mild, moderate, and severe depending upon the thickness of epithelium affected. The feature of invasion into the connective tissue is not present in dysplasia (Figure 4.17).
- **Management**: Surgical biopsy and long-term follow up. Advise patient regarding habit modification.

Squamous Cell Carcinoma
- **Clinical**: Most common type of carcinoma in the oral cavity which may present as an erythematous and/or leukoplakic patch or a non-healing indurated ulceration or mass.
- **Risk factors**: Tobacco, alcohol, radiation, areca nut, and HPV (oropharyngeal squamous cell carcinoma).
- **Diagnosis**: Biopsy and microscopic evaluation.
- **Ddx**: Non-healing ulcers may be seen in other lesions including traumatic ulcer, major aphthous ulcer, deep fungal infection, tuberculosis ulcer, and syphilitic chancre.

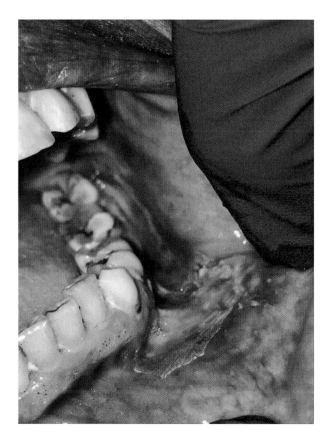

Figure 4.16 Non-homogeneous leukoplakia in mandibular vestibule from smokeless tobacco placement.

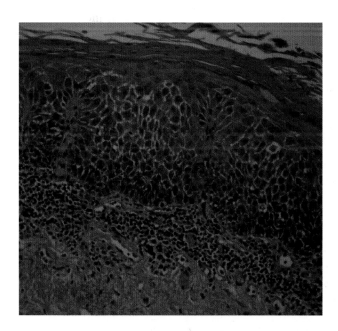

Figure 4.17 Histopathology of moderate epithelial dysplasia.

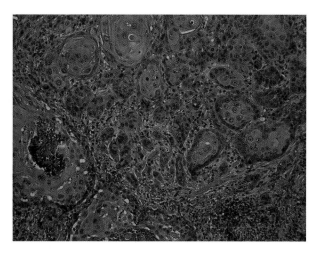

Figure 4.18 Islands of neoplastic epithelial cells infiltrating the connective tissue in squamous cell carcinoma.

- **Histopathology**: Dysplastic surface epithelium that displays invasive islands and cords of malignant epithelial cells. The neoplastic cells in the infiltrating islands show features of dyskeratosis, keratin pearl formation, nuclear/cellular pleomorphism, nuclear hyperchromatism, increased nuclear-to-cytoplasmic ratio, prominent nucleoli and increased mitotic activity with irregular mitoses (Figure 4.18).
- **Management**: Surgical excision, radiation, and chemotherapy.

Leukemia

- **Clinical**: Leukemia is a type of cancer caused by proliferation of neoplastic white blood cells. Leukemia is characterized as either acute or chronic depending upon the clinical course and as either myeloid or lymphoid depending upon the origin of the cells. Patients with leukemia present with symptoms related to anemia, neutropenia, and thrombocytopenia. Oral manifestations include gingival bleeding as a result of thrombocytopenia and gingival overgrowth due to infiltration of leukemic cells. The more common types of leukemia noted in the gingiva are the acute monocytic leukemia and the acute myelomonocytic leukemia.
- **Cause**: Neoplasia.
- **Diagnosis**: Biopsy, immunohistochemistry, and clinical features.
- **Histopathology**: Effacement of submucosal stroma by neoplastic white blood cell infiltrate.
- **Ddx**: Medication related gingival overgrowth and gingival fibromatosis.
- **Management**: Chemotherapy.

Lymphoma

- **Clinical**: Second most common type of oral malignancy which proliferates with clonal growth of neoplastic lymphocytes. Presents in the tissues of the lymph nodes or extra-nodally as an irregular mass which may be ulcerated. The most common subtype orally is the diffuse large B-cell lymphoma. The tumors have a predilection for Waldeyer's ring and may present intraosseously.
- **Cause**: Neoplasia
- **Diagnosis**: Biopsy and immunohistochemistry.
- **Histopathology**: Sheets of infiltrating neoplastic lymphocytes effacing the normal architecture.
- **Ddx**: Other malignant tumors.
- **Management**: Chemotherapy, immunotherapy.

Endocrine, Nutritional, and Metabolic Diseases

Vitamin C Deficiency (Scurvy)

- Studies have demonstrated a relationship between Vitamin C deficiency (scurvy) and increased periodontal disease. A lack of vitamin C results in defective collagen synthesis leading to effects on the extracellular matrix. In addition, immunologic and inflammatory responses are affected by a decrease in vitamin C levels. The hallmark clinical feature in scurvy is erythematous and swollen gingivae that hemorrhages with minor trauma.

Traumatic Lesions

Physical/Mechanical Insults

Frictional Keratosis

- **Clinical**: This lesion presents as a white patch and occurs in areas that are continuously subject to abrasive forces. The more common areas include edentulous ridges and the retromolar pad. Other regionally specific forms of keratosis include linea alba (buccal keratosis along the plane of occlusion), morsicatio buccarum (habitual chewing of buccal/labial mucosa), and gingival abrasion from a toothbrush.
- **Cause**: Normal hyperplastic/hyperkeratotic response to mechanical irritation.
- **Diagnosis**: Determine whether an etiology exists and remove causative factors.
- **Ddx**: Epithelial dysplasia.
- **Histopathology**: Hyperkeratosis without dysplasia (Figure 4.19).
- **Management**: The lesion should regress upon removal of irritative factors. Scalpel biopsy may be necessary if lesion does not resolve or a specific cause is difficult to pinpoint.

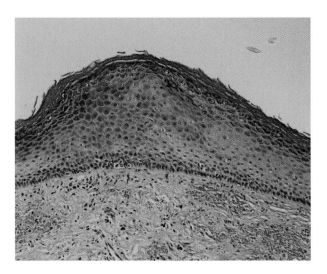

Figure 4.19 Hyperplastic epithelium with a thickened keratin layer.

Traumatic Ulcer

- **Clinical**: Traumatic ulcerations of the oral cavity have the clinical feature of a well-circumscribed area of discontinuity of epithelium surrounded by varying levels of keratosis. The ulcers can occur anywhere in the oral cavity and are most prevalent on the tongue. The floor of the ulcer is covered by a white or yellow fibrin pseudomembrane. With repeated trauma, the lesion may begin to display tumor-like growth with varying levels of induration to base and periphery. This type of lesion presents with a unique histopathologic appearance and has a specific name termed traumatic ulcerative granuloma with stromal eosinophilia (TUGSE).
- **Cause**: Physical trauma, i.e. sharp denture clasp, sharp cusp on a fractured crown, aggressive toothbrushing, and factitious injuries.
- **Diagnosis**: Determine whether recent injury occurred in the vicinity of ulcer by obtaining a thorough history.
- **Ddx**: Includes squamous cell carcinoma, major aphthous ulcer, deep fungal infection, tuberculosis ulcer, and syphilitic chancre.
- **Histopathology**: Normal stratified squamous epithelium exhibiting transition to the ulceration. The ulceration presents with a fibrin pseudomembrane scaffolding containing an infiltrate of viable and necrotic neutrophils. The TUGSE is a chronic traumatic ulcer with an inflammatory process extending deep into the submucosa accompanied by histiocyte-like cells, muscle degeneration, and numerous eosinophils.
- **Management**: Remove cause and biopsy lesion if the ulceration persists after two weeks to rule out malignancy. TUGSE may only resolve fully after biopsy procedure.

Papillary Hyperplasia of the Palate

- **Clinical**: Surface of palate displays a proliferation of multiple erythematous papules under the base of a denture. This lesion is prominent in the palatal vault under complete dentures and appears similar to the surface of raspberries. The lesion may become simultaneously infected with the fungus Candida albicans that may create a burning sensation.
- **Cause**: Unstable dentures or continuous wear of denture.
- **Diagnosis**: Lesion has a clinically distinct presentation.
- **Ddx**: N/A
- **Histopathology**: Papillary extensions on the surface mucosa which are composed of hyperplastic stratified squamous epithelium (Figure 4.20). The connective tissue displays an infiltrate of chronic inflammatory cells and occasional neutrophils. Pseudo-epitheliomatous hyperplasia (benign proliferation of squamous cells into submucosa) may also be seen.
- **Management**: Remove denture at night and consider antifungals. Lesion may not resolve completely however and requires surgical removal before the fabrication of a new denture.

Necrotizing Sialometaplasia

- **Clinical**: Initially presents as a swelling followed by a crater-like ulcer on hard palate with associated erythema. The symptoms range from painful to asymptomatic. More common in adult males older than 40. Usually unilateral but may be bilateral in presentation.
- **Cause**: Uncertain but may be a result of a local ischemic event.
- **Diagnosis**: Tissue biopsy and microscopic examination.

- **Ddx**: Squamous cell carcinoma, salivary gland tumor.
- **Histopathology**: Coagulative necrosis of minor gland acini with the preservation of the borders and lobular architecture. Pools of liberated mucin are noted in the lesion. Squamous metaplasia of the salivary ducts and pseudo-epitheliomatous hyperplasia of the mucosa may be seen. A mixed infiltrate of inflammatory cells is present.
- **Management**: If the ulcer does not show signs of resolution, a biopsy is indicated to confirm the diagnosis. After biopsy the lesion resolves on its own by filling in with granulation tissue. In some cases, spontaneous resolution may occur.

Mucocele

- **Clinical**: Dome-shaped recurrent swelling which develops as a result of rupture of a salivary gland duct and subsequent extravasation of mucin into the connective tissue stroma (Figure 4.21). Mucoceles occur more often on the lower lip of children and young adults however, they may occur anywhere minor glands are located. Variations include: (i) ranula that occurs unilaterally in the floor of the mouth and is associated with the ducts of the sublingual and submandibular gland and (ii) superficial mucocele that is common on the soft palate and retromolar pad and presents with a vesicular appearance.
- **Cause**: Pooling of mucin in connective tissue after duct is ruptured.
- **Diagnosis**: Consider history of lesion and biopsy persistent lesions.
- **Ddx**: Salivary gland tumor.
- **Histopathology**: An area of spilled mucin with surrounding granulation tissue (no epithelial lining) is

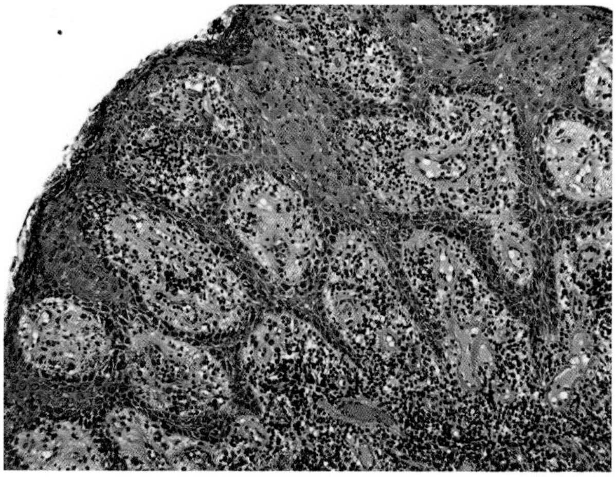

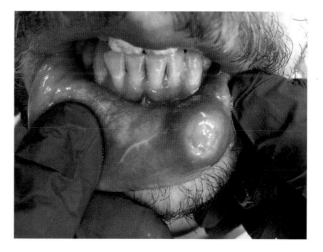

Figure 4.20 Papillary projection of squamous epithelium with a pronounced inflammatory infiltrate in the connective tissue cores.

Figure 4.21 Clinical presentation of a fluctuant swelling in the lower labial mucosa. Note the circular area of ulceration on the surface.

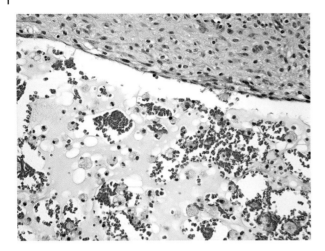

Figure 4.22 Compressed granulation tissue lining extravasated mucin. Foamy histiocytes, neutrophils and red blood cells are seen floating in the pools of mucin.

noted (Figure 4.22). The mucinous material contains neutrophils and foamy histiocytes. Superficial mucoceles present with mucin spillage near the surface epithelium that causes a lifting of the epithelium from the underlying stroma.

- **Management**: Although mucoceles may be self-limiting and rupture and heal on their own, some require local excision for treatment. Possible feeder glands adjacent to the mucocele are also removed to prevent recurrence.

Chemical/Thermal Insults

Mucosal Burn

- **Clinical**: Mucosal burns occur as a result of tissue damage when the epithelium is in contact with destructive agents. The affected tissue demonstrates the presence of a superficial white layer of necrotic tissue. When this tissue sloughs off, a corresponding area of ulceration is revealed, which starts off erythematous and exposed and becomes yellow with a fibrin membrane.
- **Cause**: Thermal or chemical injury which results in the loss of surface epithelium. The causal agent is in direct contact with the oral mucosa and causes subsequent damage. Some of the more common etiologic agents include heat from hot food or drinks, electric burns, inappropriate placement of aspirin, phenol, formocresol, eugenol, and sodium hypochlorite. Cocaine induced midline destructive lesions may cause extensive necrosis leading to palatal perforation.
- **Diagnosis**: Determine the cause of the burn and avoid exposure.
- **Ddx**: Usually the history leads to the diagnosis and the need for biopsy is rare.

- **Histopathology**: Mucosal burns demonstrate stratified squamous epithelium with a superficial necrotic layer and underlying infiltrate of inflammatory cells.
- **Management**: Provide strategies for preventing burn such as patient education regarding direct placement of aspirin. The ulcer should heal in approximately two weeks.

Nicotine Stomatitis

- **Clinical**: Nicotine stomatitis occurs more commonly in older males and presents on the hard palate. The condition is associated with the heat from pipe smoking but cigarette smoking and hot beverages are also implicated. The palatal mucosa becomes white and opacified with elevated papules containing a central erythematous dot corresponding to the opening of the minor salivary gland duct. The palatal mucosa resembles "cracked mud" with a wrinkled surface.
- **Cause**: Response to heat exposure by palatal mucosa.
- **Diagnosis**: Clinical diagnosis with a history of thermal injury to the palate by smoking or hot beverages.
- **Ddx**: Nicotine stomatitis has a distinct appearance therefore biopsy is rarely indicated.
- **Histopathology**: The epithelium displays hyperkeratosis and acanthosis with a central duct and associated chronic inflammatory infiltrate in the adjacent connective tissue. Squamous metaplasia of the duct cells may also be noted.
- **Management**: Nicotine stomatitis is reversible and the palate should return to normal after the irritant is removed.

Localized (Juvenile) Spongiotic Gingival Hyperplasia

- **Clinical**: Bright red, friable gingival overgrowth, which is painless. The surface may be finely granular.
- **Cause**: Possible association with dental plaque, trauma, orthodontic appliances, mouth breathing.
- **Diagnosis**: Biopsy with microscopic examination.
- **Ddx**: Pyogenic granuloma.
- **Histopathology**: Intercellular edema (spongiosis) with interconnecting rete pegs and exocytosis of neutrophils.
- **Management**: Excisional biopsy with follow-up. May resolve spontaneously. Scaling and removal of plaque may not improve the presentation.

Gingival Pigmentation

Post-Inflammatory Pigmentation/Smoker's Melanosis

- **Clinical**: Brown macule in an area of previous injury or inflammation. With smoker's melanosis the pigmentation is usually located on the anterior labial gingiva and most commonly affects females. Smoker's melanosis is diffuse in nature with poorly defined borders.

- **Cause**: Melanin hyperpigmentation as a result of increased melanin production in area of inflammation or exposure to chemicals in tobacco smoke.
- **Diagnosis**: Obtain history regarding previous trauma in area or manner of placement of cigarette.
- **Ddx**: Oral melanotic macule, melanocytic nevus, amalgam tattoo, melanoma, melanoacanthoma, variation of normal, drug induced pigmentation, or syndrome associated.
- **Histopathology**: Increased quantity of melanin in basal cells of epithelium (similar to melanotic macule), with associated melanin incontinence and melanophages in the superficial connective tissue.
- **Management**: If history of lesion is difficult to correlate with clinical presentation then consider biopsy to rule out other lesions especially if lesion is on hard palate or maxillary alveolar ridge (high risk sites for melanoma).

Drug-Induced Pigmentation

- **Clinical**: Varies depending upon the drug however usually presents with diffuse pigmentation.
- **Cause**: Some of the drugs implicated include minocycline, antimalarials, chemotherapeutics, and AIDS medications.
- **Diagnosis**: Clinical features and association with medication history.
- **Ddx**: Normal pigmentation of the mucosa.
- **Histopathology**: Varies depending upon medication.
- **Management**: Discontinue drug and coloration fades.

Melanotic Macule

- **Clinical**: Well-defined, brown pigmented macule usually less than 1 cm commonly noted intraorally on buccal mucosa, gingiva and palate.
- **Cause**: Unclear.
- **Diagnosis**: Biopsy and microscopic examination.
- **Ddx**: Melanocytic nevus, amalgam tattoo, melanoma, and melanoacanthoma.
- **Histopathology**: Increased melanin pigment in basal layer of normal epithelium (Figure 4.23).
- **Management**: Biopsy to confirm diagnosis.

Melanoma

- **Clinical**: Malignant tumor of melanocytes which may present in the oral cavity. Oral melanoma is noted more often in older people on the hard palate or maxillary gingiva. The lesions are typically brown and black with irregular borders however, amelanotic cases exist. Ulceration and exophytic growth may also be seen.
- **Cause**: Neoplastic proliferation of melanocytes.
- **Diagnosis**: Biopsy and microscopic examination.

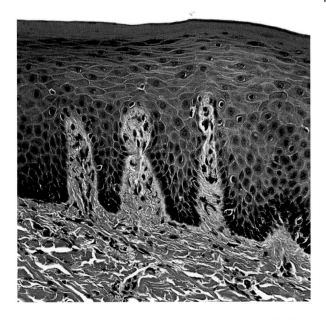

Figure 4.23 Increased melanin in basal cell layer of epithelium in melanotic macule.

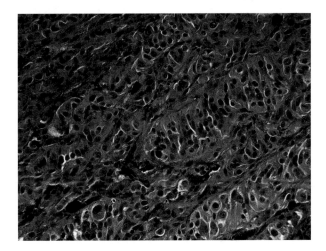

Figure 4.24 Neoplastic melanocytes with atypical features and scattered pigment in a melanoma.

- **Ddx**: Melanocytic nevus, melanotic macule, amalgam tattoo, and melanoacanthoma.
- **Histopathology**: Atypical melanocytes in epithelial and connective tissue junction. The neoplastic melanocytes are enlarged with hyperchromatic and pleomorphic nuclei (Figure 4.24).
- **Management**: Surgical excision, radiation, and immunotherapy.

Melanocytic Nevus

- **Clinical**: Well-defined black or brown pigmented macule or papule. Lesion is most commonly noted on the

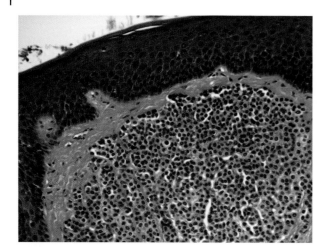

Figure 4.25 High power view of individual rounded nevus cells organized into groups or theques.

palate, mucobuccal fold, and gingiva. Some cases may lack pigmentation.

- **Cause**: Neoplastic proliferation of nevus cells.
- **Diagnosis**: Biopsy and microscopic examination.
- **Ddx**: Melanotic macule, amalgam tattoo, melanoma, and melanoacanthoma.
- **Histopathology**: Unencapsulated proliferation of nevus cells that may be organized into aggregates called theques (Figure 4.25).
- **Management**: Biopsy to confirm diagnosis.

Amalgam Tattoo/Other Tattoos

- **Clinical**: Macular area of gray-blue pigmentation as a consequence of amalgam filling material being incorporated into the oral mucosa. More common on posterior gingiva. Intentional tattoos are similar to their cutaneous counterparts and are used as a form of expression or in other cases for demonstrating landmarks.
- **Cause**: Amalgam tattoo: A couple of the mechanisms include abrasion lesions becoming secondarily implanted with amalgam particles or the spread of amalgam during an endodontic retrofill procedure. Intentional tattoos: Due to injection of permanent inks into the submucosa.
- **Diagnosis**: Periapical radiographs may show metallic fragments. If radiographs do not highlight the amalgam (due to fine particles), biopsy may be required to rule out a melanocytic lesion.
- **Ddx**: Melanocytic nevus, blue nevus, melanotic macule, melanoma, and melanoacanthoma.
- **Histopathology**: In amalgam tattoos, prominent dark brown or black particles as well as fine granules that show affinity for the reticulin fibers surrounding vascular channels and nerves are seen in the connective tissue

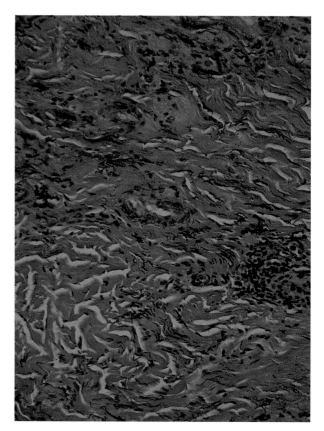

Figure 4.26 Fine amalgam particles embedded in the connective tissue and encircling vascular channels.

(Figure 4.26). Intentional tattoos display microscopic particles of ink in the submucosa.

- **Management**: Once a definitive diagnosis of amalgam tattoo is made, no further treatment is necessary. Both amalgam and intentional tattoos may be removed for cosmetic reasons either surgically or by other treatments.

Endocrine, Nutritional, and Metabolic Diseases

Genetic Disorders

Diseases Associated with Immunologic Disorders

1. Down syndrome
   Trisomy of chromosome 21 is associated with susceptibility to increased prevalence of periodontal disease. The periodontal condition is identified as severe, generalized, and of rapid progression. The etiology is associated with a problem in the immune response and not necessarily poor oral hygiene. The best treatment approach is to perform regular scaling and root planing (surgical or non-surgical) in addition to augmentation with local or systemic antibiotics.
2. Leukocyte adhesion deficiency syndrome
   Rare group of genetic disorders in the umbrella category of primary immunodeficiencies. The complications

result from the defective movement of white blood cells from the vasculature to the destination wound or infection. The consequence is susceptibility to multiple infections. The feature relevant to the periodontist is the progressive inflammation of the gingivae/periodontium which may culminate in the loss of teeth.

3. Papillon–Lefevre syndrome

Rare autosomal recessive disorder characterized by the hallmark features of palmoplantar hyperkeratosis and severe periodontitis. This condition is in the category of primary immunodeficiencies. Chemotaxis is impaired, which halts normal recruitment of neutrophils and monocytes/macrophages. The cathepsin-C gene mutation is responsible for the dysfunction.

4. Haim–Munk syndrome

Primary immunodeficiency that is a phenotypic variant of Papillon-Lefevre. The same cathepsin C gene mutation is present in this disorder. However, the Haim–Munk syndrome presents with the added features of arachnodactyly, acro-osteolysis, atrophic nail alterations, and radiographic malformation of the digits.

5. Chediak–Higashi syndrome

Rare autosomal recessive disorder in the category of primary immunodeficiency syndrome. The problem in Chediak–Higashi syndrome pertains to a defect in the lysosomal trafficking regulator protein. This leads to inadequate phagocytosis that results in constant infections. For these individuals, early onset periodontitis as well as recurrent ulcers and candidiasis are noted. Other associated conditions of note include albinism, bleeding disorders and nerve defects.

6. Severe congenital neutropenia

Pathogenesis includes an inherited condition leading to the shortage of neutrophils. This problem presents with severe bacterial/fungal infections and susceptibility to malignancy (leukemia). The oral manifestations include ulcerations, abscesses, candidiasis, desquamative gingivitis, and severe periodontitis. Routine treatment with granulocyte colony stimulating factor has improved the prognosis.

7. Primary immunodeficiency disease

Includes a large group of more than 200 uncommon conditions which are genetic or inherited in origin and lead to compromised immune systems. A number of the conditions have previously been discussed (i.e. Chediak Higashi, severe congenital neutropenia). Chronic granulomatous disease is a primary immunodeficiency disease characterized by life-threatening infections. The problem occurs due to phagocytes being unable to manage bacteria and fungi. Features noted in the oral cavity include ulcerations, gingivitis, and periodontitis. Another primary immunodeficiency,

hyperimmunoglobulin E syndrome, also presents with similar oral manifestations. The features in this condition include ligneous gingivitis, periodontitis, and susceptibility to recurrent fungal infections.

8. Cohen syndrome

Cohen syndrome is an autosomal recessive condition characterized by obesity, prominent maxilla, hypotonia, mental retardation, and abnormalities of the hands and feet. Neutropenia is also present leading to higher than normal rates of gingivitis/periodontitis and oral ulcerations.

Diseases Affecting the Oral Mucosa and Gingival Tissue

1. Epidermolysis bullosa

Rare inherited genodermatosis characterized by fragile skin/oral mucosa, which displays significant blistering and tearing upon minor manipulation. There are three major categories namely, the dystrophic form, the junctional form, and the simplex form. In all the aforementioned subtypes oral manifestations are seen, however, the generalized recessive dystrophic type presents with prominent severe bullae with scarring. As a result of this progressive scarring, there is a high propensity to develop microstomia. This subcategory also displays alterations in the tongue including loss of the papillae and ankyloglossia. Squamous cell carcinomas are also reported in adult patients with the recessive dystrophic form of this condition.

2. Plasminogen deficiency

Rare autosomal recessive systemic disease characterized by a lack of plasminogen leading to lesions on the mucous membranes. Plasminogen is the precursor of plasmin that plays a critical role in the breakdown of fibrin. As a result of this condition, deposits of excess fibrin exudate cause the expansion of the gingiva with concomitant ulceration. Ocular lesions termed ligneous conjunctivitis may also be noted.

Diseases Affecting the Connective Tissues

1. Ehlers–Danlos syndrome (Type VIII)

Group of hereditary disorders displaying a spectrum of connective tissue problems. Manifestations include joint laxity and hyperextensible skin, scarring, and bruising. Periodontal Ehlers–Danlos (previously EDS Type VIII) is an autosomal dominant form that has the defining clinical features of early severe periodontitis, joint hypermobility, and mild cutaneous findings.

2. Angioedema (C1-inhibitor deficiency)

Angioedema as a result of low levels of C1-inhibitor displays the hallmark feature of recurrent, diffuse, non-pitting edema. There is increased vascular permeability of the deeper blood vessels with leakage of plasma. This process affects the classic triad of skin, gastrointestinal tract, and larynx. There are two forms of this condition namely, the inherited and highly rare acquired form. The only difference lies in the later onset of symptoms in the acquired form.

3. Systemic lupus erythematosus (SLE)
   - Autoimmune condition (presence of antinuclear antigen-ANA, anti-double stranded DNA, anti-Sm) whereby antigen–antibody complexes become deposited in different parts of the body. This leads to an inflammatory response in a range of involved organs.
   - Oral manifestations to consider include erythematous plaque like lesions and erosive ulcerated lesions of the palate, buccal mucosa, and gingiva. The ulcerated lesions may present with white striae on the periphery in a similar manner to erosive lichen planus. Also consider possibility of a "butterfly rash" extraorally. The diagnosis is based upon clinical features, direct immunofluorescence, serology, and histopathology. Differential diagnosis includes lichen planus and lichenoid reactions. The histopathology is similar to lichen planus; however, the inflammation may extend deep into the submucosa in a perivascular fashion and keratin plugging may be present. Deposits of PAS positive material in the basement membrane may also be noted. Under direct immunofluorescence granular and linear deposits of immunoglobulin are noted along the basement membrane. Treatment for oral lesions is usually topical steroids with consideration given to immunomodulating drugs.

Metabolic and Endocrine Diseases

1. Glycogen storage disease
   This category includes a heterogeneous group of inherited disorders that presents with problems with metabolism of glycogen in the liver and muscle. The accumulation of glycogen in the specific type 1B is caused by a deficiency in glucose-6-phosphatase. This results in the inability to breakdown glycogen in cells. Other associated complications include the decrease in neutrophil migration leading to higher susceptibility to recurrent infections. Oral manifestations may consist of gingivitis/periodontitis, delayed dental maturation/eruption, and oral ulcers.

2. Gaucher disease
   Gaucher disease is an inherited autosomal recessive condition associated with problems in lipid storage. The signs and symptoms are variegated but the primary cause is the reduced or non-existent lysosomal enzyme glucocerebrosidase. This result is an accumulation of the undigested fatty macromolecule called glucocerebroside. The oral conditions that may ensue include radiolucencies in the jawbones, delayed eruption, and early onset periodontitis. Of note, the histopathology of Gaucher cells displays a characteristic "wrinkled tissue paper" appearance to the macrophage cytoplasm.

3. Hypophosphatasia
   Hypophosphatasia is a rare genetic disease characterized by problems with tooth and bone mineralization due to alkaline phosphatase deficiency. The hallmark oral feature is premature loss of deciduous teeth due to lack of normal cementum formation.

4. Hypophosphatemic rickets
   This condition was previously termed vitamin D resistant rickets and is associated with multiple inheritance patterns the most common being X-linked dominant. The levels of phosphate in the blood are decreased leading to softened bones. The dental abnormalities include large canals and large pulp chambers with heightened pulp horns. The presence of abscesses in non-carious teeth is also a feature.

5. Hajdu–Cheney syndrome (acro-osteolysis)
   Inherited disorder of bone that results in abnormal osteoporotic changes in the spinal, cranial, and facial bones and the resorption of the bone of the terminal phalanges. Several other clinical features may be noted including coarse hair and characteristic facies. Some of the oral manifestations include problems with exfoliation and eruption, underdevelopment of the alveolar process, alterations in cementum and dentin, and a rapidly progressive form of periodontitis.

6. Diabetes mellitus
   Evidence now exists for a possible two-way relationship between chronic periodontal disease and diabetes mellitus. It is already established that the abnormal glucose metabolism in diabetes mellitus contributes to the increased frequency of periodontitis. There is also emerging research that demonstrates risk and severity of both diabetes and periodontal disease are increased in a bidirectional manner. Treatment of the inflammatory periodontal condition may improve the overall health of patients with diabetes mellitus. The corollary is also true whereby glycemic control aids in periodontal status. In poorly controlled diabetics, a decrease in the function of immune cells leads to the development of persistent bacteria in the periodontal pocket. Management includes scaling and root planing with possible addition of systemic antibiotics.

7. Obesity
   Studies have shown a link between obesity and periodontal disease. There are cases that indicate greater clinical attachment loss and deeper periodontal pocket

depth in obese patients. Obesity is a complex condition with multiple variables therefore the mechanism for this connection is not fully understood.

8. Osteoporosis

There is research that supports an association between periodontitis and osteoporosis. The identification of sparse trabeculation in the alveolus may provide an indicator of low bone mineral density. Careful attention to oral hygiene measures is indicated in individuals with osteoporosis to decrease the risk of progressive periodontal disease. Consideration should also be given to the use of anti-resorptive medication and the potential for medication related osteonecrosis of the jaws.

Acquired Immunodeficiency Diseases

Acquired Neutropenia Type of neutropenia that is more common than the congenital types and may be seen in a number of settings. The scenarios include following an infection, after exposure to certain drugs, as a result of autoimmunity, nutritional deficiency, hypersplenism, or as a consequence of hematologic malignancy. The period of low neutrophil count will make the individual more liable to acquire bacterial and fungal infections. In addition, severe periodontal disease and aphthous stomatitis are prominent features of this condition.

HIV Infection Oral lesions in HIV infection are of the opportunistic type and their presence may indicate the current level of control. The more common presentations include pseudomembranous candidiasis, oral hairy leukoplakia, Kaposi sarcoma, and salivary gland disease. There is also the increase in oral warts related to possible immune-reconstitution syndrome. The periodontal lesions associated with HIV infection consist of linear gingival erythema and necrotizing periodontal diseases.

Inflammatory Diseases

Epidermolysis Bullosa Acquisita This acquired vesiculobullous disease is a subepidermal blistering condition wherein the patient possesses IgG autoantibodies to type VII collagen. Some of the oral manifestations include scarring of the mucosa and periodontal disease. The diagnostic tests used include immunofluorescence and the sodium chloride split skin method. Immunofluorescence shows a linear pattern of deposition of IgG and C3 along the epidermal basement membrane with a u-serrated pattern. Treatment includes the use of topical steroids.

Inflammatory Bowel Disease
- Term used to describe chronic inflammation in the digestive tract. The two types include ulcerative colitis

and Crohn's disease (covered earlier in granulomatous inflammatory conditions).
- Ulcerative colitis is a problem wherein ulcers are formed in the large intestine and rectum. The disease tends to undergo periods of exacerbation and remission. The oral manifestations include pyostomatitis vegetans which is characterized by erythema and edema of the mucosa with numerous small superficial yellow pustules. In addition, studies have also noted a higher risk of periodontitis in ulcerative colitis.

Osteoarthritis and Rheumatoid Arthritis
- Osteoarthritis is a chronic inflammatory disorder which causes a gradual deterioration of joint cartilage in older individuals. Patients with this condition may have difficulty with maintaining oral hygiene due to manual dexterity problems. This results in an accumulation of plaque and calculus which may create an increased likelihood of periodontal disease. Also, drugs used to treat the inflammatory condition may leave patients susceptible to infections. The temporomandibular joint may also be affected by this disease process.
- Rheumatoid arthritis is a chronic autoimmune inflammatory disorder that affects the joint cartilage of older individuals. There is a statistically significant association between periodontal disease and rheumatoid arthritis. Novel research is investigating the role of organisms such as Porphyromonas gingivalis on citrullination, and the association of periodontal disease in rheumatoid arthritis patients with seropositivity toward rheumatoid factor and the anti-cyclic citrullinated peptide antibody. The immunosuppressive drugs taken for rheumatoid arthritis may also increase the risk of opportunistic infection. In addition, patients tend to have functional limitations in the joints, which lead to difficulty with oral hygiene procedures and problems in the temporomandibular joint.

Systemic Disorders that Influence the Pathogenesis of Periodontal Disease

Emotional Stress and Depression Studies show that emotional stress and depression are risk indicators for periodontal disease. This negative impact is possibly a result of modified host defenses making an individual more susceptible to periodontal infections. However, research is still needed to fully elucidate the nature of this complex interaction.

Smoking Smoking as a risk factor in periodontal disease has been extensively researched. The prevalence and severity of this disease condition is higher in smokers. In addition, the response to periodontal therapy is adversely affected by the continued habit. Theories regarding the mechanisms of this association include an alteration in host response in the tissues and problems with wound healing. Smoking cessation, however, is also known to have a positive effect on periodontal health.

Medications Medication induced gingival overgrowth occurs as a side-effect in susceptible patients. The more common drugs associated with this enlargement include calcium channel blockers, cyclosporine and phenytoin. The management includes meticulous oral hygiene and possible substitution of the drug. Surgical management includes gingivectomy, however recurrence of the condition is a possibility.

Neoplasms

1. Oral squamous cell carcinoma
   This was already discussed in the neoplasms section.
2. Secondary metastatic neoplasms
   Metastasis to the oral cavity is a rare event which is a sign that a malignancy is in an advanced stage. The most common metastatic lesions include lung (in males) and breast (in females). In 25% of cases a biopsy in the oral cavity may serve as the first sign of malignancy. Radiographically, lytic lesions with ill-defined borders may provide hints for further evaluation. Clinical symptoms include paresthesia, swelling, pain, and loosening of teeth. The soft tissue manifestation of metastasis is noted more commonly on the gingiva and may mimic the appearance of a reactive lesion. Therefore, all atypical lesions require mandatory biopsy with microscopic evaluation.

Other Disorders

1. Granulomatosis with polyangiitis
   Rare systemic disease that results in necrotizing granulomatous inflammation of the respiratory tract, glomerulonephritis and vasculitis. Other features include ulceration of the oral/nasal mucosa and a saddle nose malformation. Oral lesions may also have the characteristic hyperplastic gingivitis or "strawberry gingivitis" appearance. These lesions may precede other manifestations of the disease. It must be noted however that the histopathology of the strawberry gingivitis specimens may not reveal typical necrotizing granulomas. The treatment is immunosuppressive therapy.
2. Langerhans cell histiocytosis
   Disorder in which Langerhans cells (cells of the immune system) accumulate in different parts of the body including the skin, bones, and lungs. This condition usually affects young children however may rarely affect adults. There are three basic clinical subtypes: (i)

acute disseminated form (multifocal multisystem), (ii) chronic disseminated form (multifocal, unisystem), (iii) Solitary eosinophilic granuloma (unifocal). Oral findings include pain, mucosal ulceration, gingival necrosis and destruction of alveolar bone with tooth mobility (which mimics periodontal disease). The radiolucencies may also display the classic "punched out" appearance. Histopathology shows sheets of large polygonal Langerhans cells with reniform nuclei with grooves and abundant eosinophils. In addition, hallmark Birbeck granules can be detected in lesional cells by electron microscopy. Treatment is guided by the extent of disease and includes surgery, chemotherapy, and radiation.

3. Central giant cell granuloma
   Lesion that presents as a non-neoplastic reactive process with an unclear etiology. The slow-growing lesion presents more commonly in young adult females in the mandible. There may be swelling and a crossing of the midline. Radiographically the central giant cell granuloma may present as a multilocular lesion; however, the unilocular presentation is also common. The histopathology consists of fibrous tissue containing mononuclear cells, clusters of multinucleated giant cells and extensive hemorrhage. These lesions need to be differentiated from the brown tumor of hyperparathyroidism and the giant cell tumors of the long bones due to similar histopathology. Treatment is excision and curettage. Other modalities include treatment with interferon-alpha-2a, corticosteroids, and calcitonin.
4. Hyperparathyroidism
   This condition is classified into three different categories namely, primary, secondary, and tertiary. In all the different presentations, the common feature is the increased production of parathyroid hormone. Hyperparathyroidism may display well-defined radiolucent lesions with bony expansion termed brown tumors. Brown tumors are named for their gross appearance, which shows features of excess vascularity, hemorrhage, and hemosiderin. Histopathologically, brown tumors appear identical to central giant cell granulomas therefore lab testing is required. Loss of lamina dura, tooth displacement, and complaints of pain and tooth mobility are noted in some cases. Renal osteodystrophy is seen in the secondary form of hyperparathyroidism and may affect 90% of patients undergoing dialysis.
5. Systemic sclerosis
   In this chronic autoimmune condition an excess production of dense extracellular collagen is noted, which results in significant fibrosis. The areas affected may include the skin, gastrointestinal tract, lungs, heart, and kidneys. There are multiple clinical presentations including a limited and diffuse form. Some of

the features related to the oral and maxillofacial area include the thickening of the skin of the face and tongue, atrophy of the alae of the nose, thinning of the lips, microstomia (leading to restricted mouth opening), osseous resorption of the mandible, and widening of the periodontal ligament space.

6. Vanishing bone syndrome (Gorham–Stout syndrome) Rare disease of unknown etiology in which the bones of the patient are replaced by a proliferation of endothelial lined vessels and fibrovascular tissue. Radiographs will demonstrate changes similar to patchy osteoporosis. Symptoms include pain and complications include chylothorax, which leads to respiratory distress. The course of this osteolytic disease is unpredictable. Treatment is still an area of ongoing research and includes surgery, radiotherapy, and pharmacotherapy.

Developmental Odontogenic Cysts

Dentigerous Cyst/Eruption Cyst
- **Clinical**: The dentigerous cyst is associated with the crown of an unerupted or impacted tooth therefore is it is only visible radiographically. This lesion is typically asymptomatic and seen in the posterior mandible associated with the third molar. The eruption cyst that is the soft tissue counterpart presents with a blue hued swelling of the gingiva overlying the erupting tooth.
- **Radiograph**: Usually unilocular well-defined, corticated radiolucent lesion around the crown of an unerupted tooth with attachment at the cemento-enamel junction.
- **Cause**: Developmental
- **Diagnosis**: Biopsy or clinical features (as in eruption cyst).
- **Ddx**: Radiographic- Odontogenic keratocyst, ameloblastoma (Figure 4.27 and 4.28), enlarged dental follicle, or other odontogenic/non-odontogenic tumors.
- **Histopathology**: Fibrous connective tissue lined by two to four layers of nonkeratinizing epithelium. If inflamed, the cyst epithelium displays irregular hyperplasia and a chronic inflammatory infiltrate in the connective tissue stroma.
- **Management**: Dentigerous cyst is treated with enucleation of the cyst with concomitant removal of tooth in most cases. Eruption cysts usually require no treatment however may perform de-roofing of the translucent swelling if needed.

Lateral Periodontal Cyst/Gingival Cyst
- **Clinical**: Developmental odontogenic cyst that forms when residual rests of odontogenic epithelium grow in excess with a characteristic histopathologic pattern. Most commonly located in the lower anterior/premolar

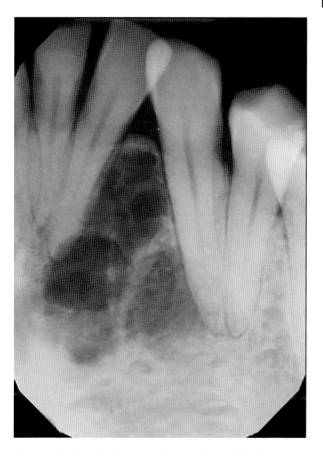

Figure 4.27 Periapical radiograph showing multilocular ameloblastoma splaying the roots of mandibular anterior teeth.

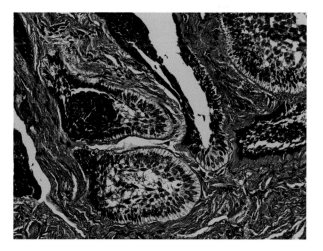

Figure 4.28 Histopathology displaying infiltrating islands of neoplastic ameloblastic epithelium with palisading of peripheral cells and reverse polarization of nuclei.

region lateral to the root surface. The lateral periodontal cyst is seen on radiographs whereas the same cyst observed clinically as a painless swelling on the gingiva is termed a gingival cyst.

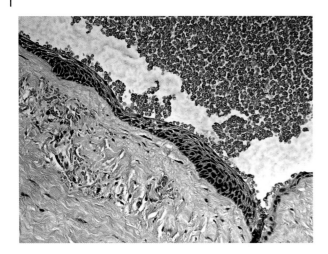

Figure 4.29 Plaque-like thickening in epithelial lining of gingival cyst.

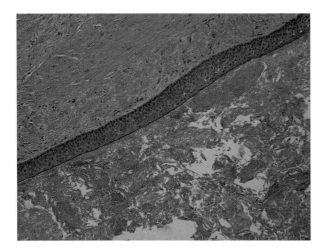

Figure 4.30 Parakeratinized epithelium with hyperchromatic and palisaded basal cells. Note extensive keratin scales in the cyst lumen.

- **Radiograph**: Well-defined corticated radiolucency lateral to a vital tooth root.
- **Cause**: Developmental.
- **Diagnosis**: Biopsy and histopathologic examination.
- **Ddx**: Lateral inflammatory cyst or other odontogenic cysts/neoplasms.
- **Histopathology**: Thin flattened epithelial lining with or without plaque-like thickenings which exhibit varying degrees of clearing or whirling (Figure 4.29).
- **Treatment**: Enucleation (lateral periodontal cyst) or surgical excision (gingival cyst).

Odontogenic Keratocyst

- **Clinical**: Asymptomatic odontogenic cyst more often noted in the posterior mandible. Multiple odontogenic keratocysts may signal presence of the Gorlin syndrome. Rarely presents in a peripheral manner on the gingival soft tissues.
- **Radiograph**: Well-defined, corticated unilocular or multilocular radiolucency. May be associated with an unerupted tooth.
- **Cause**: Developmental.
- **Diagnosis**: Biopsy and histopathologic examination.
- **Ddx**: Dentigerous cyst, ameloblastoma, inflammatory cyst or other odontogenic/non-odontogenic tumors.
- **Histopathology**: Cyst lining is composed of a "corrugated" parakeratinized stratified squamous epithelium which is 8–10 cell layers thick (Figure 4.30). The basal cells are hyperchromatic and display prominent palisading. Keratin scales may also be noted in the cyst lumen. The characteristic features are altered with inflammation.
- **Management**: Enucleation with peripheral ostectomy to prevent recurrence.

Further Reading

Al-Abeedi, F., Aldahish, Y., Almotawa, Z., and Kujan, O. (2015). The differential diagnosis of desquamative gingivitis: review of the literature and clinical guide for dental undergraduates. *J. Int. Oral Health* 7 (Suppl 1): 88–92.

Alaluusua, S., Kivitie-Kallio, S., Wolf, J. et al. (1997). Periodontal findings in Cohen syndrome with chronic neutropenia. *J. Periodontol.* 68 (5): 473–478. https://doi.org/10.1902/jop.1997.68.5.473.

Albandar, J.M., Susin, C., and Hughes, F.J. (2018). Manifestations of systemic diseases and conditions that affect the periodontal attachment apparatus: case definitions and diagnostic considerations. *J. Periodontol.* 89 (Suppl 1): S183–s203. https://doi.org/10.1002/jper.16-0480.

Al-Zahrani, M.S., Bissada, N.F., and Borawskit, E.A. (2003). Obesity and periodontal disease in young, middle-aged, and older adults. *J. Periodontol.* 74 (5): 610–615. https://doi.org/10.1902/jop.2003.74.5.610.

Antoniades, K., Kaklamanos, E., Kavadia, S. et al. (2003). Hajdu-Cheney syndrome (acro-osteolysis): a case report of dental interest. *Oral Surg. Oral Med. Oral Pathol. Oral Radiol. Endod.* 95 (6): 725–731:https://doi.org/10.1067/moe.2003.151.

Aral, C.A., Dilber, E., Aral, K. et al. (2015). Management of cyclosporine and nifedipine-induced gingival hyperplasia. *J. Clin. Diagn. Res.* 9 (12): Zd12-15:https://doi.org/10.7860/jcdr/2015/14737.6974.

Aswathyraj, S., Arunkumar, G., Alidjinou, E.K., and Hober, D. (2016). Hand, foot and mouth disease (HFMD): emerging epidemiology and the need for a vaccine strategy. *Med. Microbiol. Immunol.* 205 (5): 397–407:https://doi.org/10.1007/s00430-016-0465-y.

Auclair, P.L., Cuenin, P., Kratochvil, F.J. et al. (1988). A clinical and histomorphologic comparison of the central giant cell granuloma and the giant cell tumor. *Oral Surg. Oral Med. Oral Pathol.* 66 (2): 197–208.

Bazopoulou-Kyrkanidou, E., Vrahopoulos, T.P., Eliades, G. et al. (2007). Periodontitis associated with Hajdu-Cheney syndrome. *J. Periodontol.* 78 (9): 1831–1838:https://doi.org/10.1902/jop.2007.060385.

Bharti, P., Katagiri, S., Nitta, H. et al. (2013). Periodontal treatment with topical antibiotics improves glycemic control in association with elevated serum adiponectin in patients with type 2 diabetes mellitus. *Obes. Res. Clin. Pract.* 7 (2): e129–e138:https://doi.org/10.1016/j.orcp.2011.11.005.

Bilodeau, E.A. and Collins, B.M. (2017). Odontogenic cysts and neoplasms. *Surg. Pathol. Clin.* 10 (1): 177–222: https://doi.org/10.1016/j.path.2016.10.006.

Biosse Duplan, M., Hubert, A., Le Norcy, E. et al. (2018). Dental and periodontal manifestations of glycogen storage diseases: a case series of 60 patients. *J. Inherit. Metab. Dis.* 41 (6): 947–953: https://doi.org/10.1007/s10545-018-0182-3.

Bloch-Zupan, A. and Vaysse, F. (2017). Hypophosphatasia: oral cavity and dental disorders. *Arch. Pediatr.* 24 (5s2): 5s80-85s84:https://doi.org/10.1016/s0929-693x(18)30020-4.

Bornstein, M.M., Andreoni, C., Meier, T., and Leung, Y.Y. (2018). Squamous cell carcinoma of the gingiva mimicking periodontal disease: a diagnostic challenge and therapeutic dilemma. *Int. J. Periodont. Restor. Dent.* 38 (2): 253–259:https://doi.org/10.11607/prd.3253.

Brown, R.S. and Arany, P.R. (2015). Mechanism of drug-induced gingival overgrowth revisited: a unifying hypothesis. *Oral Dis.* 21 (1): e51–e61:https://doi.org/10.1111/odi.12264.

Bruce, A.J. and Rogers, R.S. 3rd., (2004). Oral manifestations of sexually transmitted diseases. *Clin. Dermatol.* 22 (6): 520–527:https://doi.org/10.1016/j.clindermatol.2004.07.005.

Buchner, A. and Hansen, L.S. (1980). Amalgam pigmentation (amalgam tattoo) of the oral mucosa. A clinicopathologic study of 268 cases. *Oral Surg. Oral Med. Oral Pathol.* 49 (2): 139–147.

Carneiro, T.E., Marinho, S.A., Verli, F.D. et al. (2009). Oral squamous papilloma: clinical, histologic and immunohistochemical analyses. *J. Oral Sci.* 51 (3): 367–372.

Carter, L.C., Fischman, S.L., Mann, J. et al. (1998). The nature and extent of jaw involvement in Gaucher disease: observations in a series of 28 patients. *Oral Surg. Oral Med. Oral Pathol. Oral Radiol. Endod.* 85 (2): 233–239.

Castano, A., Shah, S.S., Cicero, G., and ElChaar, E. (2017). Primary oral melanoma-A non-surgical approach to treatment via immunotherapy. *Clin. Adv. Periodont.* 7 (1): 9–17: https://doi.org/10.1902/cap.2016.160003.

Celkan, T. and Koc, B.S. (2015). Approach to the patient with neutropenia in childhood. *Turk. Pediatri. Ars.* 50 (3): 136–144:https://doi.org/10.5152/TurkPediatriArs.2015.2295.

Chi, A.C., Owings, J.R. Jr., and Muller, S. (2005). Peripheral odontogenic keratocyst: report of two cases and review of the literature. *Oral Surg. Oral Med. Oral Pathol. Oral Radiol. Endod.* 99 (1): 71–78:https://doi.org/10.1016/j.tripleo.2004.05.018.

Chi, A.C., Prichard, E., Richardson, M.S. et al. (2009). Pseudomembranous disease (ligneous inflammation) of the female genital tract, peritoneum, gingiva, and paranasal sinuses associated with plasminogen deficiency. *Ann. Diagn. Pathol.* 13 (2): 132–139:https://doi.org/10.1016/j.anndiagpath.2008.02.005.

Chue, P.W. (1975). Gonorrhea--its natural history, oral manifestations, diagnosis, treatment, and prevention. *J. Am. Dent. Assoc.* 90 (6): 1297–1301.

Cobb, C.M., Ferguson, B.L., Keselyak, N.T. et al. (2003). A TEM/SEM study of the microbial plaque overlying the necrotic gingival papillae of HIV-seropositive, necrotizing ulcerative periodontitis. *J. Periodontal. Res.* 38 (2): 147–155.

Coletta, R.D. and Graner, E. (2006). Hereditary gingival fibromatosis: a systematic review. *J. Periodontol.* 77 (5): 753–764:https://doi.org/10.1902/jop.2006.050379.

Cremonesi, I., Nucci, C., D'Alessandro, G. et al. (2014). X-linked hypophosphatemic rickets: enamel abnormalities and oral clinical findings. *Scanning* 36 (4): 456–461: https://doi.org/10.1002/sca.21141.

Crifasi, P.A., Patterson, M.C., Bonde, D., and Michels, V.V. (1997). Severe Hajdu-Cheney syndrome with upper airway obstruction. *Am. J. Med. Genet.* 70 (3): 261–266.

Demirer, S., Ozdemir, H., Sencan, M., and Marakoglu, I. (2007). Gingival hyperplasia as an early diagnostic oral manifestation in acute monocytic leukemia: a case report. *Eur. J. Dent.* 1 (2): 111–114.

Detert, J., Pischon, N., Burmester, G.R., and Buttgereit, F. (2010). The association between rheumatoid arthritis and periodontal disease. *Arthritis Res. Ther.* 12 (5): 218. https://doi.org/10.1186/ar3106.

Dionne, K.R., Warnakulasuriya, S., Zain, R.B., and Cheong, S.C. (2015). Potentially malignant disorders of the oral cavity: current practice and future directions in the clinic and laboratory. *Int. J. Cancer* 136 (3): 503–515. https://doi.org/10.1002/ijc.28754.

Ferguson, K.A. and McCormack, D.G. (1993). Tuberculosis involving the oral cavity. *Can. J. Infect. Dis.* 4 (1): 12–14.

Ferreira, R., Michel, R.C., Greghi, S.L. et al. (2016). Prevention and periodontal treatment in down syndrome patients: a systematic review. *PLoS One* 11 (6): e0158339. https://doi.org/10.1371/journal.pone.0158339.

Ficarra, G. and Carlos, R. (2009). Syphilis: the renaissance of an old disease with oral implications. *Head Neck Pathol.* 3 (3): 195–206. https://doi.org/10.1007/s12105-009-0127-0.

Fornatora, M.L., Reich, R.F., Gray, R.G., and Freedman, P.D. (2001). Intraoral molluscum contagiosum: A report of a case and a review of the literature. *Oral Surg. Oral Med. Oral Pathol. Oral Radiol. Endodontol.* 92 (3): 318–320.

Garcia-Ballesta, C., Perez-Lajarin, L., Lillo, O.C., and Bravo-Gonzalez, L.A. (2003). New oral findings in Cohen syndrome. *Oral Surg. Oral Med. Oral Pathol. Oral Radiol. Endod.* 95 (6): 681–687. https://doi.org/10.1067/moe.2003.138.

Gawron, K., Lazarz-Bartyzel, K., Potempa, J., and Chomyszyn-Gajewska, M. (2016). Gingival fibromatosis: clinical, molecular and therapeutic issues. *Orphanet. J. Rare Dis.* 11: 9. https://doi.org/10.1186/s13023-016-0395-1.

Genco, R.J., Ho, A.W., Kopman, J. et al. (1998). Models to evaluate the role of stress in periodontal disease. *Ann. Periodontol.* 3 (1): 288–302. https://doi.org/10.1902/annals.1998.3.1.288.

Gibson, C. and Berliner, N. (2014). How we evaluate and treat neutropenia in adults. *Blood* 124 (8): 1251–1258. quiz 1378. https://doi.org/10.1182/blood-2014-02-482612.

Giunta, J.L. and Fiumara, N.J. (1986). Facts about gonorrhea and dentistry. *Oral Surg. Oral Med. Oral Pathol.* 62 (5): 529–531.

Glick, M. (2015). *Burket's Oral Medicine*. Shelton, CT: People's Medical Publishing House USA.

Guevara-Canales, J.O., Morales-Vadillo, R., Sacsaquispe-Contreras, S.J. et al. (2013). Malignant lymphoma of the oral cavity and the maxillofacial region: overall survival prognostic factors. *Med. Oral Patol. Oral Cir. Bucal.* 18 (4): e619–e626.

Hadj Said, M., Foletti, J.M., Graillon, N. et al. (2016). Orofacial manifestations of scleroderma. A literature review. *Rev. Stomatol. Chir. Maxillofac. Chir. Orale* 117 (5): 322–326. https://doi.org/10.1016/j.revsto.2016.06.003.

Hakkinen, L. and Csiszar, A. (2007). Hereditary gingival fibromatosis: characteristics and novel putative pathogenic mechanisms. *J. Dent. Res.* 86 (1): 25–34. https://doi.org/10.1177/154405910708600104.

Hanisch, M., Frohlich, L.F., and Kleinheinz, J. (2016). Gingival hyperplasia as first sign of recurrence of granulomatosis with polyangiitis (Wegener's granulomatosis): case report and review of the literature. *BMC Oral Health* 17 (1): 33. https://doi.org/10.1186/s12903-016-0262-4.

Hart, T.C., Pallos, D., Bozzo, L. et al. (2000). Evidence of genetic heterogeneity for hereditary gingival fibromatosis. *J. Dent. Res.* 79 (10): 1758–1764. https://doi.org/10.1177/00220345000790100501.

Herrera, D., Retamal-Valdes, B., Alonso, B., and Feres, M. (2018). Acute periodontal lesions (periodontal abscesses and necrotizing periodontal diseases) and endo-periodontal lesions. *J. Periodontol.* 89 (Suppl 1): S85–s102. https://doi.org/10.1002/jper.16-0642.

Hirshberg, A., Shnaiderman-Shapiro, A., Kaplan, I., and Berger, R. (2008). Metastatic tumours to the oral cavity - pathogenesis and analysis of 673 cases. *Oral Oncol.* 44 (8): 743–752. https://doi.org/10.1016/j.oraloncology.2007.09.012.

Holmstrup, P., Plemons, J., and Meyle, J. (2018). Non-plaque-induced gingival diseases. *J. Periodontol.* 89 (Suppl 1): S28–s45. https://doi.org/10.1002/jper.17-0163.

Horning, G.M. (1996). Necotizing gingivostomatitis: NUG to noma. *Compend. Contin. Educ. Dent.* 17 (10): 951–954, 956, 957–958 passim; quiz 964.

Horwitz, J., Hirsh, I., and Machtei, E.E. (2007). Oral aspects of Gaucher's disease: a literature review and case report. *J. Periodontol.* 78 (4): 783–788. https://doi.org/10.1902/jop.2007.060341.

Hosur, M.B., Puranik, R.S., Vanaki, S.S. et al. (2018). Clinicopathological profile of central giant cell granulomas: an institutional experience and study of immunohistochemistry expression of p63 in central giant cell granuloma. *J. Oral. Maxillofac. Pathol.* 22 (2): 173–179. https://doi.org/10.4103/jomfp.JOMFP_260_17.

Irani, S. (2017). Metastasis to the jawbones: a review of 453 cases. *J. Int. Soc. Prev. Community Dent.* 7 (2): 71–81. https://doi.org/10.4103/jispcd.JISPCD_512_16.

Jain, P. and Jain, I. (2014). Oral manifestations of tuberculosis: step towards early diagnosis. *J. Clin. Diagn. Res.* 8 (12): Ze18-21. https://doi.org/10.7860/jcdr/2014/10080.5281.

Johnson, T.M. (2017). Smoking and periodontal disease. *US Army Med. Dep.* J(3-17): 67–70.

Kapferer-Seebacher, I., Pepin, M., Werner, R. et al. (2016). Periodontal Ehlers-Danlos Syndrome is caused by mutations in C1R and C1S, which encode subcomponents C1r and C1s of complement. *Am. J. Hum. Genet.* 99 (5): 1005–1014. https://doi.org/10.1016/j.ajhg.2016.08.019.

Kapferer-Seebacher, I., Lundberg, P., Malfait, F., and Zschocke, J. (2017). Periodontal manifestations of Ehlers-Danlos syndromes: a systematic review. *J. Clin.*

Periodontol. 44 (11): 1088–1100. https://doi.org/10.1111/jcpe.12807.

Kara, C., Demir, T., Tezel, A., and Zihni, M. (2007). Aggressive periodontitis with streptococcal gingivitis: a case report. *Eur. J. Dent.* 1 (4): 251–255.

Kasamatsu, A., Kanazawa, H., Watanabe, T., and Matsuzaki, O. (2007). Oral sarcoidosis: report of a case and review of literature. *J. Oral Maxillofac. Surg.* 65 (6): 1256–1259. https://doi.org/10.1016/j.joms.2005.09.028.

Kaur, S., Bright, R., Proudman, S.M., and Bartold, P.M. (2014). Does periodontal treatment influence clinical and biochemical measures for rheumatoid arthritis? A systematic review and meta-analysis. *Semin Arthritis Rheum.* 44 (2): 113–122. https://doi.org/10.1016/j.semarthrit.2014.04.009.

Kelsey, J.L. and Lamster, I.B. (2008). Influence of musculoskeletal conditions on oral health among older adults. *Am. J. Public Health* 98 (7): 1177–1183. https://doi.org/10.2105/ajph.2007.129429.

Kreuter, A. and Wieland, U. (2011). Oral hairy leukoplakia: a clinical indicator of immunosuppression. *CMAJ* 183 (8): 932. https://doi.org/10.1503/cmaj.100841.

Lin, T.H., Lung, C.C., Su, H.P. et al. (2015). Association between periodontal disease and osteoporosis by gender: a nationwide population-based cohort study. *Medicine (Baltimore)* 94 (7): e553. https://doi.org/10.1097/md.0000000000000553.

Lira-Junior, R. and Figueredo, C.M. (2016). Periodontal and inflammatory bowel diseases: is there evidence of complex pathogenic interactions? *World J. Gastroenterol.* 22 (35): 7963–7972. https://doi.org/10.3748/wjg.v22.i35.7963.

Ma, R., Moein Vaziri, F., Sabino, G.J. et al. (2018). Glycogen storage disease Ib and severe periodontal destruction: a case report. *Dent. J. (Basel)* 6 (4): https://doi.org/10.3390/dj6040053.

Manfredi, M., Corradi, D., and Vescovi, P. (2005). Langerhans-cell histiocytosis: a clinical case without bone involvement. *J. Periodontol.* 76 (1): 143–147. https://doi.org/10.1902/jop.2005.76.1.143.

Marshall, R.I. and Bartold, P.M. (1999). A clinical review of drug-induced gingival overgrowths. *Aust. Dent. J.* 44 (4): 219–232.

Marx, R.E. and Stern, D. (2003). *Oral and Maxillofacial Pathology: A Rationale for Diagnosis and Treatment*. Carol Stream, IL: Quintessence Publishing Co, Inc.

Menzies, S., O'Shea, F., Galvin, S., and Wynne, B. (2018). Oral manifestations of lupus. *Ir. J. Med. Sci.* 187 (1): 91–93. https://doi.org/10.1007/s11845-017-1622-z.

Mortellaro, C., Garagiola, U., Carbone, V. et al. (2005). Unusual oral manifestations and evolution in glycogen storage disease type Ib. *J. Craniofac. Surg.* 16 (1): 45–52.

Muller, S. (2018). Oral epithelial dysplasia, atypical verrucous lesions and oral potentially malignant disorders: focus on histopathology. *Oral Surg. Oral Med. Oral Pathol. Oral Radiol.* 125 (6): 591–602. https://doi.org/10.1016/j.oooo.2018.02.012.

Munde, A., Juvekar, M.V., Karle, R.R., and Wankhede, P. (2014). Malignant melanoma of the oral cavity: report of two cases. *Contemp. Clin. Dent.* 5 (2): 227–230. https://doi.org/10.4103/0976-237x.132352.

Murayama, T., Iwatsubo, R., Akiyama, S. et al. (2000). Familial hypophosphatemic vitamin D-resistant rickets: dental findings and histologic study of teeth. *Oral Surg. Oral Med. Oral Pathol. Oral Radiol. Endod.* 90 (3): 310–316. https://doi.org/10.1067/moe.2000.107522.

Myoung, H., Hong, S.P., Hong, S.D. et al. (2001). Odontogenic keratocyst: review of 256 cases for recurrence and clinicopathologic parameters. *Oral Surg. Oral Med. Oral Pathol. Oral Radiol. Endod.* 91 (3): 328–333. https://doi.org/10.1067/moe.2001.113109.

Nassef, C., Ziemer, C., and Morrell, D.S. (2015). Hand-foot-and-mouth disease: a new look at a classic viral rash. *Curr. Opin. Pediatr.* 27 (4): 486–491. https://doi.org/10.1097/mop.0000000000000246.

Neves-Silva, R., Fernandes, D.T., Fonseca, F.P. et al. (2018). Oral manifestations of Langerhans cell histiocytosis: a case series. *Spec. Care Dent.* 38 (6): 426–433. https://doi.org/10.1111/scd.12330.

Neville, B.W., Damm, D.D., Allen, C.M., and Chi, A.C. (2016). *Oral and Maxillofacial Pathology*. St. Louis, MO: Elsevier.

Nikolaou, V.S., Chytas, D., Korres, D., and Efstathopoulos, N. (2014). Vanishing bone disease (Gorham-Stout syndrome): a review of a rare entity. *World J. Orthop.* 5 (5): 694–698. https://doi.org/10.5312/wjo.v5.i5.694.

Okawa, R., Iijima, O., Kishino, M. et al. (2017). Gene therapy improves dental manifestations in hypophosphatasia model mice. *J. Periodontal. Res.* 52 (3): 471–478. https://doi.org/10.1111/jre.12412.

Palla, B., Burian, E., Fliefel, R., and Otto, S. (2018). Systematic review of oral manifestations related to hyperparathyroidism. *Clin. Oral. Investig.* 22 (1): 1–27. https://doi.org/10.1007/s00784-017-2124-0.

Papageorgiou, S.N., Hagner, M., Nogueira, A.V. et al. (2017). Inflammatory bowel disease and oral health: systematic review and a meta-analysis. *J. Clin. Periodontol.* 44 (4): 382–393. https://doi.org/10.1111/jcpe.12698.

Papapanou, P.N., Sanz, M., Buduneli, N. et al. (2018). Periodontitis: consensus report of workgroup 2 of the 2017 World workshop on the classification of periodontal and peri-implant diseases and conditions. *J. Periodontol.* 89 (Suppl 1): S173–s182. https://doi.org/10.1002/jper.17-0721.

Peacock, M.E., Arce, R.M., and Cutler, C.W. (2017). Periodontal and other oral manifestations of immunodeficiency diseases. *Oral Dis.* 23 (7): 866–888. https://doi.org/10.1111/odi.12584.

Pereira, C.M., de Andrade, C.R., Vargas, P.A. et al. (2004). Dental alterations associated with X-linked hypophosphatemic rickets. *J. Endod.* 30 (4): 241–245. https://doi.org/10.1097/00004770-200404000-00015.

Pussinen, P.J., Laatikainen, T., Alfthan, G. et al. (2003). Periodontitis is associated with a low concentration of vitamin C in plasma. *Clin. Diagn. Lab Immunol.* 10 (5): 897–902.

Ramirez-Amador, V., Anaya-Saavedra, G., Crabtree-Ramirez, B. et al. (2013). Clinical Spectrum of Oral Secondary Syphilis in HIV-Infected Patients. *J. Sex Transm. Dis.* 2013: 892427. https://doi.org/10.1155/2013/892427.

Reddy, M.S. and Morgan, S.L. (2013, 2000). Decreased bone mineral density and periodontal management. *Periodontology* 61 (1): 195–218. https://doi.org/10.1111/j.1600-0757.2011.00400.x.

Ryder, M.I., Nittayananta, W., Coogan, M. et al. (2012). Periodontal disease in HIV/AIDS. *Periodontol. 2000* 60 (1): 78–97. https://doi.org/10.1111/j.1600-0757.2012.00445.x.

Salvador, J.C., Rosa, D., Rito, M., and Borges, A. (2018). Atypical mandibular metastasis as the first presentation of a colorectal cancer. *BMJ Case Rep.* 2018: https://doi.org/10.1136/bcr-2018-225094.

Samim, F., Auluck, A., Zed, C., and Williams, P.M. (2013). Erythema multiforme: a review of epidemiology, pathogenesis, clinical features, and treatment. *Dent. Clin. N. Am.* 57 (4): 583–596. https://doi.org/10.1016/j.cden.2013.07.001.

Sapp, J.P., Eversole, L.R., and Wysocki, G.P. (2004). *Contemporary Oral and Maxillofacial Pathology*. St. Louis, MO: Mosby.

Scully, C., Gokbuget, A.Y., Allen, C. et al. (2001). Oral lesions indicative of plasminogen deficiency (hypoplasminogenemia). *Oral Surg. Oral Med. Oral Pathol. Oral Radiol. Endod.* 91 (3): 334–337. https://doi.org/10.1067/moe.2001.112158.

Scully, C., Gokbuget, A., and Kurtulus, I. (2007). Hypoplasminogenaemia, gingival swelling and ulceration. *Oral Dis.* 13 (6): 515–518. https://doi.org/10.1111/j.1601-0825.2007.01387.x.

Sharma, S.M., Mohan, M., and Baptist, J. (2014). Dental considerations in hereditary epidermolysis bullosa. *N. Y. State Dent. J.* 80 (1): 45–48.

Siegel, M.A. (1996). Syphilis and gonorrhea. *Dent. Clin. N. Am.* 40 (2): 369–383.

Silva, T.D., Ferreira, C.B., Leite, G.B. et al. (2016). Oral manifestations of lymphoma: a systematic review. *Ecancermedicalscience* 10: 665. https://doi.org/10.3332/ecancer.2016.665.

Smirani, R., Truchetet, M.E., Poursac, N. et al. (2018). Impact of systemic sclerosis oral manifestations on patients' health-related quality of life: a systematic review. *J. Oral Pathol. Med.* 47 (9): 808–815. https://doi.org/10.1111/jop.12739.

Sollecito, T.P. and Greenberg, M.S. (1992). Plasma cell gingivitis. Report of two cases. *Oral Surg. Oral Med. Oral Pathol.* 73 (6): 690–693.

Souza, M.A., Soares Junior, L.A., Santos, M.A., and Vaisbich, M.H. (2010). Dental abnormalities and oral health in patients with Hypophosphatemic rickets. *Clinics (Sao Paulo)* 65 (10): 1023–1026.

Stanko, P. and Izakovicova Holla, L. (2014). Bidirectional association between diabetes mellitus and inflammatory periodontal disease. A review. *Biomed. Pap. Med. Fac. Univ. Palacky Olomouc Czech Repub.* 158 (1): 35–38. https://doi.org/10.5507/bp.2014.005.

Staudte, H., Sigusch, B.W., and Glockmann, E. (2005). Grapefruit consumption improves vitamin C status in periodontitis patients. *Br. Dent. J.* 199 (4): 213, discussion 210–217. https://doi.org/10.1038/sj.bdj.4812613.

Thakrar, P., Aclimandos, W., Goldmeier, D., and Setterfield, J.F. (2018). Oral ulcers as a presentation of secondary syphilis. *Clin. Exp. Dermatol.* 43 (8): 868–875:https://doi.org/10.1111/ced.13640.

Thompson, G., Benwell, N., Hollingsworth, P., and McLean-Tooke, A. (2018). Two cases of granulomatosis polyangiitis presenting with Strawberry gingivitis and a review of the literature. *Semin Arthritis Rheum.* 47 (4): 520–523. https://doi.org/10.1016/j.semarthrit.2017.06.003.

Todescan, S. and Nizar, R. (2013). Managing patients with necrotizing ulcerative periodontitis. *J. Can. Dent. Assoc.* 79: d44.

Varsha, D., Kaur, M., Chaudhary, N., and Siraj, F. (2016). Solitary Langerhans cell histiocytosis of the hard palate: a diagnostic pitfall. *Ger. Med. Sci.* 14: Doc11. https://doi.org/10.3205/000238.

Varun, B.R., Varghese, N.O., Sivakumar, T.T., and Joseph, A.P. (2017). Extranodal non-Hodgkin's lymphoma of the oral cavity: a case report. *Iran J. Med. Sci.* 42 (4): 407–411.

Warren, K.R., Postolache, T.T., Groer, M.E. et al. (2014). Role of chronic stress and depression in periodontal diseases. *Periodontol. 2000* 64 (1): 127–138. https://doi.org/10.1111/prd.12036.

Wright, J.T., Fine, J.D., and Johnson, L.B. (1991). Oral soft tissues in hereditary epidermolysis bullosa. *Oral Surg. Oral Med. Oral Pathol.* 71 (4): 440–446.

XXX (1999). Position Paper: Tobacco Use and the Periodontal Patient. *J. Periodontol.* 70 (11): 1419–1427. https://doi.org/10.1902/jop.1999.70.11.1419.

Yalcin, E.D., Avcu, N., Uysal, S., and Arslan, U. (2019). Evaluation of radiomorphometric indices and bone findings on panoramic images in patients with scleroderma. *Oral Surg. Oral Med. Oral Pathol. Oral Radiol.* 127 (1): e23–e30. https://doi.org/10.1016/j.oooo.2018.08.007.

Yashoda-Devi, B., Rakesh, N., and Agarwal, M. (2012). Langerhans cell histiocytosis with oral manifestations: a rare and unusual case report. *J. Clin. Exp. Dent.* 4 (4): e252–e255. https://doi.org/10.4317/jced.50728.

Yuan, J.C., Lee, D.J., Afshari, F.S. et al. (2012). Dentistry and obesity: a review and current status in U.S. predoctoral dental education. *J. Dent. Educ.* 76 (9): 1129–1136.

Zuraw, B.L., Bernstein, J.A., Lang, D.M. et al. (2013). A focused parameter update: hereditary angioedema, acquired C1 inhibitor deficiency, and angiotensin-converting enzyme inhibitor- associated angioedema. *J. Allergy Clin. Immunol.* 131 (6): 1491–1493. https://doi.org/10.1016/j.jaci.2013.03.034.

5

Patient Examination and Initial Therapy

Claire Mc Carthy[3], Steve Engeberston[1], Edgard El Chaar[2], Mea Weinberg[1], Stuart L. Segelnick[1], and Dena M. Sapanaro[4]

[1] *Arthur Ashman Department of Periodontics and Implant Dentistry, New York University, New York, NY, USA*
[2] *Department of Periodontics, University of Pennsylvania, Dental Medicine, Philadelphia, PA, USA*
[3] *King's College, London, UK*
[4] *Department of Pediatric Dentistry, New York University, New York, NY, USA*

Medical History for the Dental Patient

The most important dental visit is the initial visit in which the dental and medical history is obtained. Presenting a case history to a colleague or instructing faculty must contain the following key pieces of information:

The **patient identifying characteristics** (Pt.ID) include sex, age, distinguishing characteristics, or whether the patient has been referred from another dentist or department within the same clinic.

The **chief concern** (CC) should be elicited describing the particular motivating factor that caused the patient to seek care at this time, ideally in the patient's own words.

The **history of the present illness** (HPI) is the history of the CC. Symptoms should be described in terms of location, quality, severity, timing (including onset duration and frequency), setting in which symptom occurs, alleviating or aggravating factors, and any associated manifestations. Medications including name dose and frequency should be determined as well as, known allergies, tobacco, alcohol, and drug use. Smoking history consists of determining whether the patient is a former, current, or never smoker and pack-years are used to quantify the smoking exposure. Alcohol use includes frequency and amount: four or more ounces for men and three ounces or more of daily alcohol intake constitute "heavy" consumption. Illicit drug use may be determined by direct questioning.

Past medical history (PMH) must include childhood illnesses, current illnesses. and their durations, hospitalizations, surgeries, obstetrics, and psychiatric treatments and diagnosis. Health maintenance including immunizations and any screening tests that have been performed should be determined.

A **family history** (FH) of illnesses of immediate family members should be included. A personal and social history (SH) should include occupation, education history, possible sources of stress, important life experiences, military service, exercise and diet, and any alternative health practices the patient may engage in.

The **review of systems** (ROS) can be thought of as a completion of any health issues that may not have arisen during the history. A "head-to-toe" scheme of questioning helps to not forget to ask anything, one possible order of questioning might begin with neurologic, then on to the skin, eyes, ears, nose, throat, neck, breasts, respiratory, cardiovascular, gastrointestinal, genitourinary, musculoskeletal, hematologic, and endocrine.

An American Society of Anesthesiologists (ASA) classification can be assessed for the patient. ASA 1 is a healthy patient, ASA 2 is a patient with mild systemic disease, ASA 3 is severe systemic disease, and ASA 4 is severe systemic disease that is a constant threat to life. ASA 5 and 6 refer to moribund and braindead patients not likely encountered in the outpatient setting.

The dentist should keep in mind that careful patient listening and asking open-ended questions will help in the collection of medical history data.

Clinical and Radiographical Examination

Clinical Examination

Healthy gingiva is normally coral pink with variations in melanin pigmentation among different ethnical groups.

The firm, pink, coronally located gingiva is distinguished from the more pliable and red mucosa seen on the maxillary buccal and on the buccal and lingual aspect of the mandibular teeth separated by a distinct line called mucogingival line. On the palatal aspect, the firm pink gingiva is continuous with the firm palatal mucosa with no demarcation line. The gingival tissue between the mucogingival line and the gingival margin is called the attached gingiva. On the surface of the oral gingiva there is a characteristic dimpled or stippled pattern formed from invaginations of the oral gingival epithelium in the underlying connective tissue.

Radiographic Examination

A thorough radiographic examination can provide an abundant information about the periodontium and past damage to periodontal structure, but cannot identify sites of ongoing periodontal destruction. In order to get an accurate measurement between the CEJ and radiographical crest, the parallel technique is recommended and the following is needed: the X-ray beam is oriented perpendicular to the bone and the film is parallel to the long axis of the tooth and adjacent bone.

When using the parallel technique for peri-apical radiographs, anatomical constraints frequently require compromise in the positioning of the film and consequently the X-ray beam.

By taking bitewing radiographs, it is possible to position the film more accurately and the X-ray beam closer to the CEJ than it is in situ. Therefore, vertical bite-wing radiographs are recommended for obtaining an anatomically correct image of the position of the alveolar bone, providing at the same time the dental anatomy relevant to periodontal assessment, i.e. crown, coronal part of the root, root trunk, furcation.

The distance between the crest of bone and the CEJ is of great significance since it allows us if bone loss exists. Hausmann et al. (1991), compared measurements taken from bite-wing radiographs in sites showing no CAL loss. They found that distance between CEJ to bone crest varied from 0.4 to 1.9 mm, and a distance >= 2 mm is considered an appropriate cut off point for bone loss.

Now that we have established the use of radiographs in diagnosis, the second most pertinent radiographical assessment is the observed intrabony defects. In 2000, Eickholz et al. explored the accuracy of radiographical measurements of a defect and found that radiographical intrabony defects were underestimated when compared to surgical measurements by 1.41 + 2.58 mm.

Radiographic Artifacts

Two radiographic artifacts have been studied in length, the crestal lamina and the furcation arrows.

For the longest time, the crestal lamina dura presence was a sign of periodontal stability as stated by Rams (1994), and negatively associated with periodontitis recurrence in cases on a maintenance program. Similarly, Carranza described a break in crestal lamina as early radiographic sign of periodontitis. Generally, presence of lamina dura indicates periodontal stability while its absence doesn't mean an active periodontal breakdown is taking place.

When radiographs of maxillary molars are observed, a small, triangular radiographic shadow is sometimes noted over either the mesial or distal roots in the proximal furcation area. In a skull study, Hardenkop found an association of the furcation arrow with Class II or III furcation involvement, which was significant when compared with uninvolved furcations. The image was equally apparent over mesial or distal furcations and was not affected by the existence of a buccal furcation involvement. However, the absence of the furcation arrow image does not necessarily indicate absence of a bony furcation involvement.

Oral Hygiene

Effective removal of oral biofilm is critical for the management of periodontal and peri-implant disease with this task resting largely with the patient and their commitment to performing regular self-care and returning to the dental office at agreed intervals. Substantial evidence supports a cause–effect relationship between biofilm accumulation and periodontal destruction and failure to follow oral hygiene regimes will certainly compromise clinical outcomes (Löe et al. 1965). Non-adherence may be partly attributed to the non-symptomatic nature of periodontal disease and inability to recognize any obvious benefits due to the subtlety of changes that occur. Complex recommendations, absence of immediate results, and unpleasant side effects are some of the other reasons for non-adherence to treatment recommendations for the management of chronic diseases.

Interproximal plaque removal is considered an essential component of periodontal therapy with substantial evidence to support the efficacy of this intervention in the reduction of plaque biofilm and gingival inflammation (Slot et al. 2008). However, this aspect of oral care is where patients are most lax.

Toothbrushing

Current recommendations for home care regarding toothbrushing include using a soft bristled manual toothbrush or powered oscillating rotating brush with small size brush head, focusing the bristles at the gum line, brushing one tooth surface at a time; use of a fluoridated toothpaste with a frequency of twice a day, morning and at night, for a minimum of two minutes.

Manual Toothbrush: Position towards gum line at 45°. Move the brush in small circles and short side to side strokes.

> **Note**: A patient's brushing method should not be altered unless there is evidence of inefficiency or of damage to the tissues. If the plaque is removed without tissue damage, then the method is correct.

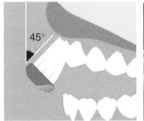 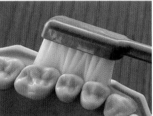

The **Modified Bass** is the most widely accepted and used brushing technique. This method of brushing requires the tufts to be pointed apically at about 45° and the ends pressed against the tooth and gingival margin to adapt the bristles to the embrasure anatomy and gingival crevice. The brush is then vibrated or moved in small circles on each surface. The brush is then moved to the next tooth/section and the technique repeated.

Power Toothbrush: Position towards gum line at approximated 80 degrees to the tooth surface. Hold brush steady on each surface. Suggest counting to 5 on each surface to ensure sufficient time to remove biofilm and stimulate the gingival tissues.

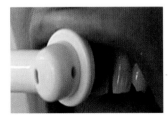 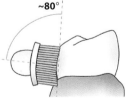

Interproximal Cleaning

Interproximal Brushes

Using specialized brushes called interproximal or interdental brushes is recommended. Patient instructions should include the following: Choose the size of brush that is a snug fit for each space (space sizes will vary). Position the brush at the gum level and push the brush into the space between your teeth. Move the brush in and out between the teeth using a back and forth (horizontal) motion. Repeat this for every space. Do this twice a day, every single day, immediately after toothbrushing.

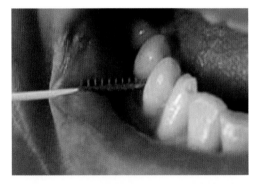

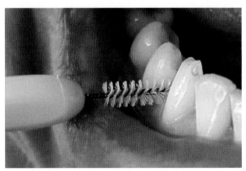

Dental Floss or Tape

Floss is designed for use in very tight spaces, with no disease, so may not be suitable for patients with significant tissue loss. It is often not as effective as interproximal brushes (discussed earlier), which remove more biofilm. The use of floss is recommended for spaces that are too tight for an interdental brush. Floss and floss holders may be used to clean between the teeth in very small tight gaps. Hold the floss taut and gently guide it between the teeth. Slide it underneath the gum and apply pressure against the tooth. Press the floss firmly against the tooth and move it along the tooth away from the gum area. Repeat this in the same space, this time cleaning the other tooth.

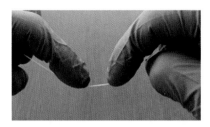

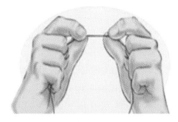

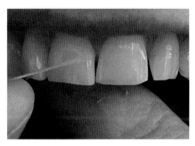

Specialized Oral Hygiene Aids

Single Tufted Brush

This is often recommended for areas that have advanced bone loss, where the roots of the teeth are visible, for deep spaces, around implants and areas of gum recession. Patients should be instructed to hold the handle as they would a pencil, position the bristles slightly beneath the gum line (on recommended area) and apply gentle pressure and rotate the bristles under the gum in small circles. This tool should be used once per day for effectiveness.

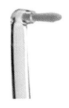

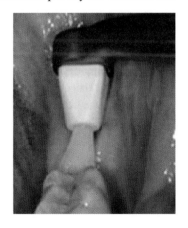

Behavior Change Techniques

Tips to help your patient get started and keep up their new homecare routine (McCarthy 2019)

1. Getting started is the hardest part.	Set a date to get started. Straight after a patient comes to see their dental professional is a good starting point, when instructions are fresh and motivation is at its highest.
2. Remembering to do it.	This can be difficult, so make it easier by setting a reminder alarm or putting a note in the bathroom or use an App to help establish this new habit.
3. Formulate a detailed plan of where the patient intends to carry out their oral hygiene routine.	Ensure you have everything you need in the right place. Ideally, you should stand in front of a mirror so you can see what you are doing and correctly target specific areas of your mouth. Decide exactly when the patient will be most likely to follow their oral care plan each day then it will start to form a routine and become a habit.
4. Ensure they know exactly how they will do each activity.	Demonstrate techniques and then observe the patient practicing so you can check they have understood your instructions correctly. Offer them positive feedback and encouragement. Record any instructions/demonstration on their mobile phone using the video feature so they can watch it at home.
5. Track your progress.	Suggest making a note of each time a patient uses their interdental brushes. This is a simple, yet effective tool that increases adherence. Use a calendar/planner, or download a toothbrushing chart from the web, or a mobile phone App that can monitor progress.
6. Make an If–Then Plan to help you achieve your goal.	It is not always easy to change the habits of a lifetime, or start doing something new, especially if it requires some time and effort. If-Then plans are a proven method to help people start and stick with new behaviors. See If–Then table in the following text.

Source: McCarthy (2019)/Springer Nature.

Some examples of **If–Then** statements, used in implementation intentions specific to oral hygiene, are as follows (Gollwitzer and Sheeran 2006).

If I am feeling too lazy to clean my teeth when I wake up in the morning, **Then** I will do it before I leave the house for work.

If I am too tired to use my interproximal brushes before I go to bed, **Then** I will use them at lunchtime everyday instead.

If I cannot remember to use my interdental brushes, **Then** I will leave them next to my toothbrush to remind me to use them immediately after I use my toothbrush.

Source: Based on Gollwitzer and Sheeran (2006).

Non-surgical Periodontal Therapy

Benefits

Non-surgical periodontal therapy (NSPT) is considered the first line of defense and a minimum standard of care in the presence of periodontal destruction. NSPT includes behavioral management to reduce and eliminate modifiable risk factors and encourage regular effective oral hygiene practices. The goal of NSPT is to reverse inflammation, eliminate edema, and bleeding and reduce plaque accumulation and probing depths by creating a biocompatible root surface environment and formation of a long junction epithelium. The patient participation including daily oral care and attendance for professional recall appointments is critical to the success of treatment.

Limitations

NSPT is a complex procedure with many clinician and patient challenges that determine the efficacy and outcome of technical and behavioral interventions. Non-surgical therapy is a closed procedure that is performed blind. Therefore, a clinical must have an experienced and detailed knowledge of root morphology and the ability to detect subgingival deposits and roughness using tactile transfer. Locating subgingival calculus requires the use of methodical, overlapping, and light strokes on the root surface using a very thin flexible exploring instrument or probe such as the ODU 11-12 Explorer.

Large bulky instruments reduce access to narrow and deep sites, furcation areas, concavities, and grooves. Dull instruments with worn cutting edges also make a complex task even more difficult. Dull instruments that have not been well maintained will increase the risk of burnishing calculus onto root surfaces, increase the number of strokes and length of time required to complete the task, and also require more force to remove deposits, thus increasing the risk of operator fatigue and injury. When choosing instruments for root surface debridement, choose instruments that are lighter in weight, with a comfortable handle, a longer terminal shank, and a miniature working end to optimize treatment outcomes. Patient tolerance and acceptance of treatment may also pose obstacles as well as unwanted side-effects of treatment that includes gingival recession, sensitivity, and change in appearance of the teeth and surrounding tissues.

Armamentarium

Hand Instruments

Universal Curettes Curettes are available in universal and area-specific designs. A **universal** curette is a debridement instrument with a rounded back and a rounded toe. Universal curettes have two cutting edges per working end and these can be applied to all tooth surfaces in both the anterior and posterior sextants of the mouth. Universal curettes are used on crown and root surfaces (supra-gingivally and sub-gingivally). Universal curettes are one of the most frequently used and versatile of all the debridement instruments. They are used for the removal of light – moderate calculus deposits located both supra and sub-gingivally.

Site-Specific Curettes A site-specific curette is a debridement instrument with a rounded back, a rounded toe, and one cutting edge. The name site-specific or area-specific signifies that each curette can be applied only to specific surfaces and areas of the mouth. For this reason, a set of curettes is required to instrument the entire dentition. Site-specific curettes are used for subgingival debridement and are the instrument of choice for deep narrow periodontal pockets with complex root morphology. They are designed especially for difficult and intricate instrumentation and are considered the "Gold Standard" for periodontal debridement.

Site-specific curettes were first developed by Dr. Clayton Gracey in the late 1930s. These curettes facilitate instrumentation of root surfaces within periodontal pockets without causing trauma to the pocket epithelium. Site-specific come in many variations such as standard design, extended shank, and miniature blade versions.

Scalers Scalers are for use on enamel surfaces as they have a sharp point and are specifically designed to remove supragingival deposits from tight contact areas, and heavy calculus deposits commonly found on the lingually of mandibular anterior teeth. Scalers are contraindicated for use on root surfaces or in periodontal sites. They typically consist of two cutting edges and thin curved shape to facilitate access to narrow interdental sites.

Powered Instruments

Ultrasonic scaling devices are widely available and are now considered acceptable for root surface debridement. Ultrasonic scalers come with a variety tip designs for supra and sub-gingival calculus deposits and site-specific options for superior adaption in furcation defects. Powered instrumentation is more ergonomic that hand instruments and less physically demanding on the clinician. Technique is still dependent on clinician skill, attention to detail, time, and tip design. Studies show no differences in clinical parameters when comparing hand and power-driven instrumentation techniques. Powered instrumentation requires less lateral pressure and therefore reduces force required to remove calculus and ultimately operator fatigue.

Techniques

The procedure should be undertaken in a methodical way, working around the mouth and around each tooth in an orderly manner. It is also important to select the correct instrument for the task you wish to carry out. Instrument selection is determined by the location of the deposit relative to the gingival margin, anterior or posterior area, mesial, distal, labial, or lingual, preference of the clinician and acceptance by the patient. NSPT consists of supragingival biofilm and calculus removal and subgingival debridement of root surfaces using a range of hand and powered devices.

Each stroke should be deliberate and effective. A firm finger rest (fulcrum) is essential for controlled use of the instrument. The movement of the instrument can be divided into two phases, the exploratory stroke – this will determine the size and location of the deposit and the working stroke – which will remove the deposit.

The working end is positioned apically until the calculus is felt. Do not press hard at this point. Slide the cutting edge over the deposit until you feel the instrument is apical to the deposit. Then press down firmly on your fulcrum finger and apply lateral pressure against the handle of the instrument with your thumb and index finger to engage the cutting edge. Ensure the terminal shank is parallel with the long axis of the tooth to establish the correct angle of the cutting edge (this is referred to as parallelism). Using lateral pressure, move the blade in a coronal direction to remove the calculus deposit in its path.

Supragingival Debridement

For supragingival calculus deposits, it is vital to establish the correct angle between the instrument face and the tooth surface. The face-to-tooth angulation for calculus removal is an angle that is greater than 45° and less than 90°. The ideal angulation for supragingival scaling or debridement is between 80° and 90° where possible.

Scalers are designed to facilitate supragingival deposit removal and they are a universal instrument with two cutting edges and the face is offset at 90° angle to the terminal shank. This makes it easier for placement and to achieve a blade to tooth angle of 90°. Common scalers for this purpose are sickle scalers such as 311-312, M23T, 204s, H6/7.

Fundamental Elements of Hand Instrumentation

There are several fundamental elements of a calculus removal stroke that a clinician should take into consideration:

1. Operator posture and seat height.
2. Patient in correct position for arch to be instrumented.
3. Correct instrument (inspect for sharpness).
4. Grasp of instrument.
5. Establish where you will position a finger rest (adjacent tooth is best where possible).
6. Mouth mirror in non-dominant hand and a finger rest for stability and control.
7. Identify the cutting edge.
8. Position the blade against the surface you wish to debride just above the gingival margin.
9. Press inward and activate the blade towards the incisal edge. This called a "Pull Stroke."
10. Relax and repeat until deposit is removed (2–3 effective strokes should be enough).
11. Check for residual calculus by drying the surface with air and using an ODU explorer 11–12.

Calculus Detection Technique

Calculus detection and tactile transfer skills are essential for complete and effective root surface debridement. The ODU 11/12 explorer is specifically designed for detailed exploration using a long, complex, fine working end with superior adaption to the anatomy of root surfaces and furcation areas. The handle is of a wide diameter to reduce risk of carpel tunnel and encourage a light grasp and is lightweight and ergonomically designed. The 11/12 explorer is used by any clinician who wants to become proficient at calculus detection and removal. The use of the explorer is taught in many programs and the ability to detect calculus is a skill that is essential for assessment and evaluation during calculus removal procedures. The explorer has a thin, tapered wire like working end with an extended complex, curved shank based on the design of a Gracey curette that will specifically adapt to narrow curved root surfaces.

ODU 11/12 Explorer: for calculus detection and root exploration

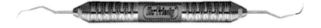

This instrument is specifically designed to adapt to the curvature of root surfaces and morphology to permit access and tactile feedback in narrow, deep, posterior sites. The working end is thin and flexible and will vibrate or "quiver" on contact with deposits. Sometimes a "click" can be heard when the instrument passes over a mineralized deposit. This instrument should be held in a relaxed, light grasp, and the leading 2 mm of the tip adapted to root surfaces and ensuring the terminal portion of the shank is parallel to the long axis of the tooth to maximize adaption of the tip.

Fulcrums

Fulcrums (finger rests) are essential when activating hand instruments. They provide stability and leverage, but also permit instrument adaption, parallelism, and access. Maintain a rest with the ring finger (4th finger) helps to steady the movement of the instrument allow for precision and safety. A finger rest will support the dominant hand as well as transmit tactile sensations to the clinician about the texture of the root surface.

The rest may be on:

1. the adjacent teeth in the same arch
2. opposite arch
3. teeth in the opposite jaw
4. the tooth being scaled (only as a last resort, as there is a risk of needle-stick injury)
5. edentulous ridges
6. external soft tissue overlying bone e.g. the patient's chin or zygomatic bone

Powered (Ultrasonic) Technique

1. Check that water is flowing through the handpiece first, then select tip and insert.
2. Adjust instrument until a fine aerosol spray of water is emitted.
3. Adjust power setting between low to medium. Medium is the maximum power recommended.
4. The instrument should be held in the pen grip with a comfortable fulcrum to support the hand
5. The tip should be inserted into the sulcus and held parallel (0° to the long axis) for biofilm disruption.
6. Tilt the tip to 15° to the long axis for calculus deposits.
7. Do not use the tip/toe of the ultrasonic perpendicular to the tooth as this will damage the surface causing grooving/pitting.
8. Continuous movement using very light pressure is important to ensure effective removal of deposits and prevent overheating.

Reevaluation of Initial Therapy

The definition of reevaluation is the action of assessing or evaluating something again or differently in order to determine if any changes have occurred and whether clinical measurement goals have been achieved. In periodontal therapy, the question arises as to when is the appropriate time to reevaluate periodontal debridement (scaling/root planning) to assess soft tissue healing. Continued assessment of the patient's progress during periodontal treatment is necessary. At the time of reevaluation, BOP, PI, CAL, PD, mobility, and furcation involvement scores are recorded. Local factors are assessed, OHI reviewed, and possible re-instrumentation also takes place. Professional judgment about continued care, modifying goals or treatment must be determined.

The ideal time to do a reevaluation of initial therapy is between four and eight weeks because it was determined that this time interval was the optimal clinical and microbiological healing time. The clinical evaluation of gingival tissues after scaling and root planing should be performed no sooner than two weeks because healing of the epithelium has not been completed and up to four to eight weeks for connective tissue collagen bundle fibers healing. Additionally, it takes approximately two months for bacteria repopulation to occur; thus, performing reevaluation after two months is not advised.

Occlusal Therapy

The correlation of occlusion and periodontal disease has been studied in length over the years. While definitive conclusion of occlusal trauma being the cause of clinical attachment has been proven invalid, the addition of occlusal trauma over an active periodontal condition with weakened periodontium can aggravate the periodontium breakdown.

A set of definitions have been established in relation to occlusal trauma:

1. Excessive occlusal force: a force that exceeds the reparative potential of the periodontium leading to occlusal trauma and/or causes tooth wear.
2. Occlusal trauma is an injury to the periodontium that can happen in an intact periodontium or reduced periodontium. It will be divided in two sub-categories:
   (i) Primary occlusal trauma is an injury leading to tissue changes in an intact periodontium
   (ii) Secondary occlusal trauma is an injury leading to tissue changes in a reduced periodontium
3. Fremitus is tooth mobility felt or observed upon chewing.
4. Bruxism is a parafunctional habit of grinding, clenching leading to damage to the tooth, the periodontium and to the temporo-mandibular joint (TMJ).
5. Non-carious cervical lesions (NCCLs): it is a loss of hard tissue on the cervical part including the root. It is generally accompanied with gingival recession. The etiology is multifactorial since abfraction, a tooth lesion caused by occlusal force, was not proven as the primary cause. The other etiologies erosion, corrosion or tooth brushing habits, eating disorders, and parafunction should be considered.

The true diagnosis of occlusal trauma is a histological one that requires sectional biopsies something unfeasible, clinicians relies on clinical and radiographical signs such as progressive mobility, discomfort upon chewing, disharmony in the teeth positions, widening of the periodontal ligaments, resorption, cemental tears, and thermal sensitivity. These symptoms are not considered by far exclusive for occlusal trauma but can be caused by different clinical conditions such as parafunction. A differential diagnosis should be considered once using these signs.

Animal studies on squirrel monkey (orthodontic-like forces), beagle dogs (high restoration), and rats (bonded wire bands or inlays), although short in duration, have shown that occlusal trauma on a healthy periodontium would not cause periodontitis, but may be a co-factor leading to further breakdown in cases where inflammation is already present.

A series of clinical studies have investigated, ranging from tooth mobility affecting clinical attachment, to effect on regenerative potential, to the relationship between cusps, occlusal disharmonies, discrepancies, different types of occlusal movements, to long-term periodontal maintenance and parafunctions. There was no conclusive evidence to support routine occlusal therapy but it showed the importance to record the patient occlusion before, during, and after treatment, which makes the occlusal treatment beneficial along the conventional periodontal therapy in periodontitis by improving the prognosis of the treated teeth through reducing the forces to become adaptive in the reduced periodontal attachment.

In regard to the studies of correlation between occlusal trauma and NCCLs and gingival recession, none was able to correlate any evidences linking the two together. In regard to the orthodontic movement, a healthy reduced periodontium, with good plaque control, can undergo tooth movement with controlled forces without compromising the periodontium, but uncontrolled orthodontic forces will lead to alveolar bone resorption and other damages such as root resorption, pulpal necrosis.

Medications and Implications for Periodontal Therapy

Medications can have a significant effect on the overall periodontal health of the patient as well as implications on periodontal/implant therapy. Table 5.1 lists various medications that either affect the periodontium or may change the course of periodontal treatment. In addition to these medications, adverse drug–drug interactions associated with medications the patient is taking must be carefully assessed before dental treatment is administered or certain drugs are prescribed or recommended.

Table 5.1 Medications that affect the periodontium or change the periodontal treatment.

- Cyclosporine A (CsA)
- Phenytoin
- Calcium channel blockers (CCBs)
- Glucocorticoids
- Alcohol
- Bisphosphonates
- Selective serotonin reuptake inhibitors (SSRIs)
- Nonsteroidal anti-inflammatory drugs (NSAIDs)
- Chemotherapy drugs
- Antiplatelets [low-dose aspirin, clopidogrel (Plavix)]
- Anticoagulants [warfarin and new oral anticoagulants (NOAC)]

Cyclosporine A (CsA), an immunosuppressant, phenytoin, anticonvulsant, and calcium channel blocker for cardiovascular conditions, can cause gingival enlargement, which has been speculated to be caused by an increased production of collagen by fibroblasts. The highest prevalence with the CCBs has been found to be with nifedipine (Procardia), amlodipine (Norvasc), and diltiazem (Cardizem). Management of these patients includes optimal plaque control and discussion with physician to change the medication.

There is still controversy whether to stop anti-platelets and anticoagulants before surgery. Most articles say not to stop. An international normalized ratio (INR) for anticoagulants is best taken on the day of periodontal debridement or surgery. The novel oral anticoagulants (NOAs) including dabigatran (Pradaxa), rivaroxaban (Xarelto), and apixaban (Eliquis) do not require an INR.

Sedation: Minimal and Moderate Sedation

Specific guidelines have been published that the periodontist must follow for safe and effective sedation and analgesia (ADA Guidelines for the Use of Sedation and General Anesthesia by Dentists 2016). The terms enteral and parenteral only indicate the route of drug administration. Since the level of sedation (minimal, moderate, deep sedation, and general anesthesia) is not dependent on the route of administration, it becomes important to have through knowledge of all drugs administered during periodontal/implant surgery besides careful monitoring of the patient. For example, administration of an oral benzodiazepine can result in different levels of sedation (e.g. minimal or moderate sedation) depending on the dose administered. If the patient is not properly monitored a parental drug intended for moderate sedation can actually push the patient into an unintentional deep sedation,

Table 5.2 Drugs: Minimal and moderate sedation.

	Sedation	Analgesia
Oral benzodiazepines	Diazepam (Valium), lorazepam (Ativan), triazolam (Halcion), and midazolam (Versed)	
Oral non-benzodiazepines	Zolpidem (Ambien) and zaleplon (Sonata)	
IV benzodiazepines	Diazepam, midazolam (Versed)	
Opioids		Fentanyl (Sublimaze)

which could be an emergency situation. It is unknown how the patient will respond. Thus, the dose required and route of administration is dependent on the clinical situation. Drugs given via the intravenous and inhalation routes can be titrated.

Table 5.2 reviews the different sedation and analgesia drugs used in periodontal practice for minimal and moderate sedation. The same drugs are used for minimal and moderate sedation, and it is just the dosing that changes depending on the length of the periodontal procedure. Pre-assessment of the patient including physical exam and classifying the ASA category of the patient is necessary before drug administration.

For sedation, usually a benzodiazepine is used either orally or intravenously for its sedative/hypnotic and anxiolytic features but without an analgesic effect. Flumazenil is the selective antagonist for benzodiazepines. For an analgesic effect usually, fentanyl is used. Fentanyl is a short-acting opioid with no amnesic effects. An advantage is that it has an immediate onset of action. Effects are reversed by naloxone. Alpha$_2$ agonists (e.g. clonidine) have sedative and anxiolytic and analgesic properties.

References

American Dental Association (2016). Guidelines for the Use of Sedation and General Anesthesia by Dentists.

Hausmann, E., Allen, K., and Clerehugh, V. (1991). What alveolar crest level on a bite-wing radiograph represents bone loss? *J. Periodontol.* 62 (9): 570–572.

Eickholz, P. and Haussman, E. (2000). Accuracy of radiographic assessment of interproximal bone loss in intrabony defects using linear measurments. *Eur. J. Oral. Sci.* 108: 70–73.

Rams, T.E., Listgarten, M.A., and Slots, J. (1994). Utility of radiographic crestal lamina dura for predicting periodontitis disease-activity. *J. Clin. Periodontol.* 21 (9): 571–576.

Gollwitzer, P.M. and Sheeran, P. (2006). Implementation intentions and goal achievement: A meta-analysis of effects and processes. *Adv. Exp. Social Psychol.* 38: 69–119.

Löe, H., Theilade, E., and Jensen, S.B. (1965). Experimental gingivitis in man. *J. Periodontol.* 36 (3): 177–187.

McCarthy, C. (2019). Closing the Gap Between Intention and Behaviour: A Clinical Application of Mental Contrasting and Intention Implementation (MCII) for Improved Adherence to Oral Health Recommendations. *Br. Dent. J.* (In Press).

Slot, D.E., Dörfer, C.E., and Van der Weijden, G.A. (2008). The efficacy of interdental brushes on plaque and parameters of periodontal inflammation: a systematic review. *Int. J. Dental Hyg.* 6 (4): 253–264.

Further Reading

Bollen, A.M., Cunha-Cruz, J., Bakko, D.W. et al. (2008). The effects of orthodontic therapy on periodontal health: a systematic review of controlled evidence. *J. Am. Dent. Assoc.* 139 (4): 413–422.

Carranza, F.A. and Newnan, M.C. (1996). *Clinical periodontology*, 8e. WB Sounders Company.

Costantinides, F., Rizzo, R., Pascazio, L., and Maglione, M. (2016). Managing patients taking novel oral anticoagulants (NOAs) in dentistry: a discussion paper on clinical implications. *BMC Oral Health* 16 (5): https://doi.org/10.1186/s12903-016-0170-7.

Dubrez, B., Graf, J.M., Vuagnat, P., and Cimasoni, G. (1990). Increase of interproximal bone density after subgingival instrumentation: a quantitative radiographical study. *J. Periodontol.* 61 (12): 725–731.

Fan, J. and Caton, J.G. (2018). Occlusal trauma and excessive occlusal forces: Narrative review, case definitions, and diagnostic considerations. *J. Periodontol.* 89: S214–S222.

Greenstein, G., Polson, A., Iker, H., and Meitner, S. (1981). Association between crestal lamina dura and periodontal status. *J. Perio.* 52: 362.

Haas, D.A. (2015). Oral sedation in dental practice. Dispatch. May/June:2–8.

Hardekop, J.D., Dunlap, R.M., Ahl, D.R., and Pelleu, G.B. Jr., (1987). The "furcation arrow" a reliable radiographic image? *J. Periodontol.* 58 (4): 258–261.

Harrel, S.K. and Nunn, M.E. (2001). The effect of occlusal discrepancies on periodontitis. II. Relationship of occlusal treatment to the progression of periodontal disease. *J. Periodontol.* 72 (4): 495–505.

Harrel, S.K. and Nunn, M.E. (2004). The effect of occlusal discrepancies on gingival width. *J. Periodontol.* 75 (1): 98–105.

Heasman, P.A. and Hughes, F.J. (2014). Drugs, medications and periodontal disease. *Br. Dent. J.* 217: 411–419.

Hersh, E.V. and Moore, P.A. (2004). Drug interactions in dentistry. The importance of knowing your CYPs. *J. Am. Dent. Assoc.* 135: 298–311.

Hersh, E.V. and Moore, P.A. (2015). Three serious drug interactions that every dentist should know about. *Compendium* 36 (6): 408–414.

Lindhe, J. and Svanberg, G. (1974). Influence of trauma from occlusion on progression of experimental periodontitis in the beagle dog. *J. Clin. Periodontol.* 1 (1): 3–14.

Ouanounou, A., Hassanpour, S., and Glogauer, M. (2016). The influence of systemic medications on osteointegration of dental implants. *J. Can. Dent. Assoc.* 82: g7.

Polson, A.M., Meitner, S.W., and Zander, H.A. (1976). Trauma and progression of marginal periodontitis in squirrel monkeys: IV. Reversibility of bone loss due to trauma alone and trauma superimposed upon periodontitis. *J. Periodontol. Res.* 11 (5): 290–298.

Segelnick, S.L. and Weinberg, M.A. (2006). Reevaluation of initial therapy: When is the appropriate time? *J. Periodontol.* 77 (9): 1598–1601.

Yagiela, J.A. (1999). Adverse drug interaction sin dental practice: interactions associated with vasoconstrictors. Part V of a series. *J. Am. Dent. Assoc.* 130: 701–709.

Part II

Principles and Practice of Periodontal Surgery

6

Surgical Anatomy and Local Anesthesia

Roya Afshar-Mohajer and Babak Hamidi

Ashman Department of Periodontology and Implant Dentistry, New York University College of Dentistry, New York, NY, USA

As dental surgeons, our main objective during the procedures we perform is to gain access to the underlying structures of the oral cavity. Whether the procedure is resective or regenerative in nature, we must be cognizant of what anatomic landmarks are present in our designated surgical site. The purpose of this chapter is to review some key anatomic landmarks that must be taken into consideration when planning a surgical procedure especially with regards to our incision, flap design, and tissue management.

The two key considerations when designing a flap is to understand the anatomy of the site and a clear goal and expected outcome. During periodontal surgery, our key objective is to have access to the underlying structures, namely, the roots and the bone. Our definitive incisions and flap reflection keeping in mind the anatomy as well as the blood supply (Figure 6.1) will lead to less tissue trauma and better tissue management. During these procedures we are often modifying the osseous architecture either in a resective manner or through regenerative modalities but ultimately leading to better hard and soft tissue contours. In turn this will lead to enhanced plaque control and long term maintenance (Rose).

To ensure an optimum outcome we must always practice atraumatic tissue techniques, which include making concise, smooth incisions with a sharp blade followed by careful flap reflection. During closure we want to avoid too much tension on a flap while suturing and making sure there is proper hemostasis. Ultimately these steps will help ensure ideal wound healing without complications.

Anatomic Landmarks

Mandible

The mandible or lower jaw is a u-shaped bony structure that is made up of different components that are important for us to be cognizant not only in terms of giving local anesthesia prior to surgery but also for proper surgical planning. It is made up of the ramus and the body and contains foramen, ridges, and concavities we need to be aware of as well as the corresponding nerves and vessels running throughout (Table 6.1; Figure 6.2).

Periodontal surgery in the posterior mandible can most often be complicated by the presence of the external oblique ridge as well as when the temporal crest and anterior border of the ramus sharply abut the most terminal mandibular molar. This makes proper re-contouring of the bone a challenge during osseous surgery or crown lengthening procedures (Figure 6.2).

The buccinator muscle, which attaches to the mandible along the molar teeth, may limit proper extension of the vestibule in the posterior mandible. This muscle forms a portion of the medial wall of the buccal space; therefore if it were damaged while elevating a buccal flap; the buccal space would be violated producing the possibility of an infection in the space. Since the buccal space communicates with the para-pharyngeal space, potential danger of the spread of a buccal space infection into other spaces of the head and neck (Clarke) (Figure 6.2).

The mental foramen that is usually located inferior to apices of mandibular premolars may become a consideration during osseous surgery where there is correction infra-bony defects or if there are muco-gingival defects that may require apically positioning the buccal flap during surgery. Damage to the mental nerve could result in temporary or possibly permanent paresthesia of the lip and gingiva (Clarke) (Figure 6.3).

While performing surgery on the lingual aspect of the mandible, we must be aware of the location of the lingual nerve, which can sometimes be positioned superficially in the area of the second and third molars. Also, anytime the attached gingiva is elevated on the lingual aspect of a mandible, or when there is a perforation in the mucosal on the floor of the mouth, the sublingual

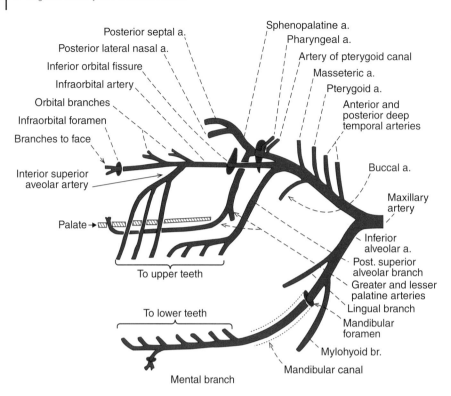

Posterior septal a.
Posterior lateral nasal a.
Inferior orbital fissure
Infraorbital artery
Orbital branches
Infraorbital foramen
Branches to face
Interior superior aveolar artery
Palate →
To upper teeth

Sphenopalatine a.
Pharyngeal a.
Artery of pterygoid canal
Masseteric a.
Pterygoid a.
Anterior and posterior deep temporal arteries
Buccal a.
Maxillary artery
Inferior alveolar a.
Post. superior alveolar branch
Greater and lesser palatine arteries
Lingual branch
Mandibular foramen
Mylohyoid br.
Mandibular canal

To lower teeth
Mental branch

Figure 6.1 Arteries supplying the maxilla and mandible.

Table 6.1 Anatomy of the mandible.

Anatomic feature	Characteristics
Alveolar process	• Forms as teeth erupt • Continuous with basal bone
Anterior border of the ramus	• Lateral to alveolar process as it extends anteriorly and inferiorly • Its anterior extension forms the external oblique ridge • Together with the temporal crest it forms the retro-molar fossa
Coronoid process	• Anterior/superior extent of the ramus • Located in infra-temporal fossa • Lateral to pterygoid plate and medial to zygomatic process of maxilla
Temporal crest	• Located medial and posterior to the anterior border of the ramus • Together with the anterior of ramus located laterally, it forms the retromolar fossa
External oblique ridge	• Formed as a continuation of the anterior border of ramus • May extend as far anteriorly as second premolar
Mylohyoid ridge	• Attachment for the mylohyoid muscle • Extends from molar region to premolars on the lingual aspect of the mandible
Genial tubercule	• Attachment for the genioglossus and geniohyoid muscles • Located at midline near inferior border of the mandible
Mental foramen	• Usually located inferior to apices of mandibular premolars yet location may vary • Transmits branches of the inferior alveolar nerve and vessels

space may be violated. If there is an infection in this space it could lead to an elevation of the tongue and respiratory problems. Such an infection may spread into the para-pharyngeal space or even produce cellulitis of the neck (Clarke).

The mentalis muscle may prevent the surgeon from adequately increasing the zone of attached gingiva or deepening the vestibule in the anterior mandible region. The elevation of this same muscle could violate the sub-mental space.

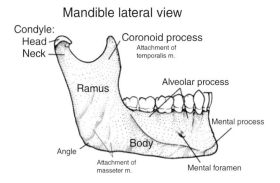

Figure 6.2 Mandible.

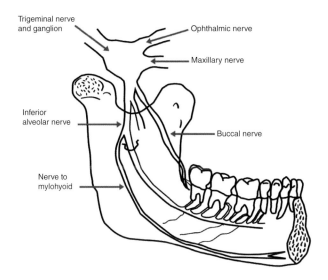

Figure 6.3 Nerve innervation of the mandible.

Since the plate of bone overlying the facial and lingual root surfaces of the mandibular anterior teeth is usually quite thin, it may be beneficial to utilize a partial thickness flap; therefore, the periosteum and connective tissue would help prevent postoperative osseous and gingival defects over these roots (Clarke).

In the anterior lingual region, the possible obstacle would be the presence of an abnormally large or high genial tubercle, which may prevent osseous re-contouring during periodontal surgery (Figure 6.2).

Anatomic Spaces

There are two categories of anatomical spaces or compartments are found in the head and neck:

- Spaces found within subcutaneous or submucosal connective tissues
- Spaces delineated by fascial membranes

These compartments are filled with loose areolar connective tissue and may be continuous with one another. Muscle groups, nerves and arteries, fat, or specific organs may be housed within such spaces. During surgery, we need to take precautions during incision and reflection to not perforate into or violate these spaces (Table 6.2).

Maxilla

The maxilla features four bony processes: the frontal, the zygomatic, the palatal, and the alveolar. For the purposes of periodontal surgery, our focus will be on the palatal processes, which form the major part of the hard palate, and the alveolar processes form the upper dental arch (Figure 6.4).

The maxillary sinus occupies much of the maxilla and its size and extent are important for us to consider when working in the area of the maxillary pre-molars and molars.

Exostoses or tori may also be found in the maxilla with the most common being the maxillary torus, which is located along the midline of the hard palate. Smaller exostoses are often observed on the buccal or palatal roots of the molars (Clarke). Prominent exostoses or a flat, shallow palatal roof make osseous re-contouring difficult to accomplish (Table 6.3).

In the maxillary anterior region, the facial bone tends to be very thin leading to the formation of a potential fenestration or dehiscence over the roots of the incisors and canines. As with mandibular anterior teeth, partial thickness flaps may be beneficial in these areas to prevent hard or soft tissue defects post-operatively.

In the posterior maxilla, the zygomatic process could form a shelf-like bony projection, which would complicate osseous re-contouring. If there is a muco-gingival defect, the buccinator muscle may also limit the apical extent to which one could move the flap to gain an adequate width of attached gingiva. Perforation of the buccinator muscle would establish entry into the buccal space and possible postoperative infection (Clarke).

Table 6.2 Anatomic spaces.

Anatomic space	Boundaries	Contents
Submental space	• Located at base of chin • Bound by the Anterior belly of digastric muscle, inferior Platysma muscle, superior Mylohyoid muscle	• Submental lymph nodes • Submental branches of facial artery and vein bilaterally
Submandibular space	• Located below the mylohyoid muscle • Boundaries: medial- mylohyoid muscle, hyoglossus muscle, and styloglossus muscle; lateral-skin; posterior-stylomandibular ligament; inferior-anterior belly of digastric; superior-mandible and mylohyoid muscle	• Submandibular gland • Lingual nerve and vessels • Mylohyoid nerve • Hypoglossal nerve • Facial artery and vein
Sublingual space	• Located in submucosal connective tissue of floor of mouth • Boundaries: medial- mylohyoid muscle, hyoglossus muscle and styloglossus muscle; anterior and lateral-lingual aspect of mandible; inferior-mylohyoid m; superior-mucosa of the floor of the mouth	• Sublingual gland • Wharton's duct
Buccal	• Lies in subcutaneous tissue of the cheek between buccinator and skin. • Boundaries: medial- buccinator muscle; lateral-skin; posterior-masseter m; zygomaticus major and depressor anguli oris muscle; superior-zygomatic arch; inferior-mandible	• Buccal fat pad • Facial artery and vein • Parotid duct
Pterygomandibular space	• Medial- medial pterygoid muscle • Lateral-ramus of mandible • Anterior-pterygomandibular raphe • Inferior -attachment of the medial pterygoid to the inferior border of the mandible	• Inferior alveolar vessels and nerve • Lingual nerve
Pterygomandibular space	• Medial- medial pterygoid muscle • Lateral-ramus of mandible • Anterior-pterygomandibular raphe • Inferior -attachment of the medial pterygoid to the inferior border of the mandible	• Inferior alveolar vessels and nerve • Lingual nerve
Parapharyngeal space	• Located at base of the skull and delineated by fascial membranes • Separated in two compartments by styloid process • Communicates anteriorly with buccal, sublingual and pterygomandibular spaces; medially with the retropharyngeal space; and inferiorly with spaces of the neck	• Anterior compartment: deep cervical lymph nodes, ascending pharyngeal artery, facial artery • Posterior compartment: carotid artery, internal jugular vein, vagus nerve, hypoglossal nerve, cervical sympathetic trunk

The palate contains several anatomic features of major importance to us during surgery especially when we are harvesting a sub-epithelial connective tissue graft for a root coverage procedure. The greater and lesser palatine nerves and blood vessels gain entrance into the palate through the greater and lesser palatine foramina. These foramina are usually located apical to the third molars. These nerves and vessels run anteriorly within a bony groove. This neuro-vascular bundle is usually located approximately 7–17 mm from the cement-enamel junctions of the maxillary premolars and molars (Reiser). Severing the greater palatine artery could lead to hemorrhage, which can sometimes be difficult to control through local clamping (Figure 6.5).

The naso-palatine nerve comes through the incisive foramen to supply the sensory innervation for the palatal mucosa from canine to canine. Surgery in this area often requires removing or undermining the incisive papilla, which could result in temporary paresthesia of the area supplied (Figure 6.5).

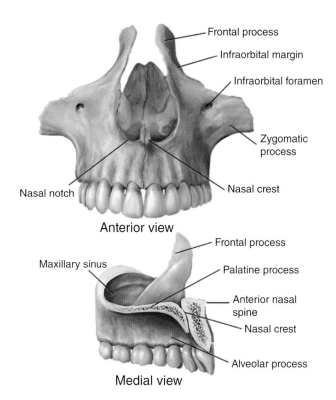

Anterior view

Medial view

Figure 6.4 Anatomy of the maxilla.

Conclusion

As surgeons working in the oral cavity, we must be cognizant of the anatomic landmarks in the surgical site. The location of nerves, vessels, and spaces as well as the bony architecture are all important to consider during the pre-operative planning phase. These considerations are key to proper tissue management, ensuring proper blood supply, hemostasis, and proper would healing.

Properties of Local Anesthesia

Local anesthesia when administered topically or by local injection will result in a temporary loss of pain or sensation without any effect on consciousness.

There are two main groups of dental anesthesia. The esters and the amides:

- The **esters** are procaine and benzocaine that are not used as injectable anesthesia. Benzocaine is used for topical anesthesia.
- **Amides** which include Lidocaine, Articaine, Prilocaine, and Mepivacaine are used as injectable anesthetics. Lidocaine is also used as a topical anesthesia.

Once local anesthetic is administered it results in blocking the operation of specialized gates called the sodium

Table 6.3 Anatomy of the maxilla.

Anatomic feature	Characteristics
Maxillary sinus	• Hollow structure occupies most of the maxilla • Extends to canine anteriorly and third molars posteriorly • Lined by the Schneiderian membrane
Zygomatico-alveolar crest	• Extends from the tip of zygomatic process to the alveolar process opposite the first and second molars • Forms the posterior border of the malar process
Palatal vault	• Formed by the palatine processes and alveolar processes of the maxilla • Shape of the palatal vault may range from wide and shallow to narrow and high
Greater (anterior) palatine foramen	• Located within the palatine bone approximately 2mm from posterior border of hard palate and 15mm from midline and superior to the second and third molars • Neurovascular bundle courses anteriorly in a groove formed at the juncture of the palatine and alveolar processes
Palatal exostoses	Midline palatine torus or palatal exostoses/ledging usually opposite the second or third molars
Incisive foramen	• Located posterior to the central incisors and deep to the incisive papilla • Contains the nasopalatine neurovascular bundle, which supplies the anterior palate from canine to canine
Alveolar process	• Forms as teeth erupt • Bone usually thinner over labial/buccal surfaces compared with palatal surfaces

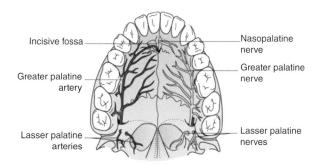

Figure 6.5 Nerve innervations and blood supply of the palate.

potential of the nerve and no nerve signals will be transmitted. Nodes of Ranvier are the only location in which the local anesthetic has access to the nerve, where multiple sodium channels exist. When nerve signal or depolarization is blocked at three uninterrupted nodes of Ranvier, the interruption of a nerve signal occurs.

Local anesthetics have vasodilation characteristics and are absorbed in the circulation. Their systemic effect is related to their blood plasma level. CNS depression, elevated heart rate, convulsions, and high blood pressure are results of local anesthetic overdose. To counteract the vasodilator action of local anesthetics, vasoconstrictors such as epinephrine and levonordefrin, are added to local anesthetics. They result in prolonging the removal of the anesthetic from the nerve and lead to longer action.

Anesthetics have different durations of action and onset of symptoms. The closer the physiologic *pH* is to the equilibrium *pH* of a given anesthetic the more rapid the onset of the anesthesia. The onset of action is slower as the acidity of a local anesthetic increases. If local anesthesia is injected at a site with infection, its effect will be delayed or there will be no effect at all. Inflammation at the site of infection will lower the normal *pH* value of (7.4), and this lower amount blocks the anesthetic action by allowing small amounts of the free base form of the anesthetic to cross the nerve sheath to allow conduction of nerve impulses.

Properties of Ideal Anesthetic

- It should not irritate the tissue to which it is applied.
- It should not make any long-lasting changes on nerve structure.
- Its systemic toxicity should be minimal.
- It must be effective regardless of whether it is injected into tissue or applied locally on mucous membrane.
- The time of onset of anesthesia should be minimal.
- Duration of action must be sufficiently long to allow the procedure to be completed but not so long as to necessitate extended recovery.
- It should have enough potency to administer full anesthesia without supplementing additional concentrated solutions that are potentially damaging.
- It should not produce allergic reaction.
- It should be stable in solution and should spontaneously undergo biotransformation in the body.
- It should be sterile or capable of being sterilized by heat without deterioration.

Techniques of Local Anesthesia

Maxillary Anesthesia

There are three major types of injections that can be performed in the maxilla for pain control.

- **Local infiltration**: This is able to be performed in the maxilla due to the thin cortical nature of the bone. It involves injecting into tissue immediately around the surgical site.

- Supraperiosteal injections
- Intraseptal injections
- Periodontal ligament injections
- **Field block**: A local anesthetic deposited near a larger terminal branch of a nerve.
  - Periapical injections
- **Nerve block**: Local anesthetic deposited near main nerve trunk and is usually distant from operation site.
  - Posterior superior alveolar
  - Middle superior alveolar
  - Anterior superior alveolar
  - Maxillary nerve block (V2 block)
  - Infraorbital
  - Greater palatine
  - Nasopalatine

Mandibular Anesthesia

This Infiltration technique does not work in the adult mandible due to the dense cortical bone.

Nerve blocks are utilized to anesthetize the inferior alveolar, lingual, and buccal nerves.

It provides anesthesia to the pulpal, alveolar, lingual, and buccal gingival tissue, and skin of lower lip and medial aspect of chin on side injected.

- *Inferior alveolar nerve block (IAN)*
  This technique involves blocking the inferior alveolar nerve prior to entry into the mandibular lingual on the medial aspect of the mandibular ramus.

  The area of insertion is the mucous membrane on the medial border of the mandible ramus at the intersection of a horizontal line (*height of injection) and vertical line (**anteroposterior plane).
  *The height of the injection should be 6–10mm above the occlusal table of the mandibular teeth.
  **The Anteroposterior plane – just lateral to the pterygomandibular raphe.
- **Akinosi technique**: Also known as the closed-mouth mandibular nerve block. It is mostly used in patients who have limited opening of the mandible or in those that have trismus; spasm of the muscles of mastication. The nerves that are anesthetized in this technique are the inferior alveolar, incisive, mental, lingual, and mylohyoid nerves.

  As Akinosi technique is an anesthetic technique that requires penetration of a significant thickness of soft tissues, a long needle is used. The needle is inserted into the soft tissue that covers the medial border of the mandibular ramus, in region of the inferior alveolar, lingual, and mylohyoid nerves. The positioning of the bevel of the needle is very important as it must be positioned away from the bone of the mandibular ramus and instead toward the midline.

- **Gow-Gates technique**: It is used to provide anesthetics to the mandible of the patient's mouth. With the aid of extra and intraoral landmarks, the needle is injected into the intraoral latero-anterior surface of the condyle, steering clear below the insertion of the lateral pterygoid muscle. The extra oral landmarks used for this technique are the lower border of the ear tragus, corners of the mouth, and the angulation of the tragus on the side of the face. All three oral sensory parts of the mandibular branch of the trigeminal nerve and other sensory nerves in the region will come in contact with the anesthetic and this reduces the need to anesthetize supplementary innervation. In comparison with other regional block methods of anesthetizing the lower jaw, the Gow-Gates technique has a higher success rate in fully anesthetizing the lower jaw. One study found that out of 1200 patients receiving injections through the Gow-Gate technique, only 2 of them did not obtain complete anesthesia.

- **Mental nerve block**

  The area of injection is the mucobuccal fold at or anterior to the mental foramen. This lies between the mandibular premolars.

  The depth of injection should be 5–6 mm.

  Inject 0.5–1.0 CC of local anesthesia.

  Massage local anesthetic into tissue to manipulate into mental foramen to anesthetize the incisive branch.

Further Reading

Rose, L., Mealey, B., and Genco, R. (2004). *Periodontics: Medicine, Surgery and Implants*, 2e. Missouri: Mosby Chapter 20.

Clarke, M.A. and Bueltmann, K.W. (1971). Anatomical considerations in periodontal surgery. *J. Periodontol.* 42: 610–625.

Reiser, G.M., Bruno, J.F., Mahan, P.E., and Larkin, L.H. (1996). The subepithelial connective tissue graft palatal donor site: anatomic considerations for surgeons. *Int. J. Periodontics Restoration Dent.* 16: 130–137.

Malamed, S.F. (ed.) (2013). Chapter 1: Neurophysiology. In: *Handbook of Local Anesthesia*, 6e, 2–24. St. Louis: Elsevier.

7

Suturing Techniques

Mea A. Weinberg[1], Stuart L. Segelnick[1], and Edgard El Chaar[2]

[1]*Arthur Ashman Department of Periodontics and Implant Dentistry, New York University, New York, NY, USA*
[2]*Department of Periodontics, University of Pennsylvania, Dental Medicine, Philadelphia, PA, USA*

Principles of Surgical Wound Closure

Wound stability, the definitive goal of wound management in periodontal surgery, is achieved primarily by wound closure without tension on the edges of the wound. There are two types of periodontal wound closure healing: primary and secondary intention. Primary wound healing occurs when there is close approximation of the wound edges with minimal formation of a blood clot or hematoma and no loss of tissue (Christgau 2004). On the contrary, during secondary wound healing the wound edges do not approximate each other delaying the healing process (Meyle 2006). Extraction sites and apically positioned flaps heal by secondary intention (Pippi 2017). There is a greater risk for infection than in primary intention healing.

Sutures stabilize the wound allowing for optimal healing and is the key to maintaining adequate postoperative wound stability (Burkhard and Lang 2000; Zuhr and Hürzeler 2017). Additionally, one of the most important aspects in achieving maximum wound stability during suturing is having less tension on the wound edges (Zuhr and Hürzeler 2017).

Periodontal surgery using magnification with a microscope has been gaining interest recently primarily because of many advantages including improved visibility to surgical site, rapid healing, and increased patient acceptance (Yadav et al. 2018). Suturing during periodontal microsurgery involves the suture needle to penetrate perpendicular to the tissues and exit the tissues at equal distance. In order to allow for appropriate wound approximation, the suture bite is about 1.5 times the tissue thickness.

Properties of Suture Materials

Basically, there are four features of suturing that should be reviewed when making a decision on surgical wound closure. These features including suture materials, suturing needles, suturing techniques, and suture thread size (refers to the diameter of the material and it ranges from the biggest, 1.0 to the smallest, 10.0) (Table 7.1). The ideal suture material should have the following properties: Christgau (2004), Koshak (2017), and Modi (2009).

(1) good tissue reaction;
(2) absent wicking effect;
(3) high tensile strength (weight required to break a suture) to hold the wound edges together during healing time;
(4) not cause tissue damage;
(5) good knotting property and security;
(6) good memory (after using the suture material it returns to its initial shape) and;
(7) good elasticity (after the suture is stretched, it should recover its original form and length).

Suture materials are classified as being absorbable or non-absorbable. Sutures are further classified based on the type: plain, chromic, braided monofilament, monofilament, or braided. Several properties of suture materials are reviewed in Table 7.2. The choice on which type of suture material as well as the technique used depends on several properties including the adequate tensile strength for wound healing, type of wound, ease of handling, length of time till suture removal, produce minimal or no inflammatory reaction, and knot security (Dennis et al. 2016;

Table 7.1 Features of the sutures.

Non Resorbable	Thread size	Resorbable	Thread size
silk	3-0,4-0,5-0	Gut	4-0
Nylon	4-0,5-0,6-0	Chromic Gut	4-0,5-0
Polypropylene	5-0,6-0	PGA	3-0,4-0,5-0
e-PTFE	4-0,5-0,6-0	PGA-dyed	3-0,4-0,5-0

Table 7.2 Properties of suturing materials.

Suture	Material	Resorption	Properties
Absorbable			
Plain surgical (cat) gut	Submucosa of sheep intestine or serosa of beef intestine. Oldest suture material	Tensile strength is maintained for 3–5 d and absorption complete within 70 d	Not flexible (difficult to be tied and knotted); weak
Chromic gut	Submucosa of sheep intestine or serosa of beef intestine; treated with a chromium salt solution to resist body enzymes	Tensile strength is maintained for 7–10 d. Prolong absorption time over 90 d	Poor knotting property; some tissue reactivity since it is natural; weak
Polyglycolic acid (PGA) (Dexon)	Braided	Via hydrolysis 28–45 d	Resists muscle pull; not for extended time; may have wicking effect
Polyglactin 910 (VICRYL)	Copolymer of glycolide and lactide with polyglactin	About 28 d; some components will have extended time to resorb	Good knotting property; strong; synthetic so less tissue reaction
Poliglecaprone 25 (MONOCRYL)	Monofilament (one strand)	High tensile strength which decreases overs 2 wk; Hydrolysis 91–119 d	Easy to handle; Slight tissue reaction; approximate without tension for extended time
Nonabsorbable			
Silk	Natural; braided; raw silk spun by silkworm and coated with wax to reduce capillary action	Has reactivity when buried in the tissue; may have a wicking effect; not strong 7 d	
Polytetrafluoroethylene (PTFE)	Synthetic; monofilament, rod shaped, and are neither expanded or dense.	No wicking effect. High tensile strength. Ideal for bone grafting, soft tissue grafting and implants. Less secure knotting. 2–4 wk	
Nylon (ETHILON)	Synthetic; polymer of polyethylene terephthalate	Better tissue reactivity than silk; poor knotting	
Polyester	Synthetic; braided	Some wicking effect because it is braided. Better tissue reactivity than silk; superior knotting	

Source: Modi (2009)/Springer Nature.

Azmat and Council 2018). Some sutures are coated on the surface allowing easy of knotting and movement through the tissues, which will reduce tissue reaction. Every case should be evaluated individually when deciding which suture material to use that will optimize healing.

Gut sutures are made from an animal collagen, which is slowly absorbed by intra-oral enzymes. They have mild to moderate tensile strength, which is lost within 48 hours. In addition, gut sutures can easily break during suturing inhibiting flap closure. Plain gut is resorbed from 3 to 5 days, while chromic gut which is coated with a chromium salt solution has a resorption time from 7 to 10 days and an extended loss of tensile strength for up to 5 days. Synthetic absorbable sutures (e.g. polyglycolic acid (PGA) is absorbed by hydrolysis and has high tensile strength, mild tissue reaction, and a resorption rate from 21 to 28 days.

Non-absorbable sutures are available as natural sutures (e.g. silk, cotton, linen) and synthetic sutures (e.g. nylon, polypropylene, polyester, ethibond, polytetrafluoroethylene [PTFE]). Additionally, silk can cause an inflammatory reaction. Advantages of using silk include easy handling and good knot security. Nylon sutures, either braided, nonbraided, monofilament, or multifilament, have good handling properties with less inflammatory reactions and greater tensile strength than silk.

The "wicking" effect of sutures allows the movement of fluids and bacteria across the suture line and up the suture, which can cause contamination of the incision and possible infection (Silverstein 2009). Although silk sutures have been implicated in having a wicking effect, some studies have not found this and reported that Dexon had a greater wicking effect (Varma et al. 2017; Grigg et al. 2004).

Suturing Techniques and Indications for Use

Surgical success of a periodontal procedure involves creation of a wound with subsequent proper closure of the wound for optimal healing to occur. There are several general suturing guidelines that should be followed (Koshak 2017; Silverstein 2009):

(1) First suture is placed in the most distal position and suturing continues in a mesial direction. For continuous sling suturing begin in the most mesial position allowing to end back in the most mesial direction.

(2) Initially suture from the mobile tissue flap to the non-mobile tissue flap.

(3) The needle should be held in the center or body of the needle, not the upper or lower third (Figure 7.1).

(4) In areas where there is limited space, use a ½ circle needle.

(5) Sutures should be placed approximately 2–3 mm apical to the flap margin to avoid tension of the margin and subsequent tearing of the flap edge.

(6) Sutures should enter at right angle to the tissue surface when entering through the tissue to avoid developing a tear.

(7) The suture knot should be tied close to where the suture first entered the tissue.

(8) The suture should not be too loose yet tight enough to ensure that the wound edges just meet without causing tissue blanching and restricting blood supply.

After selecting the appropriate suture material, the suture size and needle must be determined. In periodontal surgery the 4-0 and 5-0 thread size are commonly used (Table 7.1). A 5-0 thread diameter is usually used for soft tissue grafting and a 4-0 thread is used for most other periodontal surgical procedures. Suture needles are classified as reverse cutting, conventional cutting, or tapercut (used in periodontal plastic surgery) (Figure 7.2). Reverse cutting needles are primarily used to prevent the suture material from tearing through the papillae or flap margins (Akifuddin 2014). The 3/8 needle is commonly used in periodontal surgery and allows the needle to be passed through from the buccal surface directly through the lingual tissue in one sweep. The ½ needle is used in more restricted areas such as the maxillary facial molars and in periodontal plastic surgery procedures.

There are many different types of suturing techniques. The decision to use one type versus another depends on the ease of use while allowing for a tension free coaptation of flap margins and the type of periodontal or implant surgical procedure. For instance, interrupted sutures are most commonly used in periodontal surgery. The simple loop interrupted suture is used around implants and edentulous areas with vertical incisions and the figure-8 interrupted suture is used in flap closure especially when suturing

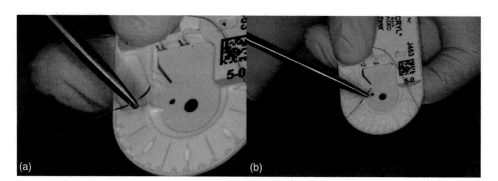

(a)   (b)

Figure 7.1 This figure shows the correct way of holding the needle in b, at a perpendicular angle.

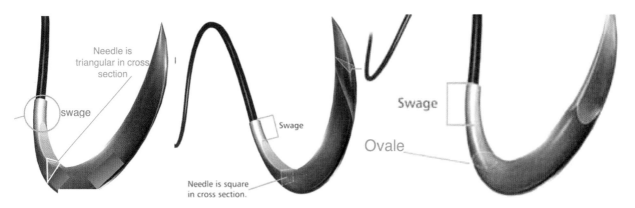

Figure 7.2 Needles can have a triangular body called "reverse cutting"; Square one called "Conventional cutting"; and an ovale body called "Tapercut".

Table 7.3 Suturing techniques and features.

Suture technique	Features	Figures
Simple loop interrupted	Most commonly used in periodontal/implant surgery; if one suture is lost there is no complete loss of suture closure. It engages the buccal side of the buccal flap and the buccal side of lingual flap	
Modified loop interrupted	Same as previous, but instead of engaging the buccal side of the lingual flap, it will engage the lingual side of it	
Periosteal	Periodontal surgery; apically position a partial thickness flap to or apical to crest of bone for pocket elimination	
Simple running or continuous	A quicker technique which distributes tension uniformly when used for long edentulous areas or for quadrant flap surgery. Only two knots are used so if there is a knot or the suture breaks the entire suture must be removed and sutured again	

(Continued)

Table 7.3 (Continued)

Suture technique	Features	Figures
Continuous locking	Same as simple continuous except passing the suture through its own loop. Edentulous regions	
Vertical mattress	Maximum tissue closure through eversion of tissue margins; reduces dead space and reduces tension across the wound	
Horizontal mattress	Maximum tissue closure through eversion of tissue margins; reduces dead space and reduces tension across the wound	
Single sling	Single tooth especially if there is a narrow interdental area which will not allow placement of single interrupted suture (e.g. soft tissue grafting procedures; GTR). It engages the buccal side from either the mesial or the distal side, wraps around the lingual coronal side of the tooth, and it re-engages the opposite side of the point of entry from the buccal side of the buccal flap	
Modified single sling	Suture designed by Dr. El Chaar, to secure a more coronal positioning of the flap. The difference from the previous, the re-engagement is from the lingual side of the buccal flap. (e.g. soft tissue grafting procedures; GTR; GBR)	

Table 7.3 (Continued)

Suture technique	Features	Figures
Bista sling suture	Suture designed by Dr. El Chaar mainly for soft tissue to accomplish a secured coronally repositioning of the flap. It engages at a mesial side of the tooth, between the tip of the buccal flap and the MGL, wraps around the lingual coronal side of the tooth, engages the lingual side of the buccal flap on the distal side at MGL and then re-enter closer to the tip of flap short 2mm and wraps again at the lingual side of the tooth ending with the knot at the mesial side	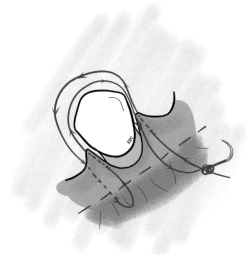
Continuous locking sling	Suture designed by Dr. El Chaar. It is recommended for periodontal surgery without GTR. The first line of suture starts from the most anterior engaging the buccal side of the buccal flap using the lingual coronal part of the tooth as an anchor and then come back re-engaging the lingual side of the flap using the buccal coronal side of each tooth as an anchor and will end the knot where we started	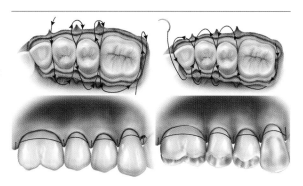
Circular suture	This is a suture technique that can to coapt to the lingual in a tight space. You engage the buccal from the mesial, engage the buccal side of the lingual, circle re-engage the lingula side of the lingual flap and come out from the lingual side of the buccal and make the knot	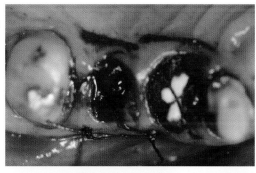
Crisscross	For an extraction socket	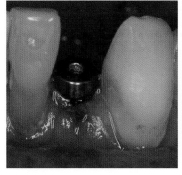 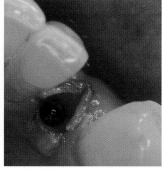

(Continued)

Table 7.3 (Continued)

Suture technique	Features	Figures
Periosteal Vertical Sling Sutures	Designed by Dr. El Chaar and Dr. Matei. This technique is very helpful for esthetic crown lengthening when the tissue is needed to be apically positioned. Engage below mucogingival one side from the buccal, come out from the inside of the flap same side 2 to 3 mm below the papillary edge of the flap. pass around the lingual of the tooth and engage the inner side of the flap from the other side, come out and re-engage 2 to 3 mm from the outside the flap, loop around the lingual of the tooth and pass from the entry side and make the knot	

Based on Dr. El Chaar manual.

the lingual aspect of mandibular molars. The vertical or horizontal mattress suture is used when Periosteal suturing utilizing the mattress technique allows for precise stable positioning of the apically positioned flap at or slightly below the alveolar crest without movement of the flap. This is accomplished by allowing the needle to slip between the bone and periosteum, thus tacking down the periosteum. Table 7.3 reviews different suturing techniques used in periodontal and implant surgery.

References

Akifuddin, S. (2014). Review on sutures in oral surgery – an update. *J. Adv. Med. Dent. Sci. Res.* 2 (3): 201–204.

Azmat, C.E. and Council, M. (2018). Wound closure techniques. In: *StatPearls*. Treasure Island, FL: StatPearls Publishing Available from: https://www.ncbi.nlm.nih.gov/books/NBK470598/.

Burkhard, R. and Lang, N.P. (2000). Influence of suturing on wound healing. *Periodontology* 2015 (68): 270–281.

Christgau, M. (2004). Wound management and postoperative cure. *Perio* 1 (4): 293–310.

Dennis, C., Sethu, S., Nayak, S. et al. (2016). Suture materials – current and emerging trends. *J. Biomed. Mater. Res. Part A* 104A: 1544–1559.

Grigg, T.R., Liewehr, F.R., Patton, W.R. et al. (2004). Effect of the wicking behavior of multifilament sutures. *J. Endod.* 30 (9): 649–652.

Koshak, H.H. (2017). Dental suturing materials and techniques. *Global J. Otolaryngol.* 12 (2): 1–11.

Meyle, J. (2006). Suture materials and suture techniques. *Perio* 3 (4): 253–268.

Modi, M. (2009). Critical evaluation of suturing materials and suturing techniques in implant dentistry. *Int. J. Clin. Implant Dent.* 1 (2): 31–40.

Pippi, R. (2017). Post-surgical clinical monitoring of soft tissue wound healing in periodontal and implant surgery. *Int. J. Med. Sci.* 14 (8): 721–728.

Silverstein, L.H. (2009). Suturing for optimal soft-tissue management. *J. Oral Implantol.* XXXV (Two): 82–90.

Varma, S., Abufanas, S., Ali, M. et al. (2017). Comparison of wicking effect of different sutures: an in vitro study. *Int. J. Curr. Res.* 9 (11): 61469–61472.

Yadav, V.S., Salaria, S.K., Bhatia, A., and Yadav, R. (2018). Periodontal microsurgery: reaching new heights of precision. *J. Indian Soc. Periodontol.* 22 (1): 5–11.

Zuhr, O. and Hürzeler, M. (2017). Wound closure and wound healing. Suture techniques in contemporary periodontal and implant surgery: Interactions, requirements, and practical considerations. *Quint. Int. Oral Surg.* 48 (8): 647–660.

8

Osseous Surgery

Thierry Abitbol

Arthur Ashman Department of Periodontics and Implant Dentistry, New York University, New York, NY, USA

Introduction

Decay and periodontal disease are the two major causes of tooth loss. As the treatment of dental caries aims at restoring teeth in form and function for the long term, so it is that periodontal treatment is intended to reduce the risk of alveolar bone loss.

To that end, periodontal probing depths or pockets have been associated with not only the likely presence of periodontitis but also the poor maintainability of such sites may be associated with progressive deterioration and attachment loss.

Typically periodontitis affects the alveolar bone crest in a manner best described as reverse architecture where the interproximal alveolar crest is found to be more apical than its vestibular counterpart; this is because the plaque front and the ensuing periodontal breakdown occurs usually, where the lesion is primarily and initially initiated.

This osseous crestal loss resulting from periodontal disease does not in turn dictate the formation of soft tissue craters. In fact the soft tissue margin, under each and all circumstances, follows the radicular anatomy, not the bone.

Specifically, the soft tissue follows either the root surface down on the convex part of the vestibular portion of the roots or up on the concave and proximal radicular surfaces.

It is these discrepancies that result in the increased periodontal probing depths where the dynamics of the soft tissue cannot conform to osseous changes resulting from periodontal deterioration.

The rational for treatment is based on the fact that deep periodontal probing depths can be the result of periodontal deterioration but also provide an environment favorable to bacterial growth.

Then one treatment alternative in the form of osseous resective surgery is a way by which periodontal tissues may be repositioned usually, as positive architecture, more apically to where it had been prior. This results in an osseous topography in harmony with soft tissue contours leading to sustainable probing depths reductions.

In order to achieve an osseous crest to a positive architecture, it should be in harmony with the soft tissue thereby resulting in a reduction in periodontal probing depths (Schluger 1949).

Material and Methods up to including flap design and osseous recontouring, as well as suturing are similar to crown lengthening.

Osseous Surgery

The technique for osseous recontouring in these cases is similar in many ways to that used for functional crown lengthening.

Following incisions and flap elevations, osteoplasty is usually implemented first to ramp the alveolar bony housing gently and coronally toward the surface of the tooth in a manner similar to the one described for a crown lengthening where a thin lip of crestal bone is left on the tooth to then be removed with sharp chisels. This avoids any unwanted nicking of the tooth with a rotary instrument. Interproximally the alveolus is handled much in the same fashion as the vestibular bone with gentle and gradual ramping to create an osseous peak just apical to the contact area. Once this is accomplished, residual osseous peaks found at transitional line angles and often referred to as widow's peaks, should be removed gently with dedicated and sharp bone chisels to achieve completely smooth contours (Friedman 1955).

As a result of this osseous recontouring a parabolic osseous crest has been created that is in harmony with the radicular anatomy and the overlying soft tissue. To be sure, the technique should be applied judiciously and on an individual basis depending on the degree of radicular curvature and other potential limiting factors to be discussed

Practical Techniques in Periodontics and Implant Dentistry, First Edition. Edited by Edgard El Chaar.
© 2023 John Wiley & Sons, Inc. Published 2023 by John Wiley & Sons, Inc.

later. There are times, for example, when the degree of osseous resection needed may in fact be modified and reduced; instead, odontoplasty is used where convexities and concavities may be modified on a case by case basis (Oschenbein 1986).

In order and for the purpose of resective surgery, furcation areas are treated much the same way as proximal surfaces as if two separate teeth were present. This conforms with the corresponding dental anatomy and prevents a furcal exposure. Bear in mind that the surgical approach should have been anticipated in the outline of the incisions and flap design.

Once the osseous surgery is done, the flap is adapted and sutured much in the same way as described in the crown lengthening section.

Post-surgical care is similar to crown lengthening.

Limitations and Contraindications to Osseous Resective Surgery

Root trunks, furcations, radicular grooves, anatomical cross sections, esthetics, degree of existing attachment loss; all are potential limiting factors for osseous surgery that the surgeon must anticipate and avoid the potential of creating an iatrogenic problem such as a furcation exposure.

One should note that when it comes to osseous resective surgery as a treatment alternative for periodontal probing depth reduction, Ochsenbein, Tibet's and their coworkers had focused their published observations on medium size interproximal osseous craters usually associated with a fairly moderate condition. As such the limiting factors discussed above were not really an issue within the context of this work. These are considerations however when such surgical techniques are applied to more severe cases (Oschenbein and Bohanan 1954; Tibetts et al. 1976; Smith et al. 1980; Olson et al. 1985).

To be sure the potential to create a positive osseous architecture surgically from the reverse osseous crest associated with periodontal deterioration is essentially limited by the anatomical factors outline earlier, where a potential iatrogenic problem results from attempts to address the actual condition. One way to stem the potential issues raised by osseous respective surgery is to have as a final objective not strictly a completely positive architecture but rather a reverse architecture with a positive flow where the osseous crest is gradually reshaped so that each proximal area is coronal only to its adjacent vestibular counterparts.

In such instances where osseous resective surgery is in fact contra indicated, decisions may be called upon to choose non-surgical or regenerative treatment alternatives described in other sections.

References

Friedman, N. (1955). Periodontal osseous surgery: osteoplasty and ostectomy. *J. Periodontol.* 26: 257–259.

Olson, C.T., Ammons, W.F., and Van Belle, G. (1985). A longitudinal study comparing apically positioned flaps with or without osseous surgery. *Int. J. Periodontics Restorative Dent.* 5 (4): 9–23.

Oschenbein, C. (1986). A primer for osseous surgery. *Int. J. Periodontics Restorative Dent.* 6: 9–47.

Oschenbein, C. and Bohanan, H.M. (1954). Palatal approach to osseous surgery. *J. Periodontol.* 35: 54–68.

Schluger, S. (1949). Osseous resection. A basic principle in periodontal surgery. *Oral Surg. Oral Med. Oral Pathol.* 2: 316–325.

Smith, D.H., Ammons, W.F., and Van Belle, G. (1980). A longitudinal study of periodontal status comparing osseous recontouring with flap curettage. Results after 6 months. *J. Periodontol.* 51 (7): 367–375.

Tibetts, L.S., Oschenbein, C., and Laughlin, D.M. (1976). Rationale for the lingual approach to osseous surgery. *Dent. Clin. N. Am.* 20: 61–78.

9

Functional Crown Lengthening

Thierry Abitbol

Arthur Ashman Department of Periodontics and Implant Dentistry, New York University, New York, NY, USA

Introduction

Broadly defined, a crown lengthening is a surgical procedure whereby additional tooth structure is exposed coronal to the free gingival margin. Indications may be functional to allow for the restoration of a severely broken-down or decayed tooth or when an improvement may be indicated in the esthetic zone. In this chapter, we will focus on the functional one.

In terms of function and the basic restoration of tooth structure, the concept of biologic width must be invoked. Specifically, roughly 2 mm of pristine unrestored tooth structure should be made available therapeutically for the connective tissue attachment to the tooth and its epithelial interface between the restorative margin and the alveolar crest. If that is not planned, then, it is likely that the resulting restorative margins will impinge on the periodontal hard and soft tissues, which would affect the long term prognosis (Cohen 1964; Schroeder and Listgarten 1971; Kois 1996; Camargo et al. 2007).

As a surgical procedure, a crown lengthening may be called upon in the esthetic zone if maxillary anterior teeth appear short either as a result of congenital or acquired excessive gingival display (Nevins and Skurow 1984; Allen 1993; Vacek et al. 1994; Herrero et al. 1995; Lanning et al. 2004; Camargo et al. 2007).

In all its indications and applications, a crown lengthening is a resective procedure where the marginal periodontium is positioned apically so that additional tooth structure is exposed supragingivally (Nevins and Skurow 1984; Parma-Benfenali et al. 1985; Wagenberg et al. 1989; Sorensen and Engelman 1990; Vacek et al. 1994).

As would be the case for any periodontal surgery, a pre-treatment checklist should be considered based on sound guiding principles and a reliable and easily reproducible road map.

Checklist

This well planned coordinated chronological checklist should include:

1. A thorough medical history.
2. A complete dental history and examination.
3. Treatment objective agreed upon by all treating dentists and clearly understood by the patient.
4. Soft tissue analysis; at the time of the relative absence of pre surgical inflammation, depth of the mucobuccal fold, width of keratinized gingiva, biotype, and periodontal probing depths. These would be significant determinants of incisions and flap designs as we will discuss later.
   Relevant considerations as to osseous anatomy: the presence or absence of bony ledges, tori, or buttressing bone.
5. Presence of periodontal disease as evidenced by deep periodontal probing depths and osseous craters. These are specifically relevant as to the nature and extent surgery planned.
6. Important aspects of dental anatomy which include proximal surfaces and vestibular convexities or lack thereof, anatomical furcations, root trunk lengths, radicular fluting, and cross section root anatomy. These considerations are relevant as to the viability and indications of the surgery in the first place and whether the tooth should even be so treated in the first place and whether the new osseous crest result in unrestorable root surfaces or furcation exposures.
7. Sterility of the surgical field. An oral antiseptic such as Chlorhexidine should be considered for rinsing during the surgery.
8. Anesthesia. Because the type of treatment involved is directed primarily at relatively superficial areas,

Practical Techniques in Periodontics and Implant Dentistry, First Edition. Edited by Edgard El Chaar.
© 2023 John Wiley & Sons, Inc. Published 2023 by John Wiley & Sons, Inc.

local infiltrations are usually sufficient to provide comfort. A fair concentration of epinephrine is recommended for adequate vasoconstriction. This helps with visualization and a more deliberate procedure.

9. Incisions. Reverse bevel or sub marginal versus intrasulcular and flap design.

   Depending on the width of keratinized tissue, this will dictate the choice of a submarginal or a reverse bevel incision where a soft tissue collar is removed, for convenience if sufficient tissue is available.

   More specifically however, with a minimal width of keratinized gingiva, an intrasulcular incision is favored. Palatal incisions however are always submarginal since, in the absence of a mucogingival junction and with a resulting ample width of keratinized tissue, the final position of the new gingival margin must be worked into the initial flap design and anticipated in that initial incision, a concept referred to as crestal anticipation.

   Releasing incisions and flap extension for access both mesiodistally and apicoronally.

   In order to have sufficient operational access and be able to a create a smooth and continuous flow in the osseous topography, one that would be compatible with a physiologic architecture, and flaps need to be designed and sufficiently extended with that purpose in mind. Within the area of osseous recontouring, the flap should logically be a full thickness elevation, partial thickness dissections to be addressed later with respect to suturing. The mesiodistal extent of soft tissue flaps should be based on passive retraction for access and instrumentation. This can be done by extending the flap sufficiently on either side beyond the operating field or by making judicious use of vertical release incisions.

   Before assigning a blanket and perhaps prejudicious appreciation of vertical releasing incisions, one should consider the fact that when such techniques are used for augmentation procedures, the vascular disruption caused by the incision itself is not easily compensated for due to tissue distention caused by the added regenerative materials; as a result, poor healing may occur; in such cases, a sufficient mesiodistal extension of the flap beyond the area of treatment may be advisable. In cases of resective procedures however, a release incision will be repositioned and the vascular disruption may not have any untoward effect on post-operative healing on the palate in the absence of mucosa, it is hard to imagine how adequate access for instrumentation can be accomplished without a vertical release. As to proper vascularization and the integrity of a flap with a vertical release, it is advisable that such incisions be placed at line angles.

Full thickness and partial thickness flaps; instances where periosteal retention of the suture for the purpose of apical positioning (Nabers 1954; Friedman 1962; Morgano and Brackett 2000).

10. Flap design is the result of the tension free access needed for instrumentation, including root surface debridement and osseous reshaping. Since it is more likely than not that osseous recontouring should be anticipated, flaps should be mostly of the full thickness design. If periosteal retention is needed for suturing purposes, however, then the apical extent of the flap may be of a partial thickness dissection variety. This is usually indicated when minimal keratinized tissue dictates a sulcular incision and the flap needs to positioned apically. A full thickness flap may be produced with the use of a blunt surgical instrument, typically a Prichard elevator. Full thickness dissections however usually commend the use of sharp instrumentation such as disposable blades or sharp surgical scissors.

    When it comes to osseous surgery, objectives should be achieved completely and yet with no iatrogenic injury. If alveolar bone is to be removed, then it should be given a final physiologic shape compatible with optimal short term healing and long term health. To that end vestibular and inter proximal bone should be give an even gradual ramp to the root surface and the interproximal area in the form of inter dental sluiceways. Residual bony ledges should be avoided and removed.

Osseous Surgery

1. Surgical Narrative

   As to osseous surgery, definitions based on the type of bone being removed are in order. Specifically it is ostectomy if supporting bone is removed, principally at the dental osseous interface and presumably for the purpose of allowing for a biologic width. Osteoplasty or the removal of non-supporting alveolar bone is instrumental for optimum and physiologic flap adaptation, optimal healing, and long term health. Often, odontoplasty should be considered and implemented judiciously when radicular irregularities, convexities, and concavities may constitute and obstacle to the objectives of the procedure (Schluger 1949; Friedman 1955; Ariaudo and Tyrell 1957; Costless et al. 1977; Garber et al. 1999; Dilbart et al. 2003).

   When removing bone at the dental interface, care should be taken to avoid the potential for iatrogenic incidents. There, osseous surgery should be done with an up and down gentle brushing motion away from the dental surface with a sharp rotary instrument. In so doing, a thin sleeve of bone usually remains on the tooth to be removed as needed with sharp chisels such as the Ochsenbein chisels, thereby avoiding the potential for nicking the tooth with a bur. As to the latter, round carbide and diamond burs should be used. For mandibular osseous surgery, a round carbide may be preferable due to the greater bone density. With the softer maxillary bone diamonds may be better for greater control. Medium size burs are recommended since larger diameters may not allow proper instrumentation and smaller burs may cause inadvertent knicks.

When using high speed instrumentation, copious irrigation is warranted to reduce the risks of traumatic overheating injuries.

When the objectives of the surgery are achieved, the passive adaptation of the soft tissue flaps, a result of initial design and incisions, is verified prior to suturing (Oschenbein 1986; Oakley et al. 1999; Pontoriero and Carnevale 2001; Dead et al. 2004).

In general, sutures may be continuous or interrupted, although an interrupted suture should be considered when periosteal retention is needed for apical positioning of the flap. Simple sutures may be sufficient but vertical mattresses may lead to better adaptation of the soft tissue to the recontoured bone (Kramer et al. 1970; Bragger et al. 1992; Lanning et al. 2003).

2. Post-operative directions should include the following:
   A period of time where tooth brushing and flossing in the area of the surgery are suspended and an antimicrobial rinse is used usually twice daily during that time. Antibiotics or analgesics are not necessarily indicated.

A period of time of about 30 days is usually allowed prior to restorative treatment for optimum healing and the reestablishment of a dentogingival interface.

The surgical principles and techniques described earlier may be applied to multiple or single units, in the esthetic zone in cases of prosthetic reconstructions or in the treatment of altered passive eruption.

For the purpose of establishing a biologically viable restorative margin and when esthetic corrections are duly called, the techniques described offer some clear and advantageous alternative. To be sure when the surgery includes the removal of supporting bone, then the following should be considered as limiting factors or potential contra indications:

– The anatomy of the treated or adjacent teeth, specifically the root trunk length or fluting and eventual restorability.
– The root trunk dimensions or the anatomical furcation in the area of treatment.
– The technique of a forced orthodontic eruption is often mentioned as an alternate to a resective surgery. In the proper and ideal clinical circumstances, it may be a bone sparing option to achieve the desired tooth surface exposure. It is often a tedious and time consuming procedure however and is not usually viable for multi-rooted teeth where the treatment is often indicated.

References

Allen, E.P. (1993). Surgical crown lengthening for function and esthetics. *Dent. Clin. N. Am.* 37 (2): 163–179.

Ariaudo, A. and Tyrell, H.A. (1957). Repositioning and increasing the zone of attached gingiva. *J. Periodontol.* 28: 106–110.

Bragger, U., Lauchenauer, D., and Lang, N.P. (1992). Surgical lengthening of the clinical crown. *J. Clin. Periodontol.* 19 (1): 58–63.

Camargo, P.M., Melnick, L.M., and Camargo, L.M. (2007). Clinical crown lengthening in esthetic zone. *J. Calif. Dent. Assoc.* 35 (7): 487–498.

Cohen, D.W. (1964). Current approaches in periodontology. *J. Periodontol.* 35: 5–18.

Costless, J.G., Vanasrsdall, R., and Weisgold, A. (1977). A diagnosis and classification of delayed passive eruption of the dentogingival junction in the adult. *Alpha Omegan* 70 (30): 24–28.

Dead, D.E., Moritz, A.J., McDonnell, H.T. et al. (2004). Osseous surgery for crown lengthening: a 6 month clinical study. *J. Periodontol.* 75 (9): 1288–1294.

Dilbart, S., Capri, D., Kachouh, I. et al. (2003). Crown lengthening in mandibular molars: a 5 year retrospective radiographic analysis. *J. Periodontol.* 74: 815–821.

Friedman, N. (1955). Periodontal osseous surgery: osteoplasty and ostectomy. *J. Periodontol.* 26: 257–259.

Friedman, N. (1962). Mucogingival surgery. The apically repositioned flap. *J. Periodontol.* 33: 328–340.

Garber, D.A., Salama, H., and Salama, M.A. (1999). Multidisciplinary cases: lessons learned. Paper Presented at the 24th Annual Meeting of the Academy of Esthetic Dentistry, Whistler, British Columbia, Canada (6 August 1999).

Herrero, F., Scott, J.B., Maropis, P.S., and Yukna, R.A. (1995). Clinical comparison desired versus actual amount of surgical crown lengthening. *J. Periodontol.* 66: 568–571.

Kois, J. (1996). The restorative-periodontal interface: biological parameters. *Periodontology* 200.

Kramer, G.M., Nevins, M., and Kohn, J.D. (1970). The utilization of periosteal suturing in periodontal surgical procedures. *J. Periodontol.* 41 (8): 457–462.

Lanning, S.K., Waldrop, T.C., Gunsolley, J.C., and Maynard, J.G. (2003). Surgical crown lengthening: evaluation of the biologic width. *J. Periodontol.* 74 (4): 468–474.

Lanning, S.K., Waldrop, T.C., Gunsolley, J.C., and Maynard, J.G. (2004). Surgical crown lengthening. Evaluation of the biologic width. *J. Periodontol.* 75 (9): 1288–1294.

Morgano, S.M. and Brackett, S.E. (2000). Foundation restorations in fixed prosthodontics: current knowledge and future needs. *J. Prosthet. Dent.* 84 (2): 169–179.

Nabers, C.L. (1954). Repositioning the attached gingiva. *J. Periodontol.* 25: 38–39.

Nevins, M. and Skurow, H.M. (1984). The intracrevicular restorative margin, the biologic width, and the maintenance of the gingival margin. *Int. J. Periodontics Restorative Dent.* 4: 31.

Nevins, M. and Skurow, H.M. (1984). The intracrevicular restorative margin, the biologic width, and the maintenance of the gingival margin. *Int. J. Periodontics Restorative Dent.* 4 (3): 30–49.

Oakley, E., Rhyu, I.C., Karatzas, S. et al. (1999). Formation of the biologic width following crown lengthening in non

human primates. *Int. J. Periodontics Restorative Dent.* 19 (6): 529–541.

Oschenbein, C.A. (1986). A primer for osseous surgery. *Int. J. Periodontics Restorative Dent.* 6 (1): 8–47.

Parma-Benfenali, S., Fugazatto, P.A., and Morris, M.P. (1985). The effect of restorative margins on the post surgical development and nature of the periodontum. Part I. *Int. J. Periodontics Restorative Dent.* 5 (6): 30–51.

Pontoriero, R. and Carnevale, G. (2001). Surgical crown lengthening: a 12 month clinical wound healing study. *J. Periodontol.* 72 (7): 841–848.

Schluger, S. (1949). Osseous resection: a basic principle in periodontal surgery. *Oral Surg. Oral Med. Oral Pathol.* 2 (3): 316–325.

Schroeder, H.E. and Listgarten, M.A. (1971). Fine structure of the developing epithelial attachment of human teeth. *Monogr. Dev. Biol.* 2: 1–134.

Sorensen, J.A. and Engelman, M.J. (1990). Ferrule design and fracture resistance of endodontically treated teeth. *J. Prosthet. Dent.* 63 (5): 529–536.

Vacek, J.S., Gher, M.E., Assad, D.A. et al. (1994). The dimensions of the human dentogingival junction. *Int. J. Periodontics Restorative Dent.* 14 (2): 154–165.

Wagenberg, B.D., Eskow, R.N., and Langer, B. (1989). Exposing adequate tooth structure for restorative dentistry. *Int. J. Periodontics Restorative Dent.* 9 (5): 322–331.

10

Root Amputation

Wayne Kye

Ashman Department of Periodontology and Implant Dentistry, New York University College of Dentistry, New York, NY, USA

Overview

Periodontitis is a chronic inflammatory condition that results in the loss of the periodontal attachment apparatus, namely, alveolar bone, cementum, and periodontal ligament. Traditional treatment modalities to manage this condition include, but are not limited to, non-surgical periodontal debridement, various pharmacotherapeutic agents, and resective and regenerative surgical procedures. It may also involve dentoalveolar extractions, with or without alveolar ridge preservation, in preparation for a subsequent implant-restoration.

Multirooted teeth often present with complex anatomical features that not only contribute to the initiation and progression of periodontal disease, but also complicate periodontal treatment and inhibit adequate patient homecare (DeSanctis and Murphy 2000; Al-Shammari et al. 2001). In their long term tooth retention study, Hirschfeld and Wasserman (1978) reported that the maxillary first and second molars are the teeth most frequently lost in the mouth. It is not a coincidence that once a tooth becomes furcally involved, the treatment becomes more complex, and the prognosis decreases. However, this is in contrast to the study by Ross and Thompson (1980), which concluded many molars with furcation involvement functioned well from 5 to 24 years and suggested that their prognosis and treatment be reconsidered. They emphasized that treatment did not include any root amputation, hemisection, osseous surgery, odontoplasty, osteoplasty, or ostectomy (Figure 10.1).

Treatment of furcation involved teeth is often dictated by the degree of furcation involvement. Root amputation was first introduced by Farrar (1884) as a "radical and heroic" treatment alternative for classes II and III furcation involved molars. Over the next century, root resection

has developed into a fundamental part of the periodontal armamentarium for the treatment of furcally involved multi-rooted teeth. However, with the advent and high success rates of dental implants, the trend in treatment selection for multi-rooted teeth with severe furcation involvement has shifted away from one of tooth preservation towards that of extraction with subsequent implant placement and restoration. Nevertheless, the periodontist, whose primary goal is to diagnose and treat periodontal disease and maintain teeth in form and function when possible, should not disregard root resection as a viable treatment alternative when indicated (Figures 10.1 and 10.2).

Terminology

Inconsistent usage of the terms root resection, root amputation, hemisection, and root separation can be found throughout the literature. Nevertheless, Shillingburg et al. (1997) has adopted the following terminology:

- **Root amputation** is defined as the surgical removal of one or more root(s) of a multi-rooted tooth, at the level of the cementoenamel junction, without the removal of the overhanging portion of the crown.
- **Root resection** is defined as the complete or partial surgical removal of a tooth root. Root resection is distinguished from root amputation in that the former provides no information regarding the crown of the root.
- **Hemisection** is defined as the surgical separation of a multi-rooted tooth (generally a mandibular molar), through the furcation thus permitting the subsequent removal of both the crown and root of the sectioned tooth as one entity.
- **Root separation** is defined as the surgical separation through a crown and root of a multi-rooted tooth without the subsequent removal of either half.

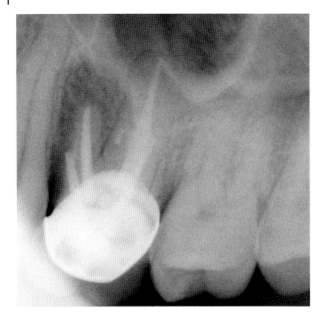

Figure 10.1 Pre-operative radiograph. Twenty-five year old healthy male presents with a chief complaint "I have a bad taste in my mouth. This tooth had a root canal over 10 years ago and was retreated 5 years later." Radiograph reveals a significant periapical radiolucent lesion approximating the mesiobuccal root. Clinical presence of a sinus tract opening noted with purulent discharge. MB probing depth of 10+mm with bleeding on probing.

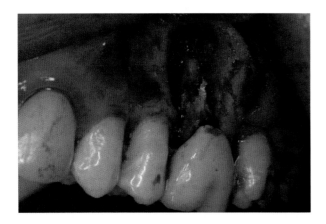

Figure 10.2 Flap reflection. Upon flap reflection, root perforation of the mesiobuccal root is confirmed. Note the complete buccal dehiscence of the distobuccal root. No clinical mobility was noted.

Indications and Contraindications

The indications and contraindications for root resection were first outlined by Basaraba (1969). Later, Minsk and Polson (2006) proposed inclusion of *teeth with high strategic value* as an additional indication. This is of particular

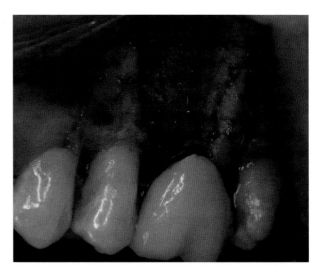

Figure 10.3 Mesiobuccal root resection. Root resection of the mesiobuccal root is completed with a rotary handpiece and surgical length cross-fissure bur. Subsequent odontoplasty completed to recontour and remove any ledges.

importance when related to sites that are unable to receive implants (Figure 10.3).

Indications Include

1. Isolated areas of severe bone loss involving an individual root
2. Fractured root
3. Failure of endodontic therapy or inoperable/calcified canals
4. Bone resorption involving the furcation of multi-rooted teeth
5. Close interdental root proximity making plaque control impossible
6. Extensive root exposure contraindicating new attachment procedures
7. Root or furcation perforation
8. Root resorption (internal and/or external)
9. Extensive caries in the furcation/roots

Contraindications Include

1. Advanced bone loss and secondary occlusal trauma
2. Individual roots fused or in close proximity
3. Remaining root cannot be restored and/or endodontically treated
4. Poor root form or length of retained roots
5. Apical location of furcation area resulting in severely compromised bone support of remaining root(s)
6. Inability to create a good post-surgical mucogingival environment with an adequate zone of attached gingiva and vestibular depth

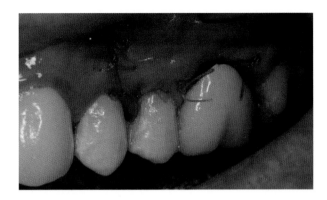

Figure 10.4 Surgical closure. Small particle cortical freeze-dried bone allograft and a resorbable Type I bovine collagen membrane were utilized to graft the socket.

7. Evidence of poor oral hygiene
8. When interdisciplinary therapy (endodontics, periodontics, restorative) is not possible due to patient's finances or medical history (Figure 10.4).

Advantages and Disadvantages

As clinicians, it's important to highlight the advantages and disadvantages for our patients so that they may make the best informed decision, based on our understanding of the evidence-based literature. Some advantages of root resective procedures may include, but are not limited to, (i) preservation of the alveolar ridge by retaining the tooth in the alveolus, (ii) financial and psychological aspects of maintaining a natural tooth, (iii) when teeth are in proximity of anatomic landmarks which prevent more invasive surgical therapies, and (iv) avoiding extensive rehabilitative and reconstructive procedures (i.e. Caldwell-Luc sinus augmentation, ridge augmentation, etc.).

One must also consider the various disadvantages, including but are not limited to (i) technique sensitive procedure which requires extensive surgical experience and skill, (ii) financial: price of endodontic, periodontic, and prosthetic treatment versus extraction and implant, and (iii) risk that procedure may ultimately fail and result in extraction.

Armamentarium

- Basic periodontal surgical kit:
  - Mirrors
  - Periodontal probe
  - Nabers probe
  - College pliers
  - Scalpel handles
  - Orban 1/2 knife
  - Chisels (i.e. Rhodes back-action, TGO)
  - Aspirating syringe
  - Iris scissors
  - Elevators (i.e. Buser, Prichard)
  - Curettes (i.e. Gracey, Prichard 1/2, Lucas 87 DE)
  - Files (i.e. Sugarman, Hirschfeld)
  - Stainless steel bowl
  - Sterile saline
  - Tissue forceps
  - Curved hemostat
  - Needle holder
- Rotary instrumentation:
  - High speed handpiece
  - Surgical length fissure cut carbide burs (for root resection)
  - Diamond rotary burs (for root resection and/or recontouring)
- Sutures
- Resorbable collagen membrane
- Bone replacement graft

Surgical Technique

After successful anesthesia has been obtained, appropriate incisions are performed and a full-thickness mucoperiosteal flap is elevated to increase visualization and obtain access to the alveolar bone and roots. Proper identification of the root(s) to be resected and confirmation of the proposed therapy is established. Utilizing a high-speed handpiece under copious irrigation, attach a bur that would most appropriately resect the root(s) without damaging the surrounding structures. Often times, a long fissure cut carbide bur (i.e. 701XL) or diamond bur can be utilized with great success. Begin the resection from the furcation area. For example, if either the mesiobuccal or distobuccal root is to be resected, begin from the buccal furcation area towards the crown, taking care not to inadvertently damage the palatal root. Continue to reduce the resected root structure in order to gain access for elevation and extraction of the intended root(s). **It is imperative to be conservative in the initial resection; further resection is always possible, if needed.** Once the resection is completed, carefully remove the resected root(s). Thoroughly degranulate the socket and furcation area of any granulomatous tissue. Undercuts, ledges and sharp corners should be recontoured accordingly. As reported by Livada et al. (2014), grafting the residual socket of the resected root is recommended. A small particle freeze-dried bone allograft with a resorbable collagen membrane is preferred. The flap is repositioned and sutured. Post-surgical instructions are

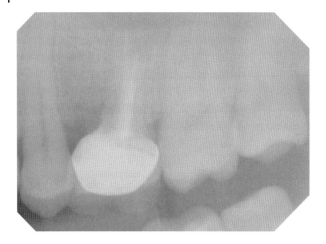

Figure 10.5 1-month post-surgical radiograph. Uneventful post-surgical healing. Radiograph suggests good consolidation of bone replacement graft.

provided verbally and in written form. Medications may include an antiseptic mouthrinse (i.e. 0.12% Chlorhexidine Gluconate), an analgesic/anti-inflammatory (non-steroidal anti-inflammatory drugs [NSAID]), and a systemic antibiotic. Radiographs can be helpful during the procedure to ensure that successful root resection has been performed. Also, it may help identify any ledges that need to be recontoured. If a bone replacement graft is utilized, a post-graft radiograph is important to obtain (Figure 10.5).

Complications

a) Incomplete removal of ledges or undercuts
b) Iatrogenic rotary instrumentation of other roots

Outcome and Follow-up

Hamp et al. treated 310 multi-rooted teeth with various degrees of furcation involvement. Treatment modalities included scaling and root planing, open flap debridement with and without odontoplasty, and/or osteoplasty for degree I furcation involvement. Degree II furcation involved teeth were treated with either root resection, tunnel preparation, or extraction. Eighty-seven teeth (39 maxillary and 44 mandibular molars, 4 premolars) were treated with root resection performed with open flap debridement. Of the 87 teeth that were root resected, 90% had probing depths less than or equal to 3 mm and 100% were maintained at five-year follow-up. The authors attribute the success to meticulous plaque control by both the patient and the clinician. Additionally, the authors propose the following factors as important when considering

which root to resect: the amount of residual supporting tissue around each root, the root and root canal anatomy as it relates to root canal treatment, the periapical condition and mobility of the remaining roots, and the amount of residual supporting tissue around each roots (Hamp et al. 1975).

In a 10-year retrospective study of 50 maxillary and 50 mandibular molars treated with root resection, Langer et al. reported survival rates of 84 and 62% at 5- and 10-year follow-up, respectively. The authors identified root fracture as the primary cause of failure (47.4%), followed by periodontal breakdown (26.3%), endodontic failure (18.4%), and cement washout (7.9%). Periodontal breakdown accounted for the majority of failures in the maxillary arch while root fracture was the primary cause of failure in the mandibular arch. Overall, greater success rates were observed in maxillary molars (Langer et al. 1981).

Results from an 11-year retrospective analysis of 488 resected molars reported greater success rates (94%) than those reported by Langer in 1981 (Carnevale et al. 1991). Of the 28 failures (5.7%), the primary cause of failure was attributed to root fracture followed by caries. In 1998, Carnevale published the results of a 10-year longitudinal study in in which the authors performed osseous recontouring and apically positioned flaps on non-furcation involved teeth. 175 teeth were subjected to root resection (test) and compared with 175 teeth without root resection (control). The reported 10-year survival rate for the root resected teeth and non-resected teeth were 93 and 99%, respectively. Endodontic complications accounted for the majority of failures (33%) followed by caries (25%), periodontal disease recurrence (25%), and root fracture (17%) (Carnevale et al. 1998).

In a 10-year retrospective study by Park et al. that included 691 root resected teeth, the authors studied the factors that influenced the outcome of root resection therapy. The factors included in the study were categorized into four groups: resection, patient, tooth, and site related factors. With respect to resection related factors, the authors reported higher survival rates for molars that underwent resection due to periodontal rather than non-periodontal reasons. Neither patient related nor tooth related factors influenced the survival rate of root resected molars. However, consistent with the results of Langer in 1981, periodontal complications were identified as the primary cause of failure in the maxillary arch, whereas root fracture and dental caries accounted for the majority of failures in the mandible. Additionally, the authors identified the amount of bone support around the remaining root(s) at the time of surgery as the sole site related factor that significantly affected the survival rate of root resected teeth resected due to periodontal causes. In fact, the authors conclude that 50% remaining bone support is required to achieve optimal results and predictability (Park et al. 2009).

A retrospective study with up to 40 years of follow-up on root resection and hemi-section outcomes by Megarbane et al. reported an overall survival rate of 94.8%. Of the 97 teeth included in the final analysis, only 5 teeth were lost during the first 5 years of follow-up, the remaining 92 teeth survived the follow-up period from 5 to 40 years. No significant differences were found between arches, molars, type of root resected, nor type of restoration. Of the 5 teeth that failed, the authors report a significant association with diabetes (Odds Ratio: 9) (Megarbane et al. 2018).

In a recent systematic review and meta-analysis on the outcome of crown and root resection, the reported weighted mean survival rate for root resected molars was 87.2%. In contrast to Langer et al. (1981), no statistically significant difference in survival rates between arches was found (Setzer et al. 2019).

While clinical outcomes appear inconsistent throughout the literature, the majority of authors agree that endodontic and technical complications such as root fracture are the most predominant complication attributed to root resection (Figure 10.6).

Given the increased susceptibility to root fracture, Gerstein (1977) advocates full coverage crowns as the restorative treatment of choice for endodontically treated root resected teeth. Final crown design and preparation of root resected teeth is complicated by the unique contours and anatomy of the remaining portion of the tooth. Thus, the crown must be designed to compensate for such variations. For example, Keough 1982 observed that root resected maxillary molars acquire an L-shaped configuration when viewed occlusally. An acute angle between the two legs of the "L" creates a cul-de-sac which, if

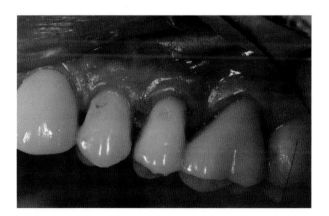

Figure 10.6 7-year follow-up (clinical). A new full-coverage ceramic restoration was fabricated and delivered three years post-surgical. There was some lapse in regular perio recall appointments.

ignored, can impair access for proper oral hygiene (Keough 1982). Additionally, both maxillary and mandibular molars present with root concavities that have to be considered when designing the outline of the final crown preparation, as they may require odontoplasty to ensure the achievement of proper contours (Bower 1979).

With regards to occlusal design, Basaraba 1969 advocates occlusal narrowing through reduction of the non-working cusps in an effort to direct forces apically and parallel along the long axis of the root resected tooth. Furthermore, complete elimination of all excursive contacts is recommended (Basaraba 1969). Abrams and Trachtenberg (1974) suggest a provisionalization phase in an effort to ensure that proper hygienic contours and line angles are achieved prior to the fabrication of the final restoration.

Implants Versus Root Resection

Root resection is a technique sensitive procedure with a complexity that may account for the variability in clinical success rates reported throughout the literature. It begs the question of whether or not root resection can provide predictable results comparable with those of implants. In 2001, Fugazzotto evaluated 701 root resected teeth and 1472 molar implants with 13 and 15 years of follow-up, respectively. Comparable survival rates were reported for both groups: 97% molar implants and 96.8% for root resected molars. The lowest success rate was reported for the resection of the distal root of mandibular molars (75%). The lowest success reported for the single molar implant was the second molar position (85%). In 2009, Zafiropoulos et al. performed a retrospective study on the long term complication and survival rates of root resected mandibular molars relative to mandibular molar implants during a maintenance care period of four years. Higher complication rates were reported for root resected molars than molar implants (32.1 versus 11.1% respectively). Root resected teeth were 3.8 times more likely to present complications compared with implants. In contrast to the majority of post-treatment complications present in the implant group, the majority of the complications present in the resected group were considered non-salvageable (Zafiropoulos et al. 2009).

Vital Root Resection

Vital root resection has been documented as a high-risk procedure and can negatively affect tooth vitality. Thus, endodontic treatment on the remaining roots is of utmost importance for the long term success of treatment (Gerstein 1977). When possible, endodontic treatment should be performed prior to root resection. However,

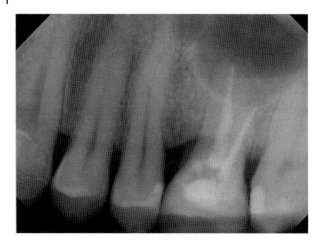

Figure 10.7 7-year follow-up (radiograph). Radiograph suggests good maturation and maintenance of bone replacement graft.

it does provide several advantages to consider (Smukler and Tagger 1976). First of all, it allows for direct surgical assessment of the root(s) to be resected. It would also avoid unnecessary endodontic treatment in cases where the procedures should be aborted (i.e. root proximity, root fusion, ankylosis). As a consequence, the absence of root canal therapy would decrease the likelihood of a root fracture. It should be noted that adverse periodontal wound healing has not been a common finding (Figure 10.7).

However, it is not always possible to predict treatment prior to surgical visualization of a defect. If resection is required at the time of surgery before the tooth has been root canal treated, vital root amputation can still be performed providing the remaining root(s) are treated endodontically within two weeks of resection (Smukler and Tagger 1976).

Several risks and/or disadvantages to consider with vital root resection include:

- Increased sensitivity during initial post-op period
- Difficulty in maintaining asepsis
- Difficulty in obtaining profound anesthesia for endodontic therapy
- Difficulty in attaining access and vision for calcium hydroxide placement
- Increases potential for internal root resorption

References

Abrams, L. and Tractenberg, D.I. (1974). Hemisection – technique and restoration. *Dent. Clin. N. Am.* 18: 415–444.

Al-Shammari, K.F., Kazor, C.E., and Wang, H.L. (2001). Molar root anatomy and management of furcation defects. *J. Clin. Periodontol.* 28: 730–740.

Basaraba, N. (1969). Root amputation and tooth hemisection. *Dent. Clin. N. Am.* 13: 121–132.

Bower, R.C. (1979). Furcation morphology relative to periodontal treatment. Furcation root surface anatomy. *J. Periodontol.* 50: 366–374.

Carnevale, G., Gianfranco, D., Tonelli, M. et al. (1991). A retrospective analysis of the periodontal prosthetic treatment of molars with interradicular lesions. *Int. J. Periodontics Restorative Dent.* 1: 189–205.

Carnevale, G., Pontoriero, R., and di Febo, G. (1998). Long-term effects of root-resective therapy in furcation-involved molars. A 10-year longitudinal study. *J. Clin. Periodontol.* 25: 209–214.

DeSanctis, M. and Murphy, K.G. (2000). The role of resective periodontal surgery in the treatment of furcation defects. *Periodontology* 2000 (22): 154–168.

Farrar, J.N. (1884). Radical and heroic treatment of alveolar abscess by amputation of roots of teeth. *Dent. Cosmos* 26: 135–139.

Fugazzotto, P. (2001). A comparison of the success of root resected molars and molar position implants in function in a private practice: results of up to 15-plus years. *J. Periodontol.* 72: 1113–1123.

Gerstein, K.A. (1977). The role of vital root resection in periodontics. *J. Periodontol.* 48: 478–483.

Hamp, S.E., Nyman, S., and Lindhe, J. (1975). Periodontal treatment of multirooted teeth. Results after 5 years. *J. Clin. Periodontol.* 2: 126–135.

Hirschfeld, L. and Wasserman, B. (1978). A long-term survey of tooth loss in 600 treated periodontal patients. *J. Periodontol.* 49 (5): 225–237.

Keough, B. (1982). Root resection. *Int. J. Periodontics Restorative Dent.* 2 (1): 17–27.

Langer, B., Stein, S.D., and Wagenberg, B. (1981). An evaluation of root resections. A ten-year study. *J. Periodontol.* 52: 719–722.

Livada, R., Fine, N., and Shiloah, J. (2014). Root amputation: a new look into an old procedure. *N. Y. State Dent. J.* 80 (4): 24–28.

Megarbane, J.M., Kassir, A.R., Mokbel, N. et al. (2018). Root resection and hemisection revisited: Part II: a retrospective analysis of 195 treated patients with up to 40 years of follow-up. *Int. J. Periodontics Restorative Dent.* 38: 783–789.

Minsk, L. and Polson, A.M. (2006). The role of root resection in the age of dental implants. *Compend Contin Educ Dent.* 27 (7): 384–388.

Park, S.Y., Shin, S.Y., Yang, S.M. et al. (2009). Factors influencing the outcome of root-resection therapy in molars: a 10- year retrospective study. *J. Periodontol.* 80: 32–40.

Ross, I.F. and Thompson, R.H. Jr., (1980). Furcation involvement in maxillary and mandibular molars. *J. Periodontol.* 51 (8): 450–454.

Setzer, F.C., Shou, H., Kulwattanaporn, P. et al. (2019). Outcome of crown and root resection: a systematic review and meta-analysis of the literature. *J. Endod.* 45 (1): 6–19.

Shillingburg, H.T., Hobo, S., Whitsett, L.D. et al. (1997). Preparations for periodontally weakened teeth. In: *Fundamentals of Fixed Prosthodontics* (ed. H.T. Shillingburg), 3e, 211–223. Chicago: Quintessence.

Smukler, H. and Tagger, M. (1976). Vital root amputation. A clinical and histological study. *J. Periodontol.* 47: 324–330.

Zafiropoulos, G.G., Hoffmann, O., Kasaj, A. et al. (2009). Mandibular molar root resection versus implant therapy: a retrospective non-randomized study. *J. Oral Implantol.* 35: 52–62.

Further Reading

Alassadi, M., Qazi, M., Ravida, A. et al. (2019). Outcomes of root resection therapy up to 16.8 years: a retrospective study in an academic setting. *J. Periodontol.* 0: 1–8.

Buhler, H. (1988). Evaluation of root-resected teeth: results after 10 years. *J. Periodontol.* 59: 805–810.

Carnevale, G., Pontoriero, R., and Hurzeler, M. (2000). Management of furcation involvement. *Periodontology* 1995 (9): 69–89.

Cassingham, R.J. and Broxson, A.W. (1979). A laboratory technique for teaching root resection. *J. Periodontol.* 50 (3): 148–150.

Derks, H., Westheide, D., Pfefferle, T. et al. (2018). Retention of molars after root-resective therapy: a retrospective evaluation of up to 30 years. *Clin. Oral Investig.* 22: 1327–1335.

Ehrlich, J., Hochman, N., and Yaffe, A. (1989). Root resection and separation of multirooted teeth: a 10-year follow-up study. *Quintessence Int.* 20: 561–564.

Haskell, E.W. and Stanley, H.R. (1982). A review of vital root resection. *Int. J. Periodontics Restorative Dent.* 6: 28–49.

Kasaj, A. (2014). Root resective procedures vs implant therapy in the management of furcation-involved molars. *Quintessence Int.* 45 (6): 521–529.

Levin, L. and Halperin-Sternfeld, M. (2013). Tooth preservation or implant placement: a systematic review of long-term tooth and implant survival rates. *J. Am. Dent. Assoc.* 144: 1119–1133.

Mokbel, N., Kassir, A.R., Naaman, N. et al. (2019). Root resection and hemisection revisited: Part I: a systematic review. *Int. J. Periodontics Restorative Dent.* 39: e11–e31.

11

Guided Tissue Regeneration

Edgard El Chaar[1] and Michael Bral[2]

[1] Department of Periodontics, University of Pennsylvania, Dental Medicine, Philadelphia, PA, USA
[2] Department of Periodontics and Implant Dentistry, New York University College of Dentistry, New York, NY, USA

Overview

Treatment of chronic periodontitis represents a significant health care challenge, especially at a time when periodontal–restorative dilemmas exist as to whether to save a tooth with limited periodontium or extract it and place a dental implant. Periodontally compromised but treated teeth are known to have survival rates equal to those of implants in well-maintained patients.

The ultimate therapeutic goal of therapy is to rebuild the tissues lost to the disease process with tissues that are structurally and functionally similar. Historically attempts to treat advanced forms of periodontitis were largely empirical and included conventional treatment that resulted in the arrest the disease but did not usually regain the bone support or connective tissue lost in the disease process. Treatment approaches were primarily resective to reduce probing depths. Formation of a long junctional epithelium is the most common form of tissue repair and typical outcome of traditional periodontal surgery.

Periodontal regeneration has been reported following a variety of approaches involving root surface biomodification, coronally advanced flaps (CAF), and use of bone grafts. However clinical situations that exhibited significant regrowth of bone often showed an epithelial lining along the root surface instead of newly formed cementum.

Guided tissue regeneration (GTR) is based on the principle that specific cells contribute to the formation of specific tissues. Exclusion of the faster-growing epithelium and connective tissue from a periodontal defect allows the slower-growing tissues to occupy the space adjacent to the tooth. Osteoblasts, cementoblasts, and periodontal ligament (PDL) cells are able to regenerate a new periodontium (new connective tissue fibers inserted into newly formed cementum and bone). The concept behind this method is that PDL and perivascular cells have the potential for regeneration of periodontium.

The concept GTR evolved over a period of years by pioneers pursuing elusive scientific evidence. Prichard's concept of interdental denudation showing new attachment in the treatment of three-wall intrabony defects was a seminal contribution. Although the concept of epithelial retardation or exclusion was not mentioned in his reports, this led to other approaches such as total removal of interdental papilla covering the defect and its replacement with a free autogenous graft from the palate with the expectation that during healing the graft epithelium necroses and is slowly replaced by proliferating epithelium from the surrounding tissue, a method that has no clinical application. Elimination of pocket or junctional epithelium from the flap margin is not sufficient because epithelium may eventually proliferate and become interposed between the connective tissue of the flap and the root surface.

The seminal work of Melcher shed light on the concept that all the periodontium's key components of the alveolar bone, cementum, and PDL play crucial roles in periodontal healing and regeneration. This notion laid the groundwork for the focus on directed wound regeneration via the exclusion of epithelium and the lamina propria of the gingiva with the progenitor cells present in the PDL.

GTR requires placement of barriers to cover furcation and intrabony defects to separate them from epithelium and gingival connective tissue allowing repopulation of the sites by cells from the PDL and bone. Non-resorbable barriers such as polytetrafluoroethylene (PTFE), that required a second procedure four to six weeks after the initial healing, are no longer used. Instead a variety of resorbable membranes are available.

Indications

Repair and Regeneration in Periodontal Defects

1. Class II furcation defects
2. Two to three walled intrabony and circumferential defects
3. Recession defects

GTR for Furcation Defects

Molar furcation involvement is one of the most common dento-alveolar sequelae of periodontal disease. The application of a specific treatment method for furcation involvement requires a thorough understanding of tooth anatomy, etiologic factors, and biologic basis for treatment modalities.

Clinical closure of furcation defects by means of GTR procedures has been extensively investigated but optimal results in all cases have been elusive. However, soft tissue closure and decrease in probing depths in class II furcations and less frequently complete regeneration have been reported. Class III furcation involved mandibular and maxillary molars have not shown any significant favorable results.

Technique

Before attempting any regenerative therapy, an initial non-surgical hygienic phase is crucial. This includes patient education on oral hygiene, scaling and root planing, anti- bacterial therapy, and removal of plaque retentive factors, all aimed to yield a good tissue response by eliminating infection and reducing the inflammatory component (Figure 11.1).

Sulcular incisions are made on the buccal (Figure 11.2). After flap reflection and thorough debridement, a prefgel

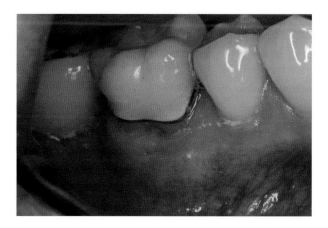

Figure 11.1 After initial therapy and resolution of inflammation.

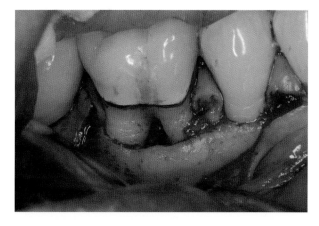

Figure 11.2 An intrasulcular incisions with papilla sparing done on the adjacent papillas and a full thickness flap was raised.

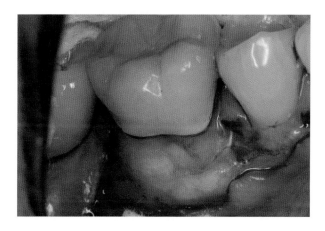

Figure 11.3 A root conditioner was applied for 2 minutes and rinsed thoroughly with saline water.

root conditioner is placed and rinsed out 2 mins after application (Figure 11.3), followed by placement of EMD (Figure 11.4) and allograft cancellous (Figure 11.5). A resorbable membrane is applied extending 2 to 3 mm past the furcation (Figure 11.6). A coronally advanced flap (CAF) is secured over with a sling suture and on this peri-acryl glue to enhance adaptation of the flap on the porcelain crown (Figure 11.7). An 11 years follow-up of the furcation shows a healthy tissue with healthy probing of 2mm (Figures 11.8 and 11.9) and the radiograph shows a good bone fill (Figure 11.10)

Factors influencing successful regeneration in furcation defects:

Cervical enamel projections and enamel pearls: These may contribute to plaque accumulation and furcal invasion and should be removed by odontoplasty during regenerative procedures.

Root/root trunk concavity and bifurcation ridges: These concavities and ridges contribute to plaque

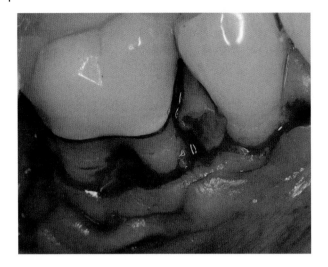

Figure 11.4 Enamel Matrix Derivative (EMD) is applied.

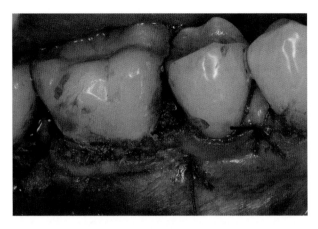

Figure 11.7 A coronally advanced flap (CAF) was put in place. The CAF was immobilized by a sling suture and secured with a peri-acryl glue over the porcelain.

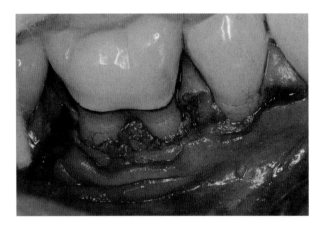

Figure 11.5 A cancellous allograft was placed in the defect.

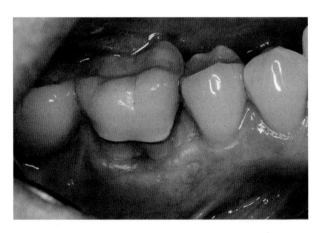

Figure 11.8 An 11-year follow-up image shows a healthy tissue.

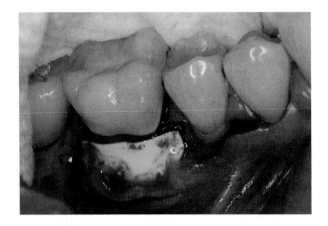

Figure 11.6 A resorbable collagenous membrane placed extending 2-3 mm from the furcation.

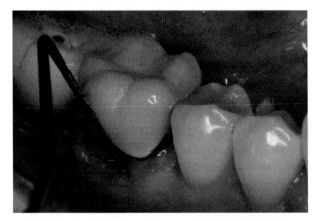

Figure 11.9 And a healthy periodontal probing of 2 mm.

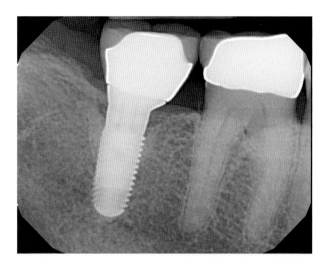

Figure 11.10 A radiograph of 11 years shows a good bony fill.

accumulation and are covered by more necrotic cementum than the adjacent sites. In addition to a direct cytotoxic effect on host cells, these surfaces may represent a poor substrate for plasma protein adsorption and subsequent fibrin adhesion.

Accessory canals: Accessory canals in the region of furcation and endodontic infections can cause periodontal disease in the furcation region of molars and impair the healing response following GTR.

Entrance of the furcation: It has been shown that the diameter of the furcation entrance in molars is smaller than the cutting width of commonly used curettes hindering effective instrumentation of these areas. Hand instrumentation alone may not be adequate for complete root surface preparation in all furcation areas and ultrasonic and rotary instruments must be used for more effective decontamination in furcation areas.

Length of root trunks: Molars with short root trunks are generally considered to be at higher risk for developing furcation involvement than teeth with long root trunks. Molars with the longest root trunks (5–6 mm) tend to respond more often with complete furcation closure following GTR therapy than teeth with shorter root trunks.

Defect morphology: The clinical success of furcation therapy is strongly related to defect morphology:

- **Root divergence**: Increases in root divergence measured at crest of bone are associated with decreases in complete furcation closure.
- **Horizontal depth of defect**: Furcation defects with a horizontal depth of 5 mm or greater measured at the level of the crest of bone demonstrated a lower probability of complete closure.
- **Distance of osseous crest to base of defect**: The deeper the vertical component, the greater the repair.

- **Distance of furcation roof to base of defect**: Increases in this measurement are associated with decreased clinical closure.
- **Distance of furcation roof to crest of the bone**: Increases in the distance of furcation roof to crest of bone are associated with a lower probability of complete furcation closure.
- **Interproximal bone height**: Teeth with interproximal bone height at the same level or superior to the roof of the furcation resolve with complete closure in a significantly higher percentage of cases.
- **Thickness of the gingival tissue**. Inadequate thickness of gingival tissue covering the membrane may result in post-treatment recession.
- **Tooth mobility**. Conflicting results exist concerning the effect that presurgical hypermobility on surgical healing and, thus, on the post-treatment clinical outcome. Although the clinical relevance of mobility in regenerative therapy has not yet been elucidated, occlusal discrepancies should be removed to minimize trauma and splinting of hypermobile teeth considered to improve patient comfort during post-therapeutic healing.

GTR in the treatment of furcations is not indicated in the following cases:

- Lack of access for adequate debridement of the furcation.
- Endodontic or prosthetic perforations in the furcation areas of the roots.
- Crown lengthening procedures that invade the furcations.
- Root proximity.
- Extensive gingival recessions.
- Deep caries involving the roots.
- Untreatable endodontic-periodontal lesions.
- Longitudinal root fractures.

Despite achieving significant positive gains in new attachment using GTR, consistently successful treatment of furcation defects with the membrane techniques remains a challenge.

GTR for Periodontal Intrabony and Circumferential Defects

Periodontal regeneration in intrabony defects is possible on previously diseased root surfaces, as evidenced by a gain in clinical attachment, decreased pocket probing depth, gain in radiographic bone height, and overall improvement in periodontal health. These clinical findings are consistent with available histologic evidence. Clinical improvements can be maintained over long periods (>10 years). While bone replacement grafts have been the most commonly investigated modality, GTR, biologics, and combination therapies have also been shown to be effective.

Techniques

- Surgical access to site by means of a mucoperiosteal flap, preferably with a modified papilla preservation technique, to achieve and maintain primary closure of the flap in the interdental space covering the membrane.
- Thorough root planning and debridement of the defects.
- Preparation of a biodegradable membrane to cover the area being treated.
- Placement of biologic agents and/or grafts as necessary.
- Suturing the membrane around the site with sling suture.
- Complete coverage of the surgical site by coronally positioning the flap (Figures 11.11–11.17).

GTR techniques in the treatment of intrabony defects are dependent on the following factors:

- Patient characteristics
- Variations in defect morphology (amount of remaining walls in the intrabony defect)
- Design of the surgical technique (Improper incisions, traumatic flap elevation, excessive surgical exposure)
- Type of barrier membrane
- Technical difficulties regarding membrane placement (inadequate barrier to root adaptation, inadequate closure, and suturing)
- Exposure and/or bacterial contamination of membrane

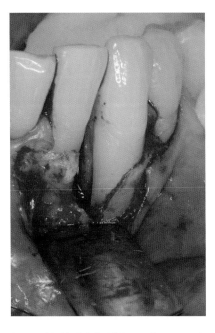

Figure 11.11 A full thickness flap was raised on tooth #22, after a thorough debridement, the tooth has a 2 wall intra-bony defect and the interesting challenge is the developmental groove on the mesial of the roots.

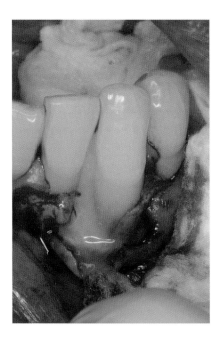

Figure 11.12 A root conditioner was applied for 2 minutes and rinsed thoroughly with saline water.

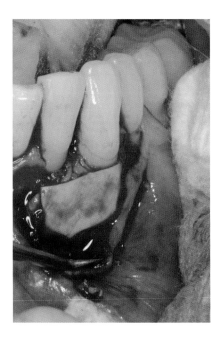

Figure 11.13 Enamel Matrix Derivative (EMD) is applied and a cancellous allograft was placed in the defect over it, followed by two resorbable collagenous membrane placed over the allograft.

- Experience of the operator
- Post-treatment plaque control and supportive care
- Susceptibility to disease recurrence
- Compliance with oral hygiene
- Smoking habits
- Age, genetics, stress levels, and unstable diabetes

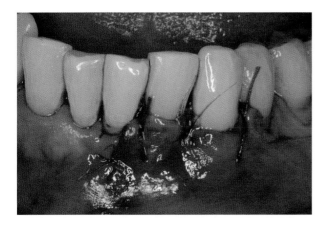

Figure 11.14 A coronally advanced flap (CAF) was put in place. The CAF was immobilized by a combination of sling suture and horizontal mattress.

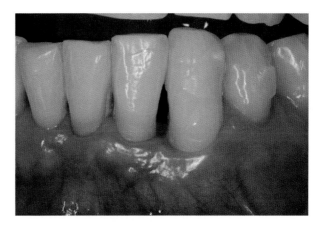

Figure 11.16 A six years follow-up image.

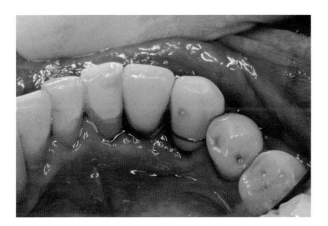

Figure 11.15 A lingual view of the closure and the sutures.

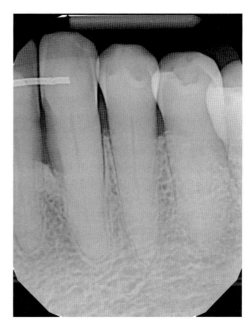

Figure 11.17 A radiograph of 6years shows a good bony fill.

GTR for the Treatment of Recession Defects

The presence of an adequate width and thickness of attached gingiva has been considered a critical component to the protective function of the mucogingival complex. Problems commonly associated with the presence of gingival recessions are undesirable aesthetics, root hypersensitivity, higher incidence of root caries, and compromised plaque control.

Treatment of gingival recession is complicated and successful outcome depends on many factors, including a complete understanding the anatomic, biologic and surgical considerations, a favorable gingival biotype, and the type of surgical technique employed.

Correction of mucogingival recession deformities with a variety of periodontal plastic surgical procedures has been described, each demonstrating variable degrees of success. Although free gingival graft (FGG) is considered a gold standard for the gingival augmentation procedures, it has several drawbacks for root coverage including inadequate

quantity, need for a second operative site, post-operative morbidity, and dual color match.

Multiple gingival recessions are more challenging to treat due to the difficulties in tissue management and wound healing. Successful results can be compromised by several factors such as variations in recession depth, the amount of existing keratinized tissue, limited blood supply and teeth position.

Among the various treatment modalities currently available, CAF are the most commonly employed for recession coverage of multiple teeth. Although CAFs can occasionally be used alone where thick and wide marginal gingiva is available, adjunctive use of connective tissue grafts (CTGs) or non-resorbable and bioresorbable membranes are more common. This involves raising a full thickness flap around the recession defect(s), placing a CTG or membrane, and covering it with a CAF. The aim of this treatment is to prevent the formation of a long junctional epithelium but instead allow normal connective tissue attachment to the exposed root surface. Bioresorbable membranes may be useful in situations where large recession defect(s) need to be treated and the available graft tissue from the palate cannot provide a sufficient volume of tissue.

Compared with the traditional grafting techniques, GTR has the advantage of eliminating the need of a second surgical site and, if non-resorbable membranes are used, a second surgical procedure. In addition to CTG other materials such as acellular dermal matrix (ADM) and Mucograft collagen matrix have been tried in periodontal plastic surgery and results have been comparable in the treatment of Miller's Classes I and II gingival recessions. Although differences between CTG and GTR in mean root coverage consistently favored the CTG procedure, the differences in measurements were not statistically significant (Figures 11.18–11.20).

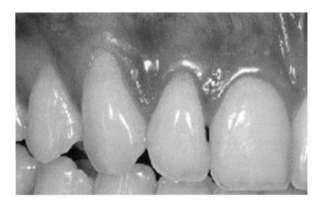

Figure 11.18 A patient with RT1 recession and a thin phenotype.

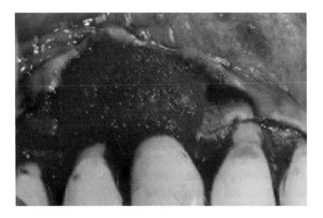

Figure 11.19 A mucoperiosteal flap with papilla sparing extending two teeth posteriorly and one tooth anteriorly.

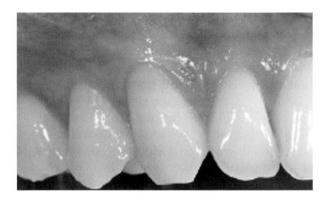

Figure 11.20 A 100 % root coverage achieved.

Following periodontal plastic surgery, the patient should be advised to avoid brushing the surgical site for at least three weeks while initial healing occurs. During this time the patient should use a 0.2% chlorhexidine gluconate mouthwash twice daily. Immediately following surgery, the patient should also be advised against lifting their lip or pulling their cheek. This can cause displacement of the tissues which have been carefully sutured into position.

Factors affecting outcome of GTR procedure in mucogingival surgery:

- Condition of root surface – presence of calculus, caries, necrotic cementum, or restorations on root surface
- Depth of vestibule
- Prominent frenal attachments
- Gingival biotype
- Size of the recession defect
- Smoking
- Poor oral hygiene

Complications following GTR procedures in the treatment of furcations, osseous lesions, and mucogingival surgery:

Pain and swelling: Majority of pain incidence originate in mandibular molar areas and disproportionately high in furcal areas. Access to furcal site often requires adjunctive debridement with ultrasonic and rotary instruments with the increased risk of accessory pulpal canal exposure after odontoplasty. The post-operative use of Medrol in a tapering dose greatly reduces the incidence of swelling especially in the mandibular posterior areas.

Membrane exposure: Membrane exposure is a major complication of GTR procedures. This is likely due to the insufficient protection of the interproximal regenerating tissue preventing its complete maturation. This can be greatly reduced using access flaps specially designed to preserve the interdental tissues such as different forms of modified papilla preservation techniques.

Bacterial contamination: Microorganisms in deep furcation areas are difficult to eradicate by mechanical means and may serve as a reservoir for bacterial recolonization. Bacterial contamination of the membrane may occur during surgery but also during the postoperative healing phase. Apical migration of epithelium on the inner surface of the covering gingival flap may allow colonization of bacteria.

Despite the use of post-operative systemic antibiotics, occurrence of post-operative wound infection cannot be totally avoided. This indicates that either the drug administered is not directed against the responsible microorganisms or the drug does not reach the infected site at a concentration sufficiently high to inhibit the target microorganisms.

Follow-up

Almost all successful GTR protocols have included a stringent post-operative regimen that called for good hygiene practices, use of daily chlorhexidine rinses, professional tooth cleaning once a week for the first month, and once every two to three weeks for at least another six months following the procedure. This regimen is seldom adhered to by many clinicians and is one of the main reasons for lack of optimum success especially in the treatment of furcation and intrabony defects.

The clinical reality of regenerative procedures validates the potential that periodontal structures lost due to chronic microbial biofilms and uncontrolled inflammation can be regenerated. This offers a strong argument for long-term tooth retention. The future suggests that new regenerative innovations built on this solid foundation can lead to greater predictability and a new era of conservative preservation of the dentition.

Further Reading

Machtei, E.E. (2001). The effect of membrane exposure on the outcome of regenerative procedures in humans: a meta-analysis. *J. Periodontol.* 72 (4): 512–516.

Machtei, E.E. and Schallhorn, R.G. (1995). Successful regeneration of mandibular Class II furcation defects: an evidence-based treatment approach. *Int. J. Periodontics Restorative Dent.* 15 (2): 146–167.

Melcher, A.H. (1976). On the repair potential of periodontal tissues. *J. Periodontol.* 42: 256.

Nyman, S., Gottlow, J., Karring, J., and Lindhe, J. (1982). A regenerative potential of the periodontal ligament: an experimental study in the monkey. *J. Clin. Periodontol.* 9: 257.

Pini Prato, G., Clauser, C., Cortellini, P. et al. (1996). Guided tissue regeneration versus mucogingival surgery in the treatment of human buccal recessions. A 4-year follow-up study. *J. Periodontol.* 67 (11): 1216–1223.

12

Esthetic Crown Lengthening
Edgard El Chaar

Department of Periodontics, University of Pennsylvania, Dental Medicine Philadelphia, PA, USA

Overview

Esthetic crown lengthening is a therapy used to elongate a particular tooth or a set of teeth either for aesthetic dentistry purpose or to correct an excess of gingival display (EGD). In the periodontal classification and conditions, this subject falls into the category of mucogingival deformities and conditions around teeth, in which we have among others, gingival excess (GE). In the GE, we can find the following:

a. Pseudo-pocket
b. Inconsistent gingival margin
c. Excessive gingival display
d. Gingival enlargement

Etiology

The etiology of GE can be due to:

a. Excessive maxillary growth (Kokich 1993)
b. Altered Passive Eruption or short tooth syndrome (STS) (Chu et al. 2004)
c. Tooth malposition (Kokich 1993)
d. Gingival enlargement due to chronic inflammation, medications such as cyclosporine, phenytoin and calcium channel blockers, hormonal (pregnancy), or hereditary gingival fibromatosis
e. Deficient maxillary lip length
f. Excessive mobility of maxillary lip (Bhola et al. 2015)

In order for a clinician to determine the appropriate etiology, the following evaluation is required:

- Facial proportions
- Lip length and smile line
- Tooth proportions
- Gingival zenith and gingival margins of adjacent teeth

These evaluations will lead to a diagnosis/etiology of GE. First, the facial proportions can be determined by taking a cephalometric radiograph. The lower anterior facial height (LAFH) should equal approximately 55% of the whole length of the profile measured from the nasion to the menton. The lip length and the smile line should be assessed to be able to determine appropriate treatment thus determining the etiology is essential. The lip length that is measured from the nasion to the middle of the vermillion border has been given numerical numbers as shown in Table 12.1 by Ahmad (2005). The interesting in this table, it quantifies not only the lip length but also the exposure of the maxillary and mandibular centrals. Garber and Salama (1996) quantified the gingival display independently of the lip length as shown in Table 12.2 with treatment modalities. The measurement of tooth proportion also is an important tool to help us determine the etiology. Magne (2003) determined the proportions of unworn and worn maxillary teeth from first premolar to first premolar as shown in Table 12.3. In order for us to define the length of the tooth we need to determine the zenith. Chu et al. (2009) defined the presence of the zenith by being at 1mm from the vertical bisected midline for the central incisor, 0.4mm for the maxillary lateral and coinciding for the maxillary canines. Once all of this has been determined, and the tooth are defined as short due to altered passive eruption, we can follow the Coslet (1977) classification, in which he divided patients in two types I and II based on the abundance of keratinized tissue from the GM to the MGL, and subdivision A and B, in which A, the bone was over 2 mm from CEJ and B the bone was at the CEJ level.

Table 12.1 Maxillary lip length in relation to anterior tooth exposure.

Maxillary lip classification	Maxillary lip length (mm)	Exposure of upper central incisor (mm)	Exposure of lower central (mm)
Short	10–15	3.92	0.64
Medium	16–20	3.44	0.77
Medium	21–25	2.18	0.98
Long	26–30	0.93	1.95
Long	31–36	0.25	2.25

Table 12.2 Gingival and mucosal display.

Degree	Gingival and mucosal display(mm)	Treatment modalities
I	2–4	Orthodontic intrusion
		Orthodontics and periodontics
		Periodontal and restorative therapy
II	4–8	Periodontal and restorative therapy
		Orthognathic surgery (Le Fort I osteotomy)
III	≥8	Orthognathic surgery with or without adjunctive periodontal and restorative therapy

Table 12.3 Teeth proportions.

	Worn	Unworn
Maxillary central	W = 9.10–9.24 mm	W = 9.10–9.24 mm
	L = 10.67 mm	L = 11.69 mm
Maxillary lateral	W = 7.07–7.38 mm	W = 7.07–7.38 mm
	L = 9.34–9.55 mm	L = 9.34–9.55 mm
Maxillary canine	W = 7.90–8.06 mm	W = 7.90–8.06 mm
	L = 9.90 mm	L = 10.83 mm
Premolars	W = 7.84 mm	W = 7.84 mm
	L = 9.33 mm	L = 9.33 mm
Percentage (W/L)	Cent = 87%	Cent = 78%
	lat = 79%	lat = 73%
	can = 81%	can = 73%
	PM = 84%	PM = 84%

Treatment

Bhola et al. (2015) divided the EGD in five different skeletal and dento-gingival etiologies (A–E). From these five categories, he proposed a decision treatment tree for the clinicians. In his article, he divided category E in three subtypes related to the lip mobility.

In his decision treatment tree, he looked at the normal clinical crown measurements, the 3 thirds of the face, gingival contour and consistency, lip length, and lip mobility. From each of these 4 questions, he correlated it to one of EGD categories proposing a treatment that has been discussed in the literature: either orthognathic surgery, aesthetic crown lengthening (based on coslet classification: osseous with gingivectomy, apically positioned flap with osseous, apically positioned flap alone, or gingivectomy alone based on the location of the CEJ to the crestal bone), oral hygiene modification, periodontal scaling and root planing, and lip treatment (specific to EGD etiology with its three different sub-classifications).

We will focus our discussion on the aesthetic crown lengthening in this chapter. The decision to perform esthetic crown lengthening using a gingivectomy procedure versus raising a flap depends on the distance between the proposed final position of the gingival margin and the underlying bone. If a gingivectomy procedure is used to remove an excessive gingival display, but the new gingival margin position is too close to the underlying bone, the biologic width will be violated and the gingival margin will usually rebound toward its original position, something we are discussing in "Post Elongation Gingival Margin Stability" section. To avoid a rebound, and re-establishing a proper biologic width, we need to resort to raising a flap.

The periodontist should establish the bone level in the initial preparation of the case. This can be done either with performing a digital intra-oral scan and a cone beam computerized tomography and combining the two files together as we will be discussing in Part III of the manual or by sounding the bone; this will allow to establish the total dento-gingival complex and biologic width for that patient. The second step is to establish the end result. If it is a case that requires a restorative treatment, the restorative team should make a wax-up, present it to the patient, and once approved, provide a surgical stent to the periodontist depicting the final margins. In case of altered passive eruption, the CEJ of the covered teeth will be used as a guide to establish the apical repositioning of the crestal bony level.

Case Surgical Description

A 20 year old male undergoing orthodontic treatment presented with excessive gingival display, abundance of melanin pigmentation. The EGD is due to an altered passive eruption (Figure 12.1a,b). Due to the abundance of melanin pigmentation, it is very critical to discuss with the patient that these pigmentations might be disappearing leaving some patches and even they might

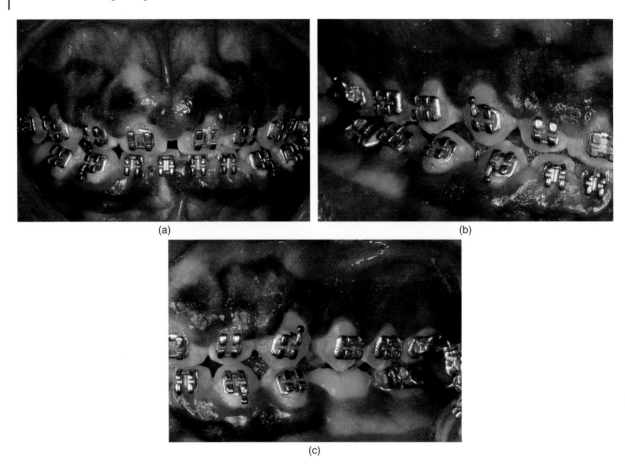

(a)   (b)

(c)

Figure 12.1 (a,b,c) A 20 year old male undergoing orthodontic treatment presented with excessive gingival display (EGD) and abundance of melanin pigmentation. The EGD is due to an altered passive eruption.

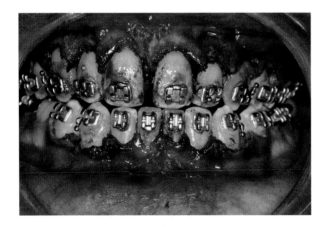

Figure 12.2 A submarginal incision was made up to the CEJ.

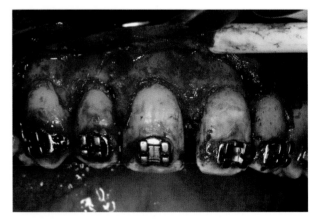

Figure 12.3 An intrasulcular incision was made buccally and a papilla sparing incision was done. A full thickness flap was raised.

re-occur. A sub-marginal incision was made up to the CEJ (Figure 12.2). An intrasulcular incision was made buccally and a papilla sparing incision was done, A full thickness flap was raised (Figure 12.3). The crest of bone is at the CEJ allowing us to confirm a Coslet classification Type I subdivision II. An ostectomy of 3 mm to re-establish the biologic width was done (Figure 12.4) and the flap was sutured with interrupted sling sutures and the aberrant frenum at the maxilla midline was excised by performing a frenectomy (Figure 12.5). A three-month follow-up showed a good marginal gingival stability (Figure 12.6).

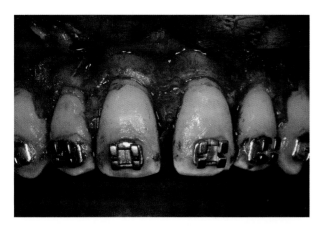

Figure 12.4 A ostectomy of 3 mm to re-establish the biologic width was done.

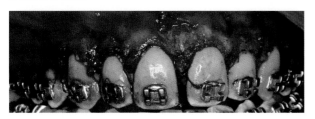

Figure 12.5 The flap was sutured with interrupted sling sutures, and the aberrant frenum at the maxilla midline was excised.

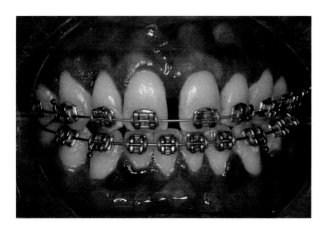

Figure 12.6 A three-month follow-up of the healing.

Post-Elongation Gingival Margin Stability

The goal is to expose a specific amount of tooth and to maintain a stable gingival margin after the surgical procedure.

Table 12.4 Mean bone removal according to clinician experience.

Experience level	Faculty	Second year graduate students	First year graduate students
Mean bone removal (mm)	1.1 ± 0.6	0.8 ± 0.5	0.0 ± 0.7

It is important to understand and recognize the morphology of the case before performing the procedure. Ochsenbein and Ross (1969) stated that thin and thick periodontium behave differently after surgery. In thin periodontium we might end up with an increased tooth exposure, which is undesirable versus in a thick periodontium a phenomenon called gingival rebound may occur.

Multiple studies have shown a rebound over time and correlate it to an insufficient bone resection. The findings are as follows:

- Pontoriero and Carnevale (2001): 1–12 months, a gingival rebound of 0.5–1.2 mm was observed. Only 8% of sites had bone resection of ≥2 mm.
- Arora et al. (2013): 64 teeth, rebound of 0.77 mm at six months, most often associated with <3 mm of reduction and thick flat biotype.
- Herrero et al. (1995): 21 teeth crown lengthened with the goal of 3 mm of biological width. A rebound of – 2.4 mm was noted. In their conclusions they stated: "although more experienced periodontists removed a larger amount of bone, the amount of root surface exposed was still short of the initially desired biologic width. Within the limits of this clinical study a 3 mm biologic width was not routinely achieved during surgical crown elongation." In that study, they quantified the difference in bone removal between experienced periodontist and students in training as shown in Table 12.4.

On the other hand, Lanning (2003) in a period of three to six months, found no significant changes in the established margins and the bone resection was ≥3 mm at 90% of sites. With that, the bone reduction is the key to keeping the newly established gingival display.

References

Ahmad, I. (2005). Anterior dental aesthetics: dental perspective. *Br. Dent. J.* 199 (3): 135.

Arora, R., Narula, S.C., Sharma, R.K., and Tewari, S. (2013). Evaluation of supracrestal gingival tissue after surgical crown lengthening: a 6-month clinical study. *J. Periodontol.* 84 (7): 934–940.

Bhola, M., Fairbairn, P.J., Kolhatkar, S. et al. (2015). LipStaT: The Lip Stabilization Technique—Indications and guidelines for case selection and classification of excessive gingival display. *Int. J. Periodontics Restorative Dent.* 35 (4).

Chu, S.J., Karabin, S., and Mistry, S. (2004). Short tooth syndrome: diagnosis, etiology, and treatment management. *CDA J.* 32 (2): 143–152.

Chu, S.J., Tan, J.H., Stappert, C.F., and Tarnow, D.P. (2009). Gingival zenith positions and levels of the maxillary anterior dentition. *J. Esthet. Restor. Dent.* 21 (2): 113–120.

Coslet, J.G., Vanarsdall, R.L., and Weisgold, A. (1977). Diagnosis and classification of delayed passive eruption of the dentogingival junction in the adult. *Alpha Omegan* 70 (3): 24–28.

Garber, D.A. and Salama, M.A. (1996). The aesthetic smile: diagnosis and treatment. *Periodontology 2000* 11 (1): 18–28.

Herrero, F., Scott, J.B., Maropis, P.S., and Yukna, R.A. (1995). Clinical comparison of desired versus actual amount of surgical crown lengthening. *Journal of periodontology.* 66 (7): 568–571.

Kokich, V.G. (1993). Esthetics and anterior tooth position: an orthodontic perspective. Part II: Vertical position. *J. Esthet. Dent.* 5 (4): 174–178.

Lanning, S.K., Waldrop, T.C., Gunsolley, J.C., and Maynard, J.G. (2003). Surgical crown lengthening: evaluation of the biological width. *Journal of periodontology.* 74 (4): 468–474.

Magne, P., Gallucci, G.O., and Belser, U.C. (2003). Anatomic crown width/length ratios of unworn and worn maxillary teeth in white subjects. *J. Prosthetic Dent.* 89 (5): 453–461.

Ochsenbein, C. and Ross, S. (1969). A reevaluation of osseous surgery. *Dent. Clin. North Am.* 13: 87–102.

Pontoriero, R. and Carnevale, J. (2001). Surgical crown lengthening: a 12 month clinical wound healing study. *J. Periodontol.* 72 (7): 841–848.

Further Reading

Johnston, D.J., Hunt, O., Johnston, C.D. et al. (2005). The influence of lower face vertical proportion on facial attractiveness. *Eur. J. Orthodont.* 27 (4): 349–354.

Kokich, V.G. (1996). Esthetics: the orthodontic-periodontic restorative connection. *Semin Orthod.* 2 (1): 21–30. Review.

Van der Velden, U. (1982). Regeneration of the interdental soft tissues following denudation procedures. *J. Clin. Periodontol.* 9: 455–459.

13

Soft Tissue Management in Natural Dentition

Edgard El Chaar

Department of Periodontics, University of Pennsylvania, Dental Medicine, Philadelphia, PA, USA

Overview

The new world workshop of 2017 has made modifications on the American Academy of Periodontology consensus of 1999 in regard to the mucogingival deformities and conditions around teeth. These modifications are the following:

1. *Periodontal biotype*
   a. *Thin scalloped*
   b. *Thick scalloped*
   c. *Thick flat*
2. Gingival/soft tissue recession
   a. Facial or lingual surfaces
   b. *Interproximal (papillary)*
   c. *Severity of recession (Cairo RT1,2,3)*
   d. *Gingival thickness*
   e. *Gingival width*
   f. *Presence of non-carious cervical lesions (NCCL)/ cervical caries*
   g. *Patient aesthetic concern (Smile Esthetics Index)*
   h. *Presence of hypersensitivity*
3. Lack of keratinized gingiva
4. Decreased vestibular depth
5. Aberrant frenum/muscle position
6. Gingival excess
   a. Pseudo-pocket
   b. Inconsistent gingival margin
   c. Excessive gingival display
   d. Gingival enlargement
7. Abnormal color

The additions included the definition of phenotype that included the gingival thickness (GT), gingival width, thickness of buccal bone, and the biotype. The presence and the absence of keratinized tissue (KT) have also been reviewed. On that latter, in 2015, both Kim et al. and Scheyer et al. concluded that lack of keratinized tissue, presence of an aberrant frenum, and lack of vestibule are not considered risk factors for gingival recession (GR) in conditions of optimum oral hygiene. However, later it was found that in the presence of gingival inflammation, lack of keratinized tissue has proven to be a predisposing factor for gingival recession (Merijohn 2016).

Also, in relation to the presence of gingival recessions a lot of the question that have been carried from the 1999 consensus have been re-examined mainly the followings: Does gingival recession worsen with time? Are there any risks or consequences associated with the presence of recession? Is tooth position a risk factor? What is the role of the periodontal phenotype, and what is its effect on the incidence of recession or its progression? And finally, should the presence of gingival recession and phenotype be considered when planning orthodontic, restorative, and implant treatment?

Gingival recession has been defined as the apical shift of the gingival margin with respect to the cemento-enamel junction (CEJ) (Pini Prato 1999). It is associated with attachment loss and exposure of the root surface to the oral environment. It is a frequent finding in adults that increases with age regardless of oral hygiene habits (Kassab and Cohen 2003). It was found that 88% of people aged ≥65 years and 50% of people aged 18–64 years have ≥1 site with gingival recession that can result in esthetic concerns and dentin hypersensitivity (Kassab and Cohen 2003). Exposing the root dentin to the oral environment can lead to carious (Nuttall et al. 2001) and NCCL, such as abrasions or erosions (Bartlett and Shah 2006; Pecie et al. 2011). Prevalence and severity of NCCL appear to increase with age (Bartlett and Shah 2006; Heasman et al. 2015; Pecie et al. 2011).

Although the etiology of gingival recessions remains unclear, several predisposing factors have been suggested (Cortellini and Bissada 2018):

a. Periodontal biotype and attached gingiva
b. The impact of toothbrushing

c. The impact of cervical restorative margins
d. The impact of orthodontics
e. Other conditions

The distinction among different biotypes that will be referred to as phenotypes, is based upon anatomic characteristics of components of the masticatory complex, including (i) gingival biotype, which includes in its definition gingival thickness (GT) and keratinized tissue width (KTW); (ii) bone morphotype (BM); and (iii) tooth dimension.

Tooth position in the alveolar process plays an important role. A buccally tilted tooth is frequently associated with thin gingiva (Cook et al. 2011) and a thin labial plate (Muller and Kononen 2005).

Thin phenotypes tend to develop greater gingival recession compared with thick phenotypes due to the presence of thin buccal bone or facial dehiscence, which influence the integrity of the periodontium, thereby constituting a risk when the tooth is subjected to orthodontic forces (Kassab and Cohen 2003; Kim and Neiva 2015; Zweers et al. 2014), restorative treatment or tooth extraction with subsequent implant placement (Cortellini and Bissada 2018; El Chaar et al. 2016a).

The presence of attached gingival tissue is considered important for maintenance of gingival health. The current consensus, based on case series and case reports (low level of evidence), is that about 2 mm of KT and about 1 mm of attached gingiva are desirable around teeth to maintain periodontal health, even though a minimum amount of keratinized tissue is not needed to prevent attachment loss when optimal plaque control is present (Kim and Neiva 2015). Furthermore, thin gingival biotype without gingival recession entails a greater risk for future development of gingival recessions, requiring an attentive follow-up from the clinicians to prevent degradation (Cortellini and Bissada 2018). With respect to these cases with severe thin gingival biotype application of mucogingival surgery in high-risk sites could be considered to prevent future mucogingival damage (Cortellini and Bissada 2018).

In 1987, Stetler and Bissada studied the effect of restorative margin placement on the periodontium and found that subgingival margin placement in patients presenting with minimal (<2 mm) or lack of gingiva resulted in greater gingival inflammation than those with a wider band of gingiva (Stetler and Bissada 1987). A recent systematic review reported clinical observations suggesting that sites with minimal or no gingiva associated with intrasulcular restorative margins were more prone to gingival recession and inflammation (Kim and Neiva 2015). Both authors recommend soft tissue augmentation to increase the width of keratinized tissue.

There is a possibility of gingival recession initiation or progression of recession during or after orthodontic treatment depending on the direction of the orthodontic movement (Bollen et al. 2008; Joss-Vassalli et al. 2010). Several authors have demonstrated that gingival recession may develop during or after orthodontic therapy (Hall 1981; Maynard 1987; Renkema et al. 2013, 2015). The direction of tooth movement and the bucco-lingual thickness of the gingiva may play important roles in soft tissue changes that occur during orthodontic treatment (Kassab and Cohen 2003; Kim and Neiva 2015).

Classifications

Proper diagnosis of gingival recession is critical for the prediction of successful treatment outcomes. In order to formulate an accurate diagnosis, it is essential to evaluate clinical measurements such as gingival recession, interdental clinical attachment level (CAL), interproximal bone level, and position of the tooth.

Measuring a gingival recession and interdental CAL rely on the detection of the CEJ. Determination of the location of the CEJ is especially important in cases presenting with previous restorations or NCCLs.

Determination of the CEJ

One of the primary goals of mucogingival surgery is to gain root coverage over areas of gingival recession. Gingival recession is defined as the apical movement of the free gingival margin (FGM) resulting in exposure of a portion of the root to the oral cavity (Cortellini and Bissada 2018). The main metric used to assess surgical success is complete root coverage (CRC), that is, the complete coverage of the exposed root surface to a point at the CEJ.

However, the CEJ is sometimes not readily detectable due to the presence of NCCLs. NCCLs may involve either the root surface, the enamel surface, or a combination of both surfaces. Should the NCCL only comprise the root surface, then mucogingival surgery alone is indicated. Should the NCCL only involve the enamel surface, restorative treatment alone is indicated. However, should the NCCL involve both surfaces, a joint restorative-periodontal approach to treatment is most appropriate. This third situation poses the greatest challenge for achieving predictable esthetic and functional results because the reference point for root coverage, i.e. the CEJ, is obscured.

Table 13.2 Miller class of recessions.

Class I	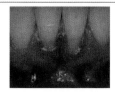	Recession that does not extend beyond the mucogingival junction with no loss of interproximal bone	Class III	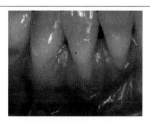	Recession that extends to or beyond the mucogingival junction with some periodontal attachment loss or malpositioning of teeth
Class II	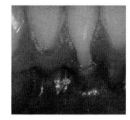	Recession that extends to or beyond the mucogingival junction with no loss of interproximal bone	Class IV	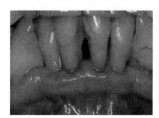	Recession that extends to or beyond the mucogingival junction with severe periodontal attachment loss and/or severe malpositioning of teeth

Most importantly, the prevalence of tooth deformities associated with gingival recessions is very high (Pini-Prato et al. 2010).

Cases in which CRC cannot be expected due to rotation, extrusion, or loss of interproximal clinical attachment (Miller III recession) are associated with greater complexity. In such cases, it may be more fruitful for the clinician and patient to anticipate maximum root coverage (MRC) versus CRC.

Utilizing MRC may also be applicable in cases of Miller I and II recession with unidentifiable CEJs. It should be noted that MRC should coincide with CRC in these cases, whereas in Miller III, MRC cannot predictably be coincident with CRC due to the presence of interproximal attachment loss.

Zucchelli et al. (2011) and coworkers have defined the level of MRC as the arc that joins the mesial and distal contact points and transitional line angles of a given tooth. In instances where the CEJ is obliterated, the line of MRC serves as a dimensional guideline to which the restorative dentist can re-create the CEJ. Should the MRC line be coronal to the CEJ, mucogingival surgery is indicated as the sole therapy. However, should the MRC line be apical to the CEJ, restoration of the tooth is indicated to the level of the MRC, followed by mucogingival surgery.

Completing the restoration prior to surgery is beneficial for both the restorative and surgical dentist. For the restorative dentist, isolation and preparation of the site are more straightforward as the entire working field is supragingival. For the surgeon, the restorative margins provide a landmark for coronal advancement of the tissue and facilitate a stable, smooth surface for flap adaptation, ultimately optimizing wound healing.

In the 2017 world workshop, the CEJ is classified based on its detection with or without steps made by the presence or absence of NCCL as shown in Table 13.1.

In 2011, Cairo et al. introduced an alternative classification for gingival recession utilizing interproximal CAL as the primary factor when defining a recession type (RT) defect rather than the location of the mucogingival line (MGL). The classification system is defined as follows:

- **Recession Type 1 (RT1)**: Gingival recession with no loss of interproximal attachment. Interproximal CEJ is clinically not detectable at both mesial and distal aspects of the tooth.
- **Recession Type 2 (RT2)**: Gingival recession associated with loss of interproximal attachment. The amount of interproximal attachment loss (measured from the interproximal CEJ to the depth of the interproximal sulcus/pocket) is less than or equal to the buccal attachment loss (measured from the buccal CEJ to the apical end of the buccal sulcus/pocket).
- **Recession Type 3 (RT3)**: Gingival recession associated with loss of interproximal attachment. The amount of interproximal attachment loss (measured from the interproximal CEJ to the apical end of the sulcus/pocket) is greater than the buccal attachment loss (measured from the buccal CEJ to the apical end of the buccal sulcus/pocket).

While the Cairo classification is today preferred over the classic Miller classification (Table 13.2) as it is considered

Table 13.1 Classification system of four different classes of root surface concavities.

CEJ	Step	Descriptors
Class A	−	CEJ detectable without step
Class A	+	CEJ detectable with step
Class B	−	CEJ undetectable without step
Class B	+	CEJ undetectable with a step

to be in greater accordance with the new advancements of root coverage therapy, it nevertheless fails to include important factors in achieving treatment success such as interproximal bone loss, tooth position (over-eruption, tilt) and root pro-eminence.

Diagnostic and Treatment Considerations Based on Classification of Periodontal Biotypes, Gingiva Recession, and Root Surface Conditions

Pursuant to the world workshop, a diagnostic table integrating recession type (RT), gingival recession (GR), keratinized tissue width (KTW), gingival thickness (GT), the detection of the CEJ and the absence or presence of concavities (Table 13.3).

This table is meant to help orient the clinician when determining the best course of treatment for a particular patient. For example, in cases that currently lack gingival recession but present with a thin phenotype thereby predisposing to future recession defects, the clinician may elect to conservatively wait and monitor the recession or to intervene by changing the phenotype especially if the patient will undergo future orthodontic treatment.

Surgical Management of Mucogingival Deficiencies

The principles that support successful surgical treatment of mucogingival deformities remain consistent regardless of

Table 13.3 Diagnostic table.

	Gingival site			Tooth site	
	REC depth	GT	KTW	CEJ(A/B)	Step(+/−)
No recession					
RT1					
RT2					
RT3					

the elected treatment modality. These fundamental principles include flap management and integrity, graft stabilization, and an understanding of wound healing.

Free Gingival Graft (FGG)

The objective of a FGG is to reduce recession and increase keratinized tissue (KT). With this procedure a great deal of controversy exists in the literature regarding the use of partial thickness flap (PTF) versus full thickness flap (FTF).

Authors Supporting FTF
- Wood (1972): Reported a mean crestal alveolar bone loss of 0.62 and 0.98 mm for FTF and PTP, respectively, thereby advocating the use of FTF.
- Dordick (1976): The authors reported less mobility, less swelling, and better hemostasis for grafts placed directly on denuded bone than those placed on periosteum.
- James and McFall (1978): In a histologic study comparing FGG placed on bone and periosteum, the authors found less shrinkage for grafts placed directly on denuded bone. The authors also reported less postoperative swelling for grafts placed on bone, though no difference in the degree of inflammation was noted.

Authors Supporting PTF
- Staffileno et al. (1966) found that periosteal retention produced minimal tissue destruction, rapid repair, slight alteration of the dentogingival junction, and maximum preservation of the periodontal supporting structures.
- Caffesse et al. (1979): reported delayed remodeling of grafts placed directly on bone.

While the FGG is one of the most well researched and documented soft tissue grafting procedures, other treatment modalities have shown greater predictability in the treatment of GR, with greater MRC and less patient morbidity.

Pedicle Soft Tissue Graft

A pedicle graft has the advantage of maintaining the blood supply from the base of the flap which thereby facilitates wound healing by providing nourishment until the re-establishment of a vascular union with the recipient site.

This procedure involves raising a flap, either PTF, FTF, or a combination of both. Vertical incisions are required to determine the width of the base.

Mormann and Ciancio (1977), recommend a 2 : 1 length to width ratio for the simple parallel pedicle flap, suggesting a broader flap base. The authors caution that minimal tension should be applied by suturing and that gentle intraoperative management of the tissue is critical. Additionally, the authors caution that the PTF covering the avascular root should maintain adequate tissue thickness to allow for a greater quantity of blood vessels to be incorporated within the flap. The apical portion of the flap should be full thickness when possible.

Histologically, Wilderman and Wentz (1965) presented the wound healing events for pedicle flaps in dogs as follows:

1. **Adaptation stage (0–4 days)**: A fibrin clot containing neutrophils is present between the flap and the crestal bone
2. **Proliferation stage (4–21 days)**: Granulation tissue invades the fibrin clot, fibroblasts are present on the root surface (6–10 days), epithelium migrates apically (10–14 days), and an average of 1 mm of crestal bone is resorbed
3. **Attachment stage (21–28 days)**: Collagen formation is visible, cementum formation occurs, and osteoblastic activity reaches its peak
4. **Maturation stage (28–180 days)**: New PDL fibers orient perpendicularly to the root surface. New attachment consisting of a combination of long junctional epithelium (2.0 mm) and connective tissue attachment (2.1 mm).

Sugarman (1969) reported three cases with human histologic evidence of the healing obtained with pedicle grafts and free soft tissue autografts. The full thickness, laterally positioned flap heal by new attachment consisting of junctional epithelium (1.0–1.6 mm), connective tissue attachment (0.1–3.2 mm), and areas of new cementum.

While the pedicle flap is a technique of the 1960–1970s, it may be a useful treatment modality in the event of sufficient width and thickness of the donor site.

Coronally Advanced Flap (CAF)

The CAF was originally introduced by Bernimoulin. After performing an FGG, the graft is then mobilized and coronally repositioned to increase RC. The technique developed over time to exclude the need for a palatal donor site. The CAF has shown to be a safe and predictable approach in cases of adequate KTW apical to the recession (>=2 mm) (Pini Prato et al. 2018) and thick gingiva (>=0.8 mm) (Baldi et al. 1999; Cairo et al. 2016), resulting in similar color, texture, and thickness to that originally present at the buccal aspect of the recessed tooth (Cairo et al. 2016). Pini Prato et al. (2011) showed that during a long-term follow-up, gingival recession recurred in 39% of the treated sites following the CAF procedure.

The factors that influence the success of the CAF are as follows:

a. **Flap tension**: Pini Prato et al. (2000) showed that tension over the flap should be less or equal to 0.4 g.
b. **Sutures**: Tatakis and Chambrone found that removal of sutures in less than 10 days, impacts negatively the success of CAF.
c. **Flap thickness**: Baldi et al. (1999), showed that the flap should be >0.8 mm to achieve success.
d. **Position of the gingival margin post-surgically**: 1.5–2 mm coronal to CEJ.
e. **No vertical release incisions**: Zucchelli et al. (2009) postulated that the envelope type of CAF with no vertical release incisions, was associated with an increased probability of achieving complete root coverage, by preserving the lateral blood supply and no Keloid formation responsible for the worst esthetic evaluation made by an independent expert periodontist. The same was reported in the literature by Fedi (1985), Bruno (1994), Joly et al. (2007), and Papageorgakopoulos et al. (2008).
f. When there is insufficient KTW and thin phenotype, Cairo et al. (2016), found sub-epithelial connective tissue graft (SCTG) with CAF to be more predictable in achieving RC.
g. The addition of EMD does not provide additional benefit (Del Pizzo et al. 2005).

Sub-epithelial Connective Tissue Graft (SCTG)

The introduction of this technique in the mid-1980s by Langer and Langer revolutionized the predictability of gingival grafting and expectations for true root coverage. The technique consists of butt joint incisions performed at the base of the adjacent papilla and vertical incisions. A PTF is reflected. Bruno modified this technique using no vertical incision to preserve the lateral blood supply and avoid keloid formation. The author uses the butt joint incision and does not require complete coverage of the SCTG.

Various techniques for harvesting the connective tissue from the palate have been described including the trap door, parallel incision or de-epithelializing of an FGG. The palatal vault plays an important role. Reiser et al. (1996) described three vaults height (shallow 7 mm, average 12 mm, and high 17 mm) affecting the width of the tissue that can be harvested. Rose and Mealey detailed the thickness of the palate as thin 0.5–0.8 mm, average 0.9–1.4 mm, and thick 1.5–2.0 mm +; and the thickness of each component of the palatal tissue: epithelium 0.3–0.6 mm, connective tissue (lamina propria) 1.25–3.0 mm, submucosa (adipose and glandular tissue). Yu et al. (2014) defined the most appropriate donor site for gingival autogenous grafting is the region 3–9 mm below the CEJ between the distal surface of the canine and the midline surface of the first molar. The clinician needs to take into consideration the pre-eminence of the palatal root on the mesial side and try to avoid thinning the tissue at that level ending with a dehiscence over that site.

The flap, as discussed prior in the CAF section, is recommended to include slicing of papilla, no vertical release and achieve a complete coverage surpassing the CEJ by 1.5–2 mm, which brings us to thickness of the harvested SCTG. Zucchelli et al. (2014), in 60 Miller classes I and II gingival recessions (GRs) (≥3 mm in depth), compared a de-epithelialized FGG of ≥2 mm thickness and the height equal to bone dehiscence; versus a thickness of <2 mm and the height of 4 mm. Results showed better color match in the thinnest graft, no statistical difference between the two groups in terms of recession reduction, CRC and increase in KTH. Greater GT increase was obtained in the thicker sites.

Stefanini et al. (2018) defined the criteria and indications of the CTG use, with CAF versus CAF alone and the outcome over three years:

a. CTG in gingival defects with a baseline keratinized tissue height (KTH) <1 mm or with KTH between 1 and 2 mm and gingival thickness <1 mm.
b. CAF alone in sites of KT band >2 mm and gingival thickness >1 mm
c. Complete root coverage (CRC) was obtained in 98.5% (CAF + CTG) and in 94.7% (CAF alone) of the sites at the one- and three-year follow-up visits, respectively.
d. No statistically significant differences in sites treated with CAF alone versus CAF + CTG at one and three years in terms of CRC and between sites belonging to the maxilla or mandible.
e. A greater increase in KTH at three years was demonstrated in sites treated with CTG. This was ascribed to the tendency of the MGL to regain its genetically pre-determined position and not to graft exposure.

Finally, El Chaar et al. in 2016b proposed in very thin biotype with noticeable pro eminent root, to add cancellous allograft to eliminate dead spaces instead of flattening the roots and to use the CTG harvested in its entirety keeping the fatty tissue as a source of fluidity needed in the first three days of healing until the vascularity has taken place. That fatty tissue should be kept facing the covering flap, which is a CAF with coverage over the CEJ of at least 1.5 mm. The flap should be stretched from the mucosa with FTF elevation to achieve CAF. If other surgeries were done in the area previously and a scare tissue is evident, a dissection of that tissue should be done by mean of parallel incision to the inner aspect of the normal flap.

Allograft

Various tissue banks supply allografts to the dental market, to cite few:

(1) Alloderm® by Life Cell distributed by BioHorizons
(2) Puros Dermis® by Tutoplast® distributed by Zimmer-Biomet
(3) DermACELL® by LifeNet Health and distributed by Straumann

The differences between the above mentioned are outlined in Tables 13.4 and 13.5.

Acellular Dermal Matrix

Originally used by plastic surgeons to treat burn victims, acellular dermal matrix (ADM), an acellular, non-immunogenic cadaveric human dermis, has been incorporated into the dental armamentarium as an alternative to the autogenous SCTG for soft tissue augmentation.

Table 13.4 Comparative description of each of the different brands.

	AlloDerm	Puros Dermis	DermACELL
Biocompatible	✓	✓	✓
Source	Human	Human	Human
Packaging	Aseptic	Sterile	Sterile
Freeze-dried	Yes	No	No
Side specific	No	No	No
Esthetic result	✓	✓	
Thickness	0.5–0.8 mm	0.3–0.8 mm	0.76–1.25 mm
	0.9–1.6 mm	0.8–1.8 mm	1.26–1.75 mm
Rehydration	15 min; 2 baths	<1 min	Comes hydrated

Table 13.5 Descriptive table of the processing methods of each of them.

Tutoplast	Life cell	Life net health
Donor selection	Donor selection	Donor selection
Donor testing	Donor testing	Donor testing
Osmotic treatment, oxidative treatment, alkaline treatment	Tissue wash (Hanks BSS), De-cellularizing (0.5% sodium dodecyl sulfate in BSS),Tissue wash ×2	ALLWASH XG® tissue sterilization, MATRACELL™
Solvent dehydration	Cryoprotection	Preservon® technique: keeps it hydrated
Sterile	Aseptic	Sterile

ADM is composed of a basal lamina for epithelial cell migration and an underlying porous dermal matrix which permits the in-growth of fibroblasts and angiogenic cells.

In 1995, Wainwright reported on the use of ADM for the treatment of full-thickness burn injuries. The author found that the use of ADM supported fibroblast infiltration, neo-vascularization, and epithelialization. In comparison with non-grafted sites, those treated with ADM showed normal dermal function exhibiting normal collagen bundle patterns and elastin at 16 days post-surgery. The authors concluded that ADM was a viable option for the early surgical management of burn victims in order to prevent scar formation and limitation in joint movement.

The results of Wainwright are consistent with those of Yim et al., who treated burn victims by stabilizing the ADM to the affected joints by means of small staples together with an overlying epithelial skin graft. The study evaluated the effect of the stabilized ADM on skin elasticity, scar thickness, trans-epidermal water loss, and melanin and erythema levels. The authors concluded that the use of stabilized Alloderm reduced scar formation and preserved normal dermal function.

Stabilization as a critical aspect of periodontal wound healing was first reported by Wikesjo and Nilvéus in 1990 (Wikesjo and Nilvéus 1990), in which the authors found greater connective tissue repair in heparin treated roots with wound stabilization using polylactic acid. Over the next 30 years, various techniques were proposed for graft stabilization including the use of suturing, tissue glue and titanium alloy tacks.

Clinical Studies Comparing Soft Tissue Allograft to the SCTG

While SCTG remains the gold standard for root coverage procedures, ADM is considered a viable treatment alternative in cases where SCTG grafts cannot be performed due to site specific and/or patient related factors.

Few studies report long term results comparing ADM and SCTG. In a retrospective study comparing ADM and SCTG for root coverage, Harris reported greater results with SCTG. While similar results were noted at the one-year post op, significant differences were detected between one and four years. Mean root coverage decreased from 93.4 to 65.8% and the mean recession increased from 0.2 to 1.1 mm in the ADM group, while the results of the SCTG group remained stable. The authors also noted greater increase in keratinized tissue with the SCTG compared to ADM at both the one year and four- to five-year follow-up. The study concluded that while ADM and SCTG exhibit comparable short-term results, SCTG is superior to ADM with respect to long

term stability and predictability of root coverage (Harris 2004).

Hirsch et al. compared the success of root coverage by means of sub-pedicle ADM and SCTG. While neither significant differences in final recession nor root coverage were found between the two groups, the SCTG resulted in significantly greater defect coverage, gain in both attachment and keratinized gingiva along with residual probing depth. Nevertheless, the authors report stable predictable results that were stable for both groups at two years post-operatively (Hirsch et al. 2005).

Schlee et al. compared human dermis graft (HDGs) with SCTG. The authors report that HDGs was an effective alternative to SCTG for root coverage and to increase soft tissue thickness, especially for the treatment of multiple recession defects within the same mouth, although HDG did provide slightly less root coverage than SCTG.

Barker et al. compared ADM with Puros Dermis (PDM), in a study in which both materials were grafted with a coronally advanced flap. The authors found neither statistical nor clinical differences in the amount of root coverage, probing neither depth nor keratinized tissue between material.

Histological Studies on Soft Tissue Allograft

In a histologic evaluation comparing autogenous SCTG and ADM in humans, the authors concluded that both SCTG and ADM are successful for root coverage with similar attachments and no adverse healing (Cummings et al. 2005).

Scarano et al. studied the histologic integration of ADM and found that after six weeks it was difficult to differentiate ADM from pre-existing collagen fibers. The substitution process was completed after 10 weeks, at which time the tissue was completely re-epithelialized with a defined basement membrane.

Clinical Case

A 41 years old female presented with an advanced RT2 (Figure 13.1) with a history of orthodontic treatment done. A connective tissue surgery was decided and a full thickness was elevated by making intra-sulcular incisions with papilla sparing (Figure 13.2).

Once the area was debrided and root scaled and root conditioned, the assessment showed that the root pro-eminence of tooth #23 is outside of the bony housing creating a significant distance from the supporting bone and the donor sub-epithelial connective tissue. A cancellous mineralized allograft was placed on the mesial

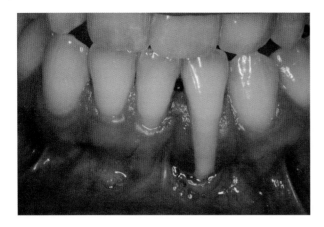

Figure 13.1 A 41 years old female presented with an advanced RT2.

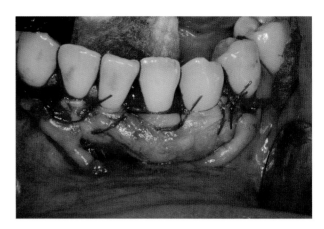

Figure 13.4 The sub-epithelial connective was placed over it and secured coronally with interrupted resorbable polyglactin sutures. The fatty part of the graft was placed towards the inner flap side.

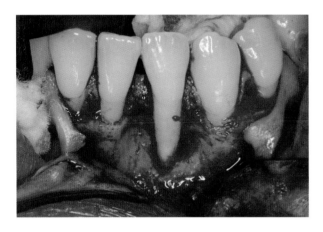

Figure 13.2 A full thickness was elevated by making intra-sulcular incisions with papilla sparing.

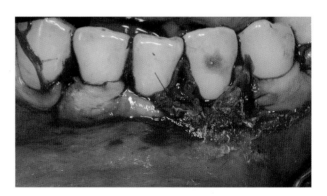

Figure 13.5 A coronally advanced flap was passivated by stretching and stabilized by one bista suture and multiple interrupted sling sutures using the resorbable polyglactin ones. Also, a peri-acrylic glue was placed at the site of #23 to reinforce the stabilization needed of the flap.

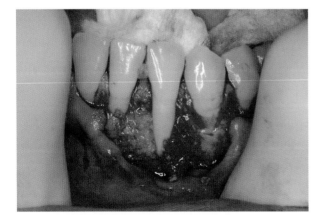

Figure 13.3 A cancellous mineralized allograft was placed on the mesial and distal of the root.

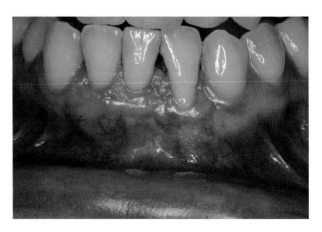

Figure 13.6 Very successful results with a 7 year follow-up.

and distal of the root (Figure 13.3) and the sub-epithelial connective was placed over it and secured coronally with interrupted resorbable polyglactin sutures. (Figure 13.4). The fatty part of the graft was placed towards the inner flap side.

A coronally advanced flap was passivated by stretching and stabilized by one bista suture and multiple interrupted

sling sutures using the resorbable polyglactin ones. Also, a peri-acrylic glue was placed at the site of #23 to reinforce the stabilization needed of the flap. (Figure 13.5).

The result were very successful initially and after 7 years. (Figure 13.6).

References

Baldi, C., Pini-Prato, G., Pagliaro, U. et al. (1999). Coronally advanced flap procedure for root coverage. Is flap thickness a relevant predictor to achieve root coverage? A 19-case series. *J. Periodontol.* 70 (9): 1077–1084.

Bartlett, D.W. and Shah, P. (2006). A critical review of non-carious cervical (wear) lesions and the role of abfraction, erosion, and abrasion. *J. Dent. Res.* 85: 306–312.

Bollen, A.M., Cunha-Cruz, J., Bakko, D.W. et al. (2008). The effects of orthodontic therapy on periodontal health: a systematic review of controlled evidence. *J. Am. Dent. Assoc.* 139: 413–422.

Bruno, J.F. (1994). Connective tissue graft technique assuring wide root coverage. *Int. J. Periodontics Restorative Dent.* 14: 126–137.

Caffesse, R.G. et al. (1979). Healing of free gingival grafts with and without periosteum. Part I. Histologic evaluation. *J. Periodontol.* 11: 586–594.

Cairo, F., Nieri, M., Cincinelli, S. et al. (2011). The interproximal clinical attachment level to classify gingival recessions and predict root coverage outcomes: an explorative and reliability study. *J. Clin. Periodontol.* 38: 661–666.

Cairo, F., Cortellini, P., Pilloni, A. et al. (2016). Clinical efficacy of coronally advanced flap with or without connective tissue graft for the treatment of multiple adjacent gingival recessions in the aesthetic area: a randomized controlled clinical trial. *J. Clin. Periodontol.* 43 (10): 849–856.

Cook, D.R., Mealey, B.L., Verrett, R.G. et al. (2011). Relationship between clinical periodontal biotype and labial plate thickness: an in vivo study. *Int. J. Periodontics Restorative Dent.* 31: 345–354.

Cortellini, P. and Bissada, N.F. (2018). Mucogingival conditions in the natural dentition: narrative review, case definitions, and diagnostic considerations. *J. Periodontol.* 89 (Suppl 1): S204–S213.

Cummings, L.C., Kaldahl, W.B., and Allen, E.P. (2005 Feb). Histologic evaluation of autogenous connective tissue and

acellular dermal matrix grafts in humans. *J. Periodontol.* 76 (2): 178–186.

Del Pizzo, M., Zucchelli, G., Modica, F. et al. (2005). Coronally advanced flap with or without enamel matrix derivative for root coverage: a 2-year study. *J. Clin. Periodontol.* 32 (11): 1181–1187.

Dordick, B., Coslet, J.G., and Seibert, J.S. (1976). Clinical evaluation of free autogenous gingival grafts placed on alveolar bone. Part I. Clinical predictability. *J. Periodontol.* 47 (10): 559–567.

El Chaar, E., Oshman, S., and Fallah, P.A. (2016a). Single-rooted extraction sockets: classification and treatment protocol. *Compend. Contin. Educ. Dent.* 37 (8): 537–541.

El Chaar, E.S., Oshman, S., Danesh-Sani, S.A. et al. (2016b). Increasing contact between soft tissue graft and blood supply. journal of cosmetic. *Dentistry* 32 (3): 52–66.

Fedi, P. (1985). *Periodontic Syllabus*. Philadelphia: Lea & Febiger.

Hall, W.B. (1981). The current status of mucogingival problems and their therapy. *J. Periodontol.* 52: 569–575.

Harris, R.J. (2004). A short term and long term comparison of root coverage with an acellular dermal matrix and a subepithelial graft. *J. Periodontol.* 75 (5): 734–743.

Heasman, P.A., Holliday, R., Bryant, A., and Preshaw, P.M. (2015). Evidence for the occurrence of gingival recession and non-carious cervical lesions as a consequence of traumatic toothbrushing. *J. Clin. Periodontol.* 42 (Suppl 16): S237–S255.

Hirsch, A., Goldstein, M., Goultschin, J. et al. (2005). A 2-year follow-up of root coverage using subpedicle acellular dermal matrix allografts and subepithelial connective tissue autografts. *J. Periodontol.* 76 (8): 1323–1328.

James, W.C. and McFall, W.T. Jr. (1978). Placement of free gingival grafts on denuded alveolar bone. Part I: clinical evaluations. *Journal of Periodontology* 49 (6): 283–290.

Joly, J.C., Carvalho, A.M., da Silva, R.C. et al. (2007). Root coverage in isolated gingival recessions using autograft versus allograft: a pilot study. *J. Periodontol.* 78: 1017–1022.

Joss-Vassalli, I., Grebenstein, C., Topouzelis, N. et al. (2010). Orthodontic therapy and gingival recession: a systematic review. *Orthod. Craniofacial Res.* 13: 127–141.

Kassab, M.M. and Cohen, R.E. (2003). The etiology and prevalence of gingival recession. *J. Am. Dent. Assoc.* 134: 220–225.

Kim, D.M. and Neiva, R. (2015). Periodontal soft tissue non-root coverage procedures: a systematic review from the AAP regeneration workshop. *J. Periodontol.* 86 (S2): S56–S72.

Maynard, J.G. (1987). The rationale for mucogingival therapy in the child and adolescent. *Int. J. Periodontics Restorative Dent.* 7: 36–51.

Merijohn, G.K. (2016). Management and prevention of gingival recession. *Periodontology* (71): 228–242.

Mormann, W. and Ciancio, S.G. (1977). Blood supply of human gingiva following periodontal surgery. *J. Periodontol.* 48: 681–692.

Muller, H.P. and Kononen, E. (2005). Variance components of gingival thickness. *J. Periodontol. Res.* 40: 239–244.

Nuttall, N.M., Steele, J.G., Pine, C.M. et al. (2001). The impact of oral health on people in the UK in 1998. *British Dental Journal* 190 (3): 121–126.

Papageorgakopoulos, G., Greenwell, H., Hill, M. et al. (2008). Root coverage using acellular dermal matrix and comparing a coronally positioned tunnel to a coronally positioned flap approach. *J. Periodontol.* 79 (6): 1022–1030.

Pecie, R., Krejci, I., Garcia-Godoy, F., and Bortolotto, T. (2011). Noncarious cervical lesions – a clinical concept based on the literature review. Part 1: prevention. *Am. J. Dent.* 24: 49–56.

Pini Prato, G.P. (1999). Mucogingival deformities. *Ann. Periodontol.* 4: 1–6.

Pini Prato, G., Pagliaro, U., Baldi, C. et al. (2000). Coronally advanced flap procedure for root coverage. Flap with tension versus flap without tension: a randomized controlled clinical study. *J. Periodontol.* 71 (2): 188–201.

Pini Prato, G., Rotundo, R., Franceschi, D. et al. (2011 Aug). Fourteen-year outcomes of coronally advanced flap for root coverage: Follow-up from a randomized trial. *J. Clin. Periodontol.* 38 (8): 715–720.

Pini Prato, G.P., Magnani, C., and Chambrone, L. (2018). Long-term evaluation (20 years) of the outcomes of coronally advanced flap in the treat-ment of single recession-type defects. *J. Periodontol.* 89: 265–274.

Pini-Prato, G., Franceschi, D., Cairo, F. et al. (2010). Classification of dental surface defects in areas of gingival recession. *J. Periodontol.* 81: 885–890.

Reiser, G.M., Bruno, J.F., Mahan, P.E., and Larkin, L.H. (1996). The subepithelial connective tissue graft palatal donor site: anatomic considerations for surgeons. *Int. J. Periodontics Restorative Dent.* 16 (2): 130–137.

Renkema, A.M., Fudalej, P.S., Renkema, A.A.P. et al. (2013). Gingival labial recessions in orthodontically treated and untreated individuals – a pilot case–control study. *J. Clin. Periodontol.* 40: 631–637.

Renkema, A.M., Navratilova, Z., Mazurova, K. et al. (2015). Gingival labial recessions and the post-treatment proclination of mandibular incisors. *Eur. J. Orthod.* 37: 508–513.

Staffileno, H., Levy, S., and Gargiulo, A. (1966). Histologic study of cellular mobilization and repair following a periosteal retention operation via split thickness mucogingival flap surgery. *J. Periodontol.* 37: 117–131.

Stefanini, M., Zucchelli, G., Marzadori, M., and de Sanctis, M. (2018). Coronally advanced flap with site specific application of connective tissue graft of connective tissue graft for the treatment of multiple adjacent gingival recessions: a 3 year follow-up case series. *Int. J. Periodontics Restorative Dent.* 38: 25–33.

Stetler, K.J. and Bissada, N.F. (1987). Significance of the width of keratinized gingiva on the periodontal status of teeth with submarginal restorations. *J. Periodontol.* 58 (10): 696–700.

Sugarman, E.F. (1969 Jul). A clinical and histological study of the attachment of grafted tissue to bone and teeth. *J. Periodontol.* 40 (7): 381–387.

Wikesjo, U.M. and Nilvéus, R. (1990). Periodontal repair in dogs: effect of wound stabilization on healing. *Journal of Periodontology* 61 (12): 719–724.

Wilderman, M.N. and Wentz, F.M. (1965). Repair of a dentogingival defect with a pedicle flap. *J. Periodontol.* 36 (3): 218–231.

Wood, D.L., Hoag, P.M., Donnenfeld, O.W., and Rosenfeld, L.D. (1972). Alveolar crest reduction following full and partial thickness flaps. *J. Periodontol.* 43 (3): 141–144.

Yu, S.K., Lee, M.H., Kim, C.S. et al. (2014). Thickness of the palatal masticatory mucosa with reference to autogenous grafting: a cadaveric and histologic study. *Int. J. Periodontics Restorative Dent.* 34: 115–121.

Zucchelli, G., Mele, M., Mazzotti, C. et al. (2009). Coronally advanced flap with and without vertical releasing incisions for the treatment of multiple gingival recessions: a comparative controlled randomized clinical trial. *J. Periodontol.* 80 (7): 1083–1094.

Zucchelli, G., Gori, G., Mele, M. et al. (2011). Non-carious cervical lesions associated with gingival recessions: a decision-making process. *J. Periodontol.* 82: 1713–1172.

Zucchelli, G., Mounssif, I., Mazzotti, C. et al. (2014). Does the dimension of the graft influence patient morbidity and root coverage outcomes? A randomized controlled clinical trial. *J. Clin. Periodontol.* 41 (7): 708–716.

Zweers, J., Thomas, R.Z., Slot, D.E. et al. (2014). Characteristics of periodontal biotype, its dimensions, associations and prevalence: a systematic review. *Journal of clinical periodontology* 41 (10): 958–971.

Further Reading

Ahmad, I. (2005). Anterior dental aesthetics: gingival perspective. *Br. Dent. J.* 199: 195–202.

Allen, E.P. and Miller, P.D. (1989). Coronal positioning of existing gingiva: short term results in the treatment of shallow marginal tissue recession. *J. Periodontol.* 60: 316–319.

Barker, T.S. et al. (2010). A comparative study of root coverage using two different acellular dermal matrix products. *J. Periodontol.* 81: 1596–1603.

Bernimoulin, J.P., Luscher, B., and Muhlemann, H.R. (1975). Coronally repositioned periodontal flap. Clinical evaluation after one year. *J. Clin. Periodontol.* 2: 1–13.

Bignozzi, I., Littarru, C., Crea, A. et al. (2013). Surgical treatment options for grafting areas of gingival recession association with cervical lesions: a review. *J. Esthet. Restor. Dent.* 25: 371–382.

Chambrone, L. and Tatakis, D.N. (2015). Periodontal soft tissue root coverage procedures: a systematic review from the AAP regeneration workshop. *J. Periodontol.* 86 (S2): S8–S51.

Cairo, F., Pagliaro, U., and Nieri, M. (2008). Treatment of gingival recession with coronally advanced flap procedures: a systematic review. *J. Clin. Periodontol.* 35 (S8): 136–162.

De Sanctis, M. and Zucchelli, G. (2007). Coronally advanced flap: a modified surgical approach for isolated recession-type defects: three-year results. *J. Clin. Periodontol.* 34: 262–268.

Guiha, R., el Khodeiry, S., Mota, L., and Caffesse, R. (2001). Histological evaluation of healing and revascularization of the subepithelial connective tissue graft. *J. Periodontol.* 72 (4): 470–478.

Johal, A., Katsaros, C., Kiliaridis, S. et al. (2010). Orthodontic therapy and gingival recession: a systematic review. *Orthod. Craniofacial Res.* 13: 127–141.

Kois, J.C. (2001). Predictable single tooth peri-implant esthetics: five diagnostic keys. *Compend. Contin. Educ. Dent.* 22: 199–206.

Löe, H., Ånerud, Å., and Boysen, H. (1992). The natural history of periodontal disease in man: prevalence, severity, and extent of gingival recession. *J. Periodontol.* 63: 489–495.

Matas, F., Sentís, J., and Mendieta, C. (2011). Ten-year longitudinal study of gingival recession in dentists. *J. Clin. Periodontol.* 38: 1091–1098.

Miller, P. (1987). Root coverage with the free gingival graft: factors associated with incomplete coverage. *J. Periodontol.* 58 (10): 674–681.

Pini Prato, G.P., Baldi, C., Nieri, M. et al. (2005). Coronally advanced flap: the post-surgical position of the gingival margin is an important factor for achieving complete root coverage. *J. Periodontol.* 76 (5): 713–722.

Scarano, A., Barros, R.R., Iezzi, G. et al. (2009). Acellular dermal matrix graft for gingival augmentation: a preliminary clinical, histologic, and ultrastructural evaluation. *J. Periodontol.* 80 (2): 253–259.

Scheyer, E.T., Sanz, M., Dibart, S. et al. (2015). Periodontal soft tissue non–root coverage procedures: a consensus report from the AAP regeneration workshop. *J. Periodontol.* 86: S73–S76.

Schlee, M. and Esposito, M. (2011). Human dermis graft versus autogenous connective tissue grafts for thickening soft tissue and covering multiple gingival recessions: 6-month results from a preference clinical trial. *Eur. J. Oral Implantol.* 4 (2): 119–125.

Senna, P., Del Bel, C.A., and Rosing, C. (2012). Non-carious cervical lesions and occlusion: a systematic review of clinical studies. *J. Oral Rehabil.* 39: 450–462.

Serino, G., Wennstrom, J., Lindhe, J., and Eneroth, L. (1994). The prevalence and distribution of gingival recession in subjects with a high standard of oral hygiene. *J. Clin. Periodontol.* 21: 57–63.

Tatakis, D.N. and Chambrone, L. (2016). The effect of suturing protocols on coronally advanced flap root-coverage outcomes: a meta-analysis. *J. Periodontol.* 87 (2): 148–155.

Vanarsdall, R.L. and Corn, H. (1977). Soft-tissue management of labially positioned unerupted teeth. *Am. J. Orthod.* 72: 53–64.

Wennstrom, J.L. and Pini Prato, G.P. (1997). Mucogingival therapy. In: *Clinical Periodontology and Implant Dentistry* (ed. J. Lindhe, T. Karring and N.P. Lang), 550–596. Copenhagen: Munksgaard.

Wennstrom, J.L. and Zucchelli, G. (1996). Increased gingival dimensions. A significant factor for successful outcome of root coverage procedures? A 2-year prospective clinical study. *J. Clin. Periodontol.* 23: 770–777.

Zucchelli, G. and De Sanctis, M. (2000). Treatment of multiple recession type defects in patients with aesthetic demands. *J. Periodontol.* 71: 1506–1514.

Zucchelli, G. and De Sanctis, M. (2005). Long-term outcome following treatment of multiple Miller class I and II recession defects in esthetic areas of the mouth. *J. Periodontol.* 76: 2286–2292.

Zucchelli, G. and Mounssif, I. (2015). Periodontal plastic surgery. *Periodontology* 68 (1): 333–368.

Zucchelli, G., Amore, C., Sforza, N.M. et al. (2003). Bilaminar techniques for the treatment of recession-type defects. A comparative clinical study. *J. Clin. Periodontol.* 30 (10): 862–870.

Zucchelli, G., Testori, T., and De Sanctis, M. (2006). Clinical and anatomical factors limiting treatment outcomes of gingival recession: a new method to predetermine the line of root coverage. *J. Periodontol.* 77 (4): 714–721.

Part III

Principles and Practice of Implant Dentistry

14

Principles of Implant Dentistry

Edgard El Chaar[1] and Aikaterini Georgantza[2]

[1]*Department of Periodontics, University of Pennsylvania, Dental Medicine, Philadelphia, PA, USA*
[2]*Ashman Department of Periodontology and Implant Dentistry, New York University College of Dentistry, New York, NY, USA*

Introduction

Historically, the interest in dental implants started in the late 1800s. Not until the late 1950s that some pioneers made either a subperiosteal implants or blade implants that get some successful results. The restoration over the blade implants used to be connected to natural teeth in most of the cases. When those implants failed, they led to a drastic damage in the supporting bone leading to an extensive bony defect.

In the early 1960s, Brånemark developed a novel implant, a root form, for clinical function depending on direct bone anchorage calling it osseointegration. He was able later to confirm his theory by an animal experiment in 1969 (Brånemark et al. 1969). This concept was further documented in the first clinical report published in 1977 (Branemark 1977). This bone anchorage has been independently proven by Schroeder (Schroeder et al. 1976; Schroeder et al. 1981) through histological proof, using new histological techniques at that time, by cutting through undecalcified bone and implant without previous separation of the anchorage. A 100% bone connection to the implant does not occur, for that reason the definition of osseointegration has been based on clinical stability instead of histologic criteria: "A process whereby clinically asymptomatic rigid fixation of alloplastic material is achieved, and maintained, in bone during functional loading" (Zarb and Albrektsson 1991).

Steps for Implant Success

In order for a dental implant to be successful, three goals need to be achieved:

1. Initial Objective: Primary stability
2. The Challenge: Secondary stability ⟶ Wound healing
3. Ultimate goal: Long term function ⟶ Osseointegration
   ⟶ Peri-implant health

Primary stability is defined as the Initial mechanical fixation and absence of mobility upon insertion (O'Sullivan et al. 2000). The primary stability can be achieved differently in a healed site versus an immediate implant placement. In the first, it's a locking effect between the implant and the avascular cortical bone of the crest and in the latter, in the apical portion, passing the apex of the socket by 3–4 mm (El-Chaar 2011) in what is called the primary stability rectangle.

The second goal which is the challenge, which is the process of wound healing around the dental implant. During site preparation and implant placement, bone trabeculae are dislocated into the marrow space, blood vessels are severed and bleeding occurs leading to a blood clot formation. The blood clot is also formed between the implant body and the host bone, definitely the more trabecular bone the more blood will be perfused and the more blood clot will form versus, the more cortical avascular bone is present, the less blood perfusion thus less blood clot formation.

After the blood clot formation, the wound will go through phases remodeling, leading to granulation tissue that replaces the blood clot, to woven bone leading to trabecular/lamellar bone at the latest phases of the healing, which has a good potential to take up and distribute the load when the implant is in function by creating bridging between the trabeculation inserting into the outer cortex.

This process takes time:

Primitive bone tissue forms (four to six weeks)
Bone adaptation to load (at two months)

Bone remodeling (at three months and ongoing)

The latter constitute the ultimate goal of long-term function which is a successful osseointegration (Schenk and Buser 1998).

Factors Affecting the Implant Success

Bone Quality Classification

When almost the entire jaw is composed of homogenous cortical bone (type 1), a thick layer of cortical bone that surrounds a central part of dense trabecular bone (type 2), a thin layer of cortical bone that surrounds dense trabecular bone of favorable strength (type 3), and a thin layer of cortical bone that surrounds low density trabecular bone (type 4) (Lekholm and Zarb 1985).

Placing implants into type 1 to type 3 bone leads to good clinical outcomes, whereas type 4 is linked with a lower success rate that is related to the lack of adequate provision of implant primary stability to attain successful osseointegration (Martinez et al. 2001).

In addition to the ratio between cortical and trabecular bone, the latter hold information with regard to bone quality. Trabecular bone is filled with bone marrow, the source of osteoblasts and osteoclasts, and has therefore a higher turnover than cortical bone (Manolagas and Jilka 1995).

Bone to Implant Contact

Studies show that smooth titanium surfaces have less percentage of bone implant contact when compared with rough titanium surfaces (Bowers et al. 1992; Wennerberg et al. 1996; Alsaadi et al. 2007; Baffin and Berman 1991). Albrektsson stated that bone ingrowth in turned titanium surfaces does not occur in spaces smaller than $100\,\mu$ (Albrektsson et al. 1981). However, Wennerberg (Wennerberg et al. 1996) found that bone ground substance will adapt to surface irregularities in the $1-100\,\mu$, and the roughening of the implant surface by $25\,\mu$ by blasting them with aluminum oxide increased the bone to implant contact. Thus, a specific surface roughness on the endosseous section of the implant enhances the regeneration potential at the interface, thus improving clinical implant osseointegration. This opened up the dental implant to a whole variety of surface topography that will be discussed later.

Transmucosal Attachment Around Dental Implants

Eleven different gingival fibers makes up the supra-crestal connective tissue attachment around natural tooth: dentogingival, alveolo-gingival, interpapillary, transgingival, circular, semicircular, dentoperiosteal, transseptal, periosteogingival, intercircular, and inter-gingival fibers. Six of them insert in the cementum dentogingival dentoperiosteal, transseptal, circular, semi-circular, and transgingival (Hassell 1993). Only two are found around the dental implants circular and periosteogingival (Schroeder et al. 1976).

A comparison of clinically healthy marginal tissue around teeth and dental implants had revealed the presence of connective tissue and a junctional epithelium of a length of 2 mm. Collagen fibers around teeth are fan-shaped having the acellular cementum as a center. Around implants they are parallel to the implant surface originating from the bone (Bauman et al. 1993; Berglundh et al. 1991).

In an animal study, the blood vessels of the peri-implant mucosa were found to be terminal branches of larger vessels originating from the periosteum of the bone of the implant site. The microscopic examinations further revealed that in both the gingiva and in the peri-implant mucosa, the blood vessels lateral to the junctional epithelium formed a characteristic "crevicular plexus." While, however, the supracrestal connective tissue lateral to the root cementum was found to be richly vascularized, the corresponding site in the peri-implant tissue was almost devoid of vascular supply (Berglundh et al. 1994).

Probing Around Dental Implants

In animal study on beagle dogs, it was observed that the resistance offered by the gingiva to probing was greater than that offered by the peri-implant mucosa, and consequently the probe penetration became more advanced at implants than at teeth (Ericsson and Lindhe 1993).

In another animal study (Lang et al. 1994) with the purpose to determine the histological level of probe penetration in healthy and inflamed mucosal tissues around implants using probes inserted at 0.2 N Probe penetration increased with the degree of inflammation and in the peri-implantitis group the probe exceeded the connective tissue level by a mean 0.52 mm (mean histological probing depth (HPD): 3.8 mm).

Probing depth measurements at implant and teeth yielded different information, small alterations in probing depth at implants may reflect changes in soft tissue inflammation rather than loss of supporting tissues (Schou et al. 2002).

It was reported that probing with a force of 0.2 N resulted in a probe penetration that was similar at implants and teeth. Probing inflamed tissues at both tooth and implant sites will, however, result in a more advanced probe penetration and the tip of the probe may come closer to the bone crest (Abrahamsson and Soldini 2006).

In a human study (Mombelli et al. 1997), a variety probing depth values were determined at different force levels ranging from 0.25,0.50, 0.75, 1.00, and 1.25 N. Curve analysis of depth force patterns showed that a change in probing force had more impact on the depth reading in the peri-implant than in the periodontal situation. The mean distance between the probe tip and the peri-implant bone crest amounted to 0.75 ± 0.60 mm at 0.25 N probing force. It is concluded that peri-implant probing depth measurements are more sensitive to force variation than periodontal pocket probing. In another study (Gerber et al. 2009), bleeding upon probing (BOP) with different probing forces is analyzed. It showed that 0.15 N might represent the threshold pressure to be applied to avoid false positive BOP readings around oral implants. Hence, probing around implants demonstrated a higher sensitivity compared with probing around teeth. Furthermore, It is not possible to define a range of probing depth compatible with peri-implant health (Caton et al. 2018).

In summary, factors influencing probing depth around implant are as follows:

a. **Inflammation**: will lead to greater numbers than around natural teeth (Lang et al. 1994; Schou et al. 2002; Abrahamsson and Soldini 2006).
b. **Probing force**: a force varying between 0.20–0.25 N should be the one used. Which clinically is very difficult to do (Mombelli et al. 1997; Gerber et al. 2009).
c. **Implant/crown design** (Misch 2014): can affect the accuracy and reproducibility of the probing measurement (Misch 2014).
d. A physiologic probing depth (PD) can't be established (Caton et al. 2018).

Biological Width Around Implants

In 1996, Berglundh and Lindhe (Berglundh and Lindhe 1996) performed an animal study, where on side they did the abutment connection at three month after placement (control side) and on test side, critical amount of connective tissue on the inside of the flap was excised, abutment connection performed, and the trimmed flaps sutured. After a six-month period of plaque control, the animals were sacrificed and biopsies sampled and processed for light microscopy. The length of the junctional epithelium varied within a rather narrow-range: 2.1 mm (control side) and 2.0 mm (test side). The height of the supra bony connective tissue in this model varied between 1.3 ± 0.3 mm (test side) and 1.8 ± 0.4 mm (control side). At sites where the ridge mucosa prior to abutment connection was made thin (≤ 2 mm), wound healing consistently included bone

resorption. This implies that a certain minimum width of the peri-implant mucosa may be required, and that bone resorption may take place to allow a stable soft tissue attachment to form. This was replicated later, the authors found that the thickness of the soft tissue of ≤ 2 mm did influence the crestal bone stability regardless the implant position supracrestal or crestal (Linkevicius et al. 2009; Puisys and Linkevicius 2015).

In another animal study, it was found that dis/reconnection of the abutment resulted in a more apical connective zone attachment and led to bone resorption, postulating that it is due to "biologic width" formation (Abrahamsson et al. 1997). The latter, was confirmed, that a biologic width exists around unloaded and loaded non-submerged one-part titanium implants and that this is a physiologically formed and stable dimension as is found around teeth (Cochran et al. 1997).

The Microgap: Interface Between Implant and Abutment

The location of the microgap has a significant effect on marginal bone formation as evaluated by standardized longitudinal radiography. Bone remodeling occurs rapidly during the early healing phase after implant placement for non-submerged implants and after abutment connection for submerged implants (Hermann et al. 1997).

Jansen et al. (1997) found that the microgap between the implant and the abutment act as a trap for bacteria, possibly can cause inflammatory reactions in the peri-implant soft tissues, these gaps are inevitable and the width of the marginal gaps measured by a scanning electron microscope, was < than 10 microns. In another study by other authors, a significant crestal bone loss occurred in two-piece implant configurations even with the smallest-sized microgaps (<10 microns) possibly due to the movements between implant components (Hermann et al. 2001).

Platform Switching

3I implant innovations introduced the wide diameter implant in 1991. At this time, they didn't have matching abutments; they used the abutments for 4.1 mm diameter platforms. After 13 years review of these cases, the typical pattern of crestal bone resorption was not observed radiographically. They called it "platform switching" and reported it in the literature (Lazzara and Porter 2006).

Canullo in 2007 explained the possible reasons for bone preservation with platform switching is due to the alteration of the microgap location inward and the stress concentration area between the implant and bone (Canullo and Rasperini 2007).

In an experimental study made on a canine model, it was shown that the marginal fBIC (first radiographical Bone to Implant Contact) level was located between 0.37 and 0.52 mm apical to implant–abutment interface using a two-piece implant with non-matching implant and abutment diameters (Berglundh et al. 2005).

Implants with non-matching implant–abutment diameters demonstrated some bone loss; however, it was a small amount. There was no clinically significant difference between submucosal and transmucosal approaches (Jung et al. 2008).

In a retrospective radiographic analysis of 70 platform switched implants placed less than 1.5 mm from an adjacent tooth, findings of this study suggested that implants can be placed 1 mm away from a natural tooth without affecting bone level of the tooth and maintaining the peak of bone in a platform switched implants used as two pieces (Vela et al. 2012).

A systematic review on that subject found that based on the current evidence, the use of abutments with a smaller diameter than their corresponding implant platforms seems to exert beneficial effects on peri-implant marginal bone. Some potential confounding factors, for example, the apico-coronal position of the implant in relation to crestal bone, the presence of various implant micro-textures, the degree of platform switch, and the reliability of examination methods, should be considered when interpreting the present results (Al-Nsour et al. 2012).

Fundamental Criteria in Implant Placement: Healed Ridges

In order to place the dental implant properly, a set of criteria has to be followed:

- Submucosal positioning of the implant shoulder
- Adequate three-dimensional implant positioning
- Long-term stability of esthetic and peri-implant soft tissue contours
- Symmetry of clinical crown volumes between the implant site and contra-lateral teeth

A surgical guide should be made of the wax-up of the anticipated final restoration. A channel will be made for the implant bur to fit in and achieve the osteotomy based on the following:

1. The depth of the osteotomy should be 3–4 mm from the zenith of the anticipated final restoration (Esposito et al. 1993; Buser et al. 2004).
2. The implant shoulder should be 1.5 mm away from the adjacent tooth (Al-Nsour et al. 2012; Grunder et al. 2005).
3. The implant shoulder bucco-lingually should be 1 mm palatal to the point of emergence at adjacent teeth (Esposito et al. 1993).
4. To achieve hard and soft tissue stability a buccal thickness of 2 mm is needed (Choquet et al. 2001).
5. In regard to achieve a papilla between an implant and natural tooth, a distance of 5 mm from the implant shoulder to the contact point is necessary (Tarnow et al. 2000).

In the case of two adjacent implants, a 3 mm distance between the implants is needed (Grunder et al. 2005).

Implant Surface Topography

Implant Topography on Wound Healing

Implant Materials

The ideal implant material on a broad level should be biocompatible i.e. have optimal qualities regarding mechanical aspects, physicochemical stability, absence of toxicity and immunogenicity and under no circumstances intervene with the normal tissue healing. The modern concept of biocompatibility however is defined also by the ability of the material to perform a specific function. The surface of dental implants for that reason must allow the adsorption of specific proteins to trigger the mechanisms involved in ossointegration.

Traditionally, implants are made out of metals ranging from titanium, titanium alloys, gold alloys, etc. and are now being fabricated by polymers such as Polytetrafluoroethylene (PTFE), Polyetheretherketone (PEEK) and even ceramics such as zirconia. It was noted that pure titanium limited the mechanical strength, justifying the use of titanium alloys. The major implant companies in use today use either pure grade titanium or a titanium alloy.

Bone Healing

What makes Titanium biocompatible is its *oxide surface layer. Titanium forms spontaneously a very thin oxide film on its surface at the room temperature that continues to grow at a rate of few nanometers per year. It is through this film that the contact between the implant and the body is established.*

The placement of an implant also initiates a cascade of wound healing inflammatory cell responses and release of TNF-1alpha, and IL-1. By activating their target cells, these cytokines produce a second wave of cells response by releasing chemokines (MCP-1 family). At the in vivo bone implant interface, cellular attachment is mediated via the oxide layer and a protein rich layer to which cells adhere using a variety of surface receptors, mainly from the integrin family. The healing around the implant is characterized by an increase in bone-implant contact starting at the implantation, while the biomechanical stability slightly decreases over the first weeks.

The implant to bone interface provides two theories on healing after implant placement: Fibro-osseous integration, and osseointegration (Newman and Takei 2014). Fibro-osseous integration is defined as tissue to implant contact with healthy dense collagenous tissue between the implant and bone. Osseointegration, a concept introduced by Branemark (1985) is defined as a direct functional and structural connection between living bone and the surface of a load carrying implant.

Generally rough metal surfaces osseointegrate whereas smooth metal surfaces tend to fibrointegrate (Ricci et al. 1991).

Principles of Surface Treatment, Topographies, and Roughness

Implant Design

Regardless of design or size, the surgical success rate of implants is quoted to be higher than 98%. Macroscopic design considerations include the gross body design and thread geometry. Endosseous implants, which are utilized today, have a unique history starting with the advent of hollow cylindrical implants.

Threads or a screw shape was added to the body of the cylinder to achieve initial stability and increase the implant surface area. These threading systems have varying numbers of threads, distance between threads, and unique surface topography. Early endosseous implants also had parallel walls which have now made way to the tapered wall to help distribute compressive forces placed on the implant. Thread geometry describes the pitch, depth, and configuration of threads on a specific implant and can play an important role in stress distribution to the implant and bone. Common shapes of threads include the V-shape, square, buttress, revers buttress, and spiral.

Implant Surface Topography

First generation implants were machine washed with a smooth surface, successfully used in clinical trials for 50 years, and selected due to their mechanical properties and corrosion resistance under physiological conditions. Machined surfaces, used by Branemark, were considered to be minimally rough (Sa 0f .3-1 micrometer) (Wennerberg and Albrektsson 2000).

Since varying surfaces materials and roughness have an effect on the osseointegration of an implant, biomaterial scientists started to modify the surface topography

of the implants to reduce healing and loading time and increase primary stability. The second generation implants saw a large variation in surface properties. Structural and chemical compositions such as mechanical blasting with or without etching, bioactive coatings, anodized surfaces, and laser modifications were all introduced. These modifications can be either additive or subtractive, but ultimately aim to increase surface roughness. The objectives of surface roughness are: increased surface area of implant adjacent to bone (Wennerberg and Albrektsson 2000). A moderately rough surface (Sa 1.0–2.0 μm) is a major key to success of the implant from a surface topography point of view because it shows stronger bone responses than smoother or rougher surfaces (Albrektsson and Wennerberg 2004). Implant surface topography modification can accelerate and improve implant osseointegration by playing an important role in molecular interactions and cellular responses (Ito et al. 1991).

Implant Surface Specificities: Advantages and Disadvantages

Morphological methods may be additive or subtractive in nature. Sand blasting is an example of a subtractive method in which implants are blasted with varying particle sizes to produce a small, medium, or large grit. Particle collision with the implant surface produces craters. Roughness of the implant is dictated by particle size, time of blasting, and distance from the source of particles to the implant surface. The goal of sand blasting is to clean surface contaminants, roughen the surface, and produce surface compressive residual stress.

A second subtractive method for modifying implant topography is chemical etching. In this case, the metallic implant is submerged into an acidic solution which erodes its surface by removing grains and grain boundaries, creating pits of specific diameter. Certain impurities are more sensitive to etching resulting in a selective removal of material. The bulk material, surface microstructure, concentration of the acidic solution, soaking time, and temperature are all factors determining the result of chemical attack and microstructure alterations on the surface of the implant.

The two previous techniques can be used together for an implant that is sand blasted and acid etched. These surfaces are produced by a large grit sand blasting process followed by etching with hydrochloric or sulfuric acid. The resulting topography is a dual surface roughness, and additionally removes all embedded blasting particles.

Much more recently, additional modifications have been made to these sand blasted and etched surfaces, giving birth to the concept of SLActive. Rinsing SLA implants in a nitrogen rich atmosphere and storing in saline solution until installation, the amount of carbon communication can be reduced, improving the hydrophilicity of the implant surface. Studies show that SLActive hydrophilic implants achieve higher bone contact stability at earlier time points when compared to SLA implants, and dramatically reduced healing times. "The two previous techniques can be used together for an implant that is sand blasted and acid etched" the words producing a surface that is called SLA (sand blasted large grid acid etched).

Continuing with subtractive methods, the next topography results from anodized surfaces, e.g. TiUnite implant surface. A voltage is applied on the titanium implant immersed in electrolyte resulting in micro-pores of varying diameter that demonstrate lack of cytotoxicity and show increased cell attachment and proliferation.

The last subtractive method to be discussed is laser modification of implants. High intensity Nano-seconds of laser light beam strike the ablative surface and generate short lived plasma which causes a shock wave to travel the implant. The shock waves induce compression residual stress that penetrated beneath the surface and strengthens the implant resulting in improvement in fatigue life and retarding the stress corrosion cracking occurrence. In laser modifications there is no contact of the implant with anything, so it is a contamination free peening method.

The first additive method or coating to be discussed is plasma spray. Plasma spraying is one of the most common methods for surface modification using hydroxyapatite.

Plasma spraying is used for the application of both titanium of hydroxyapatite on metallic cores. Plasma coating can increase the surface area of bone implant interfaces by 600%. Several documented disadvantages do exist with plasma spray including poor long-term adherence of the coating to substrate, non-uniformity of thickness, and variations in crystallinity and composition of the coating. Additional additive methods include sputtering deposition, porous sintering, and chemical surface additive modifications (Pilliar 1998).

Although some attempts have been made to mathematically describe the ideal surface morphology, there is currently no consensus on the degree of the roughness that is optimum for bone cell attachment. The majority of the commercially available implants are moderately rough (Raghavendra et al. 2005).

To summarize the advantages of rough surfaces that have been extensively documented in the literature are the following:

- Enhanced bone-to-implant contact and increased removal torque forces
- Improved cell attachment
- Increased biomechanical interaction of the implant with bone
- Better early bone-to-implant contact

For the aforementioned reasons moderately rough hydrophilic implant surfaces are the preferred ones especially in suboptimal situations, e.g. sinus grafts, areas of poor bone quality and immediate placed implants.

References

Abrahamsson, I. and Soldini, C. (2006). Probe penetration in peri-odontal and peri-implant tissues: an experimental study in the beagle dog. *Clin. Oral Implants Res.* 17: 601–605.

Abrahamsson, I., Berglundh, T., and Lindhe, J. (1997). The mucosal barrier following abutment dis/reconnection: an experimental study in dogs. *J. Clin. Periodontol.* 24 (8): 568–572.

Albrektsson, T., Brånemark, P.I., Hansson, H.A., and Lindström, J. (1981). Osseointegrated titanium implants: requirements for ensuring a long-lasting, direct bone-to-implant anchorage in man. *Acta Orthop. Scand.* 52 (2): 155–170.

Al-Nsour, M.M., Chan, H.L., and Wang, H.L. (2012). Effect of the platform-switching technique on preservation of peri-implant marginal bone: a systematic review. *Int. J. Oral Maxillofac. Implants* 27 (1).

Alsaadi, G., Quirnynen, M., Michiels, K. et al. (2007). A biomechanical assessment of the relation between the oral implant stability at insertion and subjective bone quality assessment. *J. Clin. Periodontal.* 34: 359–366.

Baffin, R.A. and Berman, C.L. (1991). The excessive loss of Branemark fixtures in type IV bone: A 5-year analysis. *J. Periodontal.* 62: 2–4.

Bauman, G.R., Rapley, J.W., Hallmon, W.W., and Mills, M. (1993). The peri-implant sulcus. *Int. J. Oral Maxillofac. Implants* 8 (3).

Berglundh, T. and Lindhe, J. (1996). Dimension of the periimplant mucosa: biological width revisited. *J. Clin. Periodontol.* 23 (10): 971–973.

Berglundh, T., Lindhe, J., Ericsson, I. et al. (1991). The soft tissue barrier at implants and teeth. *Clin. Oral Implants Res.* 2 (2): 81–90.

Berglundh, T., Lindhe, J., Jonsson, K., and Ericsson, I. (1994). The topography of the vascular systems in the periodontal and peri-implant tissues in the dog. *J. Clin. Periodontol.* 21 (3): 189–193.

Berglundh, T., Abrahamsson, I., and Lindhe, J. (2005). Bone reactions to longstanding functional load at implants: an experimental study in dogs. *J. Clin. Periodontol.* 32 (9): 925–932.

Bowers, K.T., Keller, J.C., Randolph, B.A. et al. (1992). Optimization of surface micromorphology for enhanced osteoblast responses in vitro. *Int. J. Oral Maxillofac. Implants* 7: 302–310.

Branemark, P.I. (1977). Osseointegrated implants in the treatment of the edentulous jaw. Experience from a 10-year period. *Scand. J. Plast. Reconstr. Surg. Suppl.* 16.

Brånemark, P.I., Breine, U., Adell, R. et al. (1969). Intra-osseous anchorage of dental prostheses: I. Experimental studies. *Scand. J. Plast. Rreconstr. Surg.* 3 (2): 81–100.

Buser, D., Martin, W., and Belser, U.C. (2004). Optimizing esthetics for implant restorations in the anterior maxilla: anatomic and surgical considerations. *Int. J. Oral Maxillofac. Implants* 19 (7).

Canullo, L. and Rasperini, G. (2007). Preservation of peri-implant soft and hard tissues using platform switching of implants placed in immediate extraction sockets: a proof-of-concept study with 12-to 36-month follow-up. *Int. J. Oral Maxillofac. Implants* 22 (6).

Newman, M.G. and Takei, H. (ed.) (2014). *Carranza's Clinical Periodontology*, 12e.

Caton, J., Armitage, G., Berglundh, T. et al. (2018). A new classification scheme for periodontal and peri-implant diseases and conditions- Introduction and key changes from the 1999 classification. *J. Periodontol.* 89 (Suppl 1): S1–S8.

Choquet, V., Hermans, M., Adriaenssens, P. et al. (2001). Clinical and radiographic evaluation of the papilla level adjacent to single-tooth dental implants. A retrospective study in the maxillary anterior region. *J. Periodontol.* 72 (10): 1364–1371.

Cochran, D.L., Hermann, J.S., Schenk, R.K. et al. (1997). Biologic width around titanium implants. A histometric analysis of the implanto-gingival junction around unloaded and loaded nonsubmerged implants in the canine mandible. *J. Periodontol.* 68 (2): 186–197.

El-Chaar, E.S. (2011). Immediate placement and provisionalization of implant-supported, single-tooth restorations: a retrospective study. *Int. J. Periodont. Restor. Dent.* 31 (4).

Ericsson, I. and Lindhe, J. (1993). Probing depth at implants and teeth: an experimental study in the dog. *J. Clin. Periodontol.* 20 (9): 623–627.

Esposito, M., Ekestubbe, A., and Gröndahl, K. (1993). Radiological evaluation of marginal bone loss at tooth

surfaces facing single Brånemark implants. *Clin. Oral Implants Res.* 4 (3): 151–157.

Gerber, J.A., Tan, W.C., Balmer, T.E. et al. (2009). Bleeding on probing and pocket probing depth in relation to probing pressure and mucosal health around oral implants. *Clin. Oral Implants Res.* 20 (1): 75–78.

Grunder, U., Gracis, S., and Capelli, M. (2005). Influence of the 3-D bone-to-implant relationship on esthetics. *Int. J. Periodont. Restor. Dent.* 25 (2): 113–119.

Hassell, T.M. (1993). Tissues and cells of the periodontium. *Periodontology 2000* 3 (1): 9–38.

Hermann, J.S., Cochran, D.L., Nummikoski, P.V., and Buser, D. (1997). Crestal bone changes around titanium implants. A radiographic evaluation of unloaded nonsubmerged and submerged implants in the canine mandible. *J. Periodontol.* 68 (11): 1117–1130.

Hermann, J.S., Schoolfield, J.D., Schenk, R.K. et al. (2001). Influence of the size of the microgap on crestal bone changes around titanium implants. A histometric evaluation of unloaded non-submerged implants in the canine mandible. *J. Periodontol.* 72 (10): 1372–1383.

Ito, Y., Kajihara, M., and Imanishi, Y. (1991). Materials for enhancing cell adhesion by immobilization of cell-adhesive peptide. *J. Biomed. Mater. Res. Part A* 25: 1325–1337.

Jansen, V.K., Conrads, G., and Richter, E.J. (1997). Microbial leakage and marginal fit of the implant-abutment interface. *Int. J. Oral Maxillofac. Implants* 12 (4).

Jung, R.E., Jones, A.A., Higginbottom, F.L. et al. (2008). The influence of non-matching implant and abutment diameters on radiographic crestal bone levels in dogs. *J. Periodontol.* 79 (2): 260–270.

Lang, N.P., Wetzel, A.C., Stich, H., and Caffesse, R.G. (1994). Histologic probe penetration in healthy and inflamed peri-implant tissues. *Clin. Oral Implants Res.* 5 (4): 191–201.

Lazzara, R.J. and Porter, S.S. (2006). Platform switching: a new concept in implant dentistry for controlling postrestorative crestal bone levels. *Int. J. Periodont. Restor. Dent.* 26 (1).

Lekholm, U. and Zarb, G. (1985). Patient selection and preparation. In: *Tissue-Integrated Prostheses: Osseointegration in Clinical Dentistry*. Chicago: Quintessence (ed. P.I. Branemark, G.A. Zarb and T. Albrektsson), 199–209.

Linkevicius, T., Apse, P., Grybauskas, S., and Puisys, A. (2009). The influence of soft tissue thickness on crestal bone changes around implants: a 1-year prospective controlled clinical trial. *Int. J. Oral Maxillofac. Implants* 24 (4).

Manolagas, S.C. and Jilka, R.L. (1995). Bone marrow, cytokines, and bone remodeling. Emerging insights into the pathophysiology of osteoporosis. *N. Engl. J. Med.* 332: 305–311.

Martinez, H., Davarpanah, M., Missika, P. et al. (2001). Optimal implant stabilization in low density bone. *Clin. Oral Implants Res.* 12: 423–432.

Misch, C.E. (2014). An implant is not a tooth: a comparison of periodontal indices. In: *Dental Implant Prosthetics* E-Book, 46.

Mombelli, A., Muumlhle, T., Brägger, U. et al. (1997 Dec). Comparison of periodontal and peri-implant probing by depth-force pattern analysis. *Clin. Oral Implants Res.* 8 (6): 448–454.

O'Sullivan, D., Sennerby, L., and Meredith, N. (2000). Measurements comparing the initial stability of five designs of dental implants: a human cadaver study. *Clin. Implant Dent. Relat. Res.* 2: 85–91.

Pilliar, R.M. (1998). Overview of surface variability of metallic endosseous dental implants: textures and porous surface structured designs. *Implant Dent.* 7 (4): 305–314.

Puisys, A. and Linkevicius, T. (2015). The influence of mucosal tissue thickening on crestal bone stability around bone-level implants. A prospective controlled clinical trial. *Clin. Oral Implants Res.* 26 (2): 123–129.

Raghavendra, S., Wood, M.C., and Taylor, T.D. (2005). Early wound healing around endosseous implants: A review of literature. *Int. J. Oral Maxillofac. Implants* 20: 425–431.

Ricci, J.L., Spivak, J.M., Blumenthal, N.C., and Alexander, H. (1991). *The Bone-Biomaterial Interface* (ed. J.E. Davies), 334–349. Toronto, Ont. Canada.: University of Toronto Press.

Schenk, R.K. and Buser, D. (1998). Osseointegration: a reality. *Periodontology 2000* (17): 22–35.

Schou, S., Holmstrup, P., Stolze, K. et al. (2002). Probing around implants and teeth with healthy or inflamed marginal tissues. A histologic comparison in cynomolgus monkeys (*Macaca fascicularis*). *Clin. Oral Implants Res.* 13: 113–126.

Schroeder, A., Pohler, O., and Sutter, F. (1976). Tissue reaction to an implant of a titanium hollow cylinder with a titanium surface spray layer. *Schweiz. Monatsschr. Zahnheilkund.* 86 (7): 713–727.

Schroeder, A., van der Zypen, E., Stich, H., and Sutter, F. (1981). The reactions of bone, connective tissue, and epithelium to endosteal implants with titanium-sprayed surfaces. *J. Maxillofac. Surg.* (9): 15–25.

Tarnow, D., Cho, S.C., and Wallace, S.S. (2000). The effect of inter-implant distance on the height of inter-implant bone crest. *J. Periodontol.* 71 (4): 546–549.

Vela, X., Méndez, V., Rodríguez, X. et al. (2012). Crestal bone changes on platform-switched implants and adjacent teeth when the tooth-implant distance is less than 1.5 mm. *Int. J. Periodont. Restor. Dent.* 32 (2): 149.

Wennerberg, A. and Albrektsson, T. Suggested Guidelines for the Topographi(2000). Evaluation of implant surfaces. *Int. J. Oral Maxillofac. Implants* 15: 331–344.

Wennerberg, A., Albrektsson, T., and Andersson, B. (1996). Bone tissue response to commercially pure titanium implants blasted with fine and coarse particles of aluminum oxide. *Int. J. Oral Maxillofac. Implants* 11 (1).

Zarb, G.A. and Albrektsson, T. (1991). Osseointegration: a requiem for the periodontal ligament. *Int. J. Periodont. Restor. Dent.* 11 (1): 88–91.

Further Reading

Albrektsson, T. and Wennerberg, A. (2004). Oral implant surfaces: Part 1-Review focusing on topographic and chemical properties of different surfaces and in vivo responses to them. *Int. J. Prosthodont.* 17 (5): 536–543.

Ballo, A.M., Omar, O., Xia, W., and Palmquist, A. (ed.) (2011). *Dental Implant Surfaces - Physicochemical Properties, Biological Performance, and Trends*. IntechOpen.

Heimke, G. and Stock, D. (1984). Clinical application of ceramic osseo – or soft tissue - integrated implant. *Orthop. Ceram. Implants* 4: 1–19.

Spray, J.R., Black, C.G., Morris, H.F., and Ochi, S. (2000). The influence of bone thickness on facial marginal bone response: stage 1 placement through stage 2 uncovering. *Ann. Periodontol.* 5 (1): 119–128.

15

Examination and Diagnosis
Zahra Bagheri

Ashman Department of Periodontology and Implant Dentistry, New York University College of Dentistry, New York, NY, USA

Radiographic Examination

In addition to an accurate and thorough clinical examination, a radiographic analysis of each patient is warranted in order to provide a catered diagnosis. Diagnostic imaging modalities help to develop and implement cohesive and comprehensive implant treatment plans. Selection of proper imaging modalities is important to both limit radiation to the patient and accurately diagnose.

Cone Beam Computed Tomography

Cone beam computed tomography (CBCT) provides a diagnostic and measurable three-dimensional interpretation of bone and soft tissue. This allows the practitioner to localize anatomic features for implant placement and avoid delicate structures such as nerves, arteries, etc. X-ray beams in this tool are divergent, forming a cone. Originally designed and used in the medical field, advances in the limitations of radiation dosage have allowed the CBCT to be used in dental offices. During the CBCT, the machine rotates around the patient's head while obtaining hundreds of images. This set of images is referred to as the volumetric data set. The scanning software analyzes and interprets this data to reconstruct a three-dimensional image of the hard and soft tissue (Pal et al. 2010). While the CBCT shares many similarities to the tradition CT scan used in medicine, there are many differences in the reconstruction of the image. A CBCT alone does not provide the exact position and orientation of a prosthetically driven implant; however, in conjunction with diagnostic templates, this precision may be achieved. Types of diagnostic templates include: Vaquform, acrylic, templates fabricated with radiopaque denture teeth, complex tomography, and panoramic radiography (Misch 2014). Vaquform templates are used on a diagnostic cast with wax-up. The material uses barium sulfate which will be radiopaque on the CBCT.

This method of template production allows the visualization of restorations and tooth borders, however does not indicate the exact position nor orientation of the proposed implant. This method can further be altered by drilling a 2 mm channel through the ideal prosthetic position of the implant crown. This will align with the implants ideal position, and be visible on the CT examination. The second modality of template production is an acrylic template. Similar to the Vaquform method, this allows for drilling of a channel and filling this void with gutta percha to visualize the ideal position of the implant on the scan (Asher et al. 1999). The third technique includes using radiopaque denture teeth. An additional advantage of denture teeth is that the template/stent can be modified for use as a surgical stent. Lastly, the complex tomography, and panoramic radiography techniques can be utilized. They involve placing ball bearings to align with the implant positions and curvature of the arch (Shannoun et al. 2008). These modalities are seldom used, however are available.

Clinical Parameters

Patients never really want implants. What is truly desired is the most convenient, safe, and predictable way to restore oral function AND in most cases oral facial esthetics. In the case of implant dental reconstruction, in order to obtain the most satisfactory outcome for the patient and dentist, this requires absolute prioritization of what the patient wants and how they look at themselves during and after treatment. Thus, it is imperative to provide patients with all information pertaining to treatment considerations and procedures. In order to predictably accomplish this, the relevant medical and dental history, physical examination, especially critical anatomic and physiological parameters, and understanding of the benefits and limitations of each implant system and method are essential.

Clinical Examination

Esthetics naturally remains one if not the major concern for a patient and can be extremely challenging considering the effects of aging, post-dental tooth loss resorption, and anatomic and medical considerations. For the population seeking permanent fixture options, often the best esthetic and functional result may not be the most complex or necessitate absolute replacement of each lost tooth with an implant fixture. Rather, the intrinsic mechanics of occlusal forces and restoration of hard and soft tissues is more important. Also, since implant procedures are costly and time consuming this aspect of treatment is often most perplexing for the patient and the dental provider. Accurate and reliable evidence-based decisions along with immediate and long-term risks and benefits are often excluded or not fully understood and can lead to dissatisfaction and/or further oral health deterioration.

Factors Influencing Surgical Management

Prior to initiation of therapy it is crucial to evaluate whether the patient is healthy enough to undergo and tolerate implant rehabilitation. Accurate and up-to-date health history, current medications, prior surgeries, allergies, and any habits must be known. For example, bleeding or hepatic disorders can affect blood clotting, resulting in complications during a procedure and severely affect post implant surgery recovery. Further, bone physiology and healing ability leading to predictable osseointegration will be aggravated by chronic or systemic diseases including cardiovascular diseases, osteoporosis, diabetes, severe periodontal disease, chemo- or radiotherapy, immunodeficiency, chronic infections, pregnancy or lactation, or even prior large bone reconstructions that may interfere with bone regeneration and integration (Davies et al. 2002). Post-menopausal women may have affected bone regeneration capacity. Therefore, it is always necessary to be aware, prior to any procedure, of such conditions which affect fixture healing and gear our decision making as to whether to proceed with implant reconstruction, or not accordingly.

Habits, i.e. smoking affects wound healing in several ways. It reduces migration capacity of stromal cells around implant surface during osseointegration, directly irritates soft tissues healing, and prevents mucosal seal after osseointegration. Suggest quitting smoking. Bruxism is a common parafunctional habit, which induces damage of dental surfaces and results in loss of dental tissues, occurrence of wear facets, loss of vertical dimension, temporomandibular joint disorders, neuromuscular pain, and perhaps most importantly, excessive mechanical overloading leading to ultimate mechanical and biological failures (Juodzbalys and Kubilius 2013). These and many other personal habits heavily impact implant success and must be mitigated appropriately and respectfully before dental implant delivery.

Following careful consideration of the medical/dental history the next step is the clinical and anatomical investigation. Implant success highly depends on a sophisticated clinical examination and a prescribed or guided planning approach. The clinical examination provides a clear-cut difference between the dos and don'ts of the procedure and the structural and functional demands.

A complete understanding of the anatomy is vital and anatomical anomalies should always be considered. Relationship of the anticipated implants with the maxillary sinuses, trigeminal nerve, facial/skeletal arteries, and veins should be mastered for any type of implant placement. There should be adequate interdental and inter-occlusal space for implant restoration to avoid unnecessary damage or injury to healthy teeth or prime surrounding locations.

Other critical factors include the quantity and quality of bone, type of prosthesis chosen, and the occlusal loads which will ultimately decide the position and number of implants needed (Misch 2014).

Once conditions are deemed favorable for the procedure, guided treatment planning is highly advised. Guided planning ensures smooth execution of the procedure and multidisciplinary coordination. Post-implant recovery time is slow and requires careful follow up. When multiple health professionals are working together, it is vital to plan each step to avoid unnecessary delays or missed opportunities. Moreover, it is essential to plan the procedure in a way that it does not interfere with a patient's social and private life because it might lead to either making the patient feel depressed or socially isolated. Ultimately, the patient must be completely aware of the intricacies and adjustments of the treatment. They must know the importance of keeping up to their appointments and not terminating treatment halfway, which might be more deleterious than not receiving treatment. In summary, complete medical, dental history, and physical examination are the foundation upon which dental restoration with implant fixtures and prosthetics may proceed.

Factors Influencing Prosthetic Parameters

A number of factors influence the prosthetic parameters of implants and their subsequent crowns. Among these are the availability of bone, density of bone, and force factors related to the patient. Additional considerations are to be made based on the number of teeth to be restored, and whether the prosthesis is fixed or removable.

Bone availability may the most significant predisposing factor to influence implant placement. Previously, implants were placed in native bone and as a result the prosthesis would have large cantilever forces or poor esthetics. As we advance in the dental field, a new system of setting a prosthetic goal and working backwards has developed. These circumstances require grafting and other augmentation procedures first in order to place a prosthetically driven implant (Misch 2014). Prosthetic options for replacing missing teeth can be divided into fixed and removable options. Within the fixed options there are three subgroups: (i) Prosthesis that only replaces the crown and appears like a natural tooth, (ii) prosthesis to replace the crown and portion of the root. The crown contour in these scenarios appears normal in the occlusal half, but may be elongated or over-contoured in the cervical half. (iii) A prosthesis to replace both missing crowns and gingiva. The removable subset has two groups including a removable prosthesis completely supported by implant or a prosthesis supported by both implants and soft tissue.

Bone density should also be considered in the prosthetic and implant treatment planning process. The densest bone is found in the mandibular anterior region and gradually becomes less dense moving posteriorly. The maxilla is less dense than the mandible and also become less dense as we move posterior in the arch (Kim et al. 2012). The strength of the bone supporting an endosteal implant is directly related to the density of that bone (Misch 2014). To compensate for poor quality bone, prosthetic design must be considered. Implants should be placed such that the angle of load on the implant should be in an axial direction, narrower occlusal tables should be designed, splinting of crowns of adjacent implants may be considered, and the use of night guards is likely indicated (Davies et al. 2002; Vasconcellos et al. 2011; Yuan and Sukotjo 2013).

Force factors are one last consideration to be made when considering prosthetic options for patient treatment. The extent, distribution, duration, type, and direction of these forces can impact implant and prosthetic components (Vasconcellos et al. 2011). Parafunctional habits, load forces, and nature of the opposing arch can influence the stress environment of the implant and prosthesis (Kim et al. 2012). To combat these factors a number of modifications can be made including elimination of premature contacts and fabrication of a night guard.

References

Asher, E.S., Evans, J.H., Wright, R.F., and Wazen, J.J. (1999). Fabrication and use of a surgical template for placing implants to retain an auricular prosthesis. *J. Prosthet. Dent.* 81: 228–233.

Davies, S.J., Gray, R.J., and Young, M.P. (2002). Good occlusal practice in the provision of implant borne prostheses. *Br. Dent. J.* 192: 79–88.

Juodzbalys, G. and Kubilius, M. (2013). Clinical and radiological classification of the jawbone anatomy in endosseous dental implant treatment. *J. Oral Maxillofac. Res.* 4: e2.

Kim, H.J., Yu, S.K., Lee, M.H. et al. (2012). Cortical and cancellous bone thickness on the anterior region of alveolar bone in Korean: a study of dentate human cadavers. *J. Adv. Prosthodont.* 4: 146–152.

Misch, C.E. (2014). *Dental Implant Prosthetics*, 2e. Amsterdam, Netherlands: Elsevier Health Sciences.

Pal, U.S., Chand, P., Dhiman, N.K. et al. (2010). Role of surgical stents in determining the position of implants. *Natl. J. Maxillofac. Surg.* 1: 20–23.

Shannoun, F., Blettner, M., Schmidberger, H., and Zeeb, H. (2008). Radiation protection in diagnostic radiology. *Dtsch. Ärztebl. Int.* 105: 41–46.

Vasconcellos, L.G., Nishioka, R.S., Vasconcellos, L.M., and Nishioka, L.N. (2011). Effect of axial loads on implant-supported partial fixed prostheses by strain gauge analysis. *J. Appl. Oral Sci.* 19: 610–615.

Yuan, J.C. and Sukotjo, C. (2013). Occlusion for implant-supported fixed dental prostheses in partially edentulous patients: a literature review and current concepts. *J. Periodontal Implant Sci.* 43: 51–57.

Further Reading

Dursun, E. et al. A comparison of esthetic features of pre-existing natural tooth versus post-implant restoration in the esthetic zone: a retrospective 12-month follow-up. *Int. J. Oral Maxillofac. Implants* 33 (4): 919–928. https://doi.org/10.11607/jomi.6465.

Kazuhiro, K. (2017). Potentially risk factors of remaining tooth extraction in long term cases of implant therapy: retrospective study in 10 years follow up patients. *Clin. Oral Implants Res.* 28: 378. https://doi.org/10.1111/clr.376_13042.

Linetskiy, I. et al. (2017). Impact of annual bone loss and different bone quality on dental implant success – a finite element study. *Comput. Biol. Med.* 91: 318–325. https://doi.org/10.1016/j.compbiomed.2017.09.016.

Ibbetson, R., Hemmings, K., and Harris, I. (2017). The British society for restorative dentistry: guidelines for crowns, fixed bridges and implants. *Dent. Update* 44 (5): 374-6, 378-80, 382-4, 386.

16

Prosthetic Considerations
Zahra Bagheri

Ashman Department of Periodontology and Implant Dentistry, New York University College of Dentistry, New York, NY, USA

Review of the Esthetic Parameters

When considering the natural aesthetics in patient treatment, there are a number of components to be considered. These include extra-oral, intra-oral, and indirect components. Extra-oral components are comprised of the face and smile line. An adequate facial analysis will address issues such as any midline deviations and occlusal plane discrepancy. It has been noted that the mean threshold for acceptable dental midline deviation was 2.2 ± 1.5 mm (Beyer and Lindauer 1998). Furthermore, natural and subtle asymmetry is often unimportant in judging the facial attractiveness, so much so that beautiful faces may be functionally asymmetrical (Zaidel and Cohen 2005). In addition to a midline analysis, the planes of the inter-pupillary line and frontal occlusal plane are assessed. In an ideal situation these two lines are parallel to one another and perpendicular to the midline. Phonetics is also addressed. The second portion of the extra-oral evaluation is the smile line. Tjan et al. (1984) evaluated the smiles of 454 dental hygiene students 20–30 years old and defined a standard of normalcy for the esthetic smile. A high smile line (10.57%) was defined as revealing the total cervico-incisal length of the maxillary anterior teeth and a contiguous band of gingiva. Average smiles (68.94%) revealed 75–100% of the maxillary anterior teeth and only interproximal gingiva. Low smiles (20.48%) displayed less than 75% of the anterior teeth (Tjan et al. 1984). In addition to evaluating the amount of maxillary teeth and gingiva showing, they also assessed the curvature of the incisal edges in relationship to the lower lip finding that 84.8% had a parallel curve, 13.88% showed a straight curve, and only 1.32% have a reverse curve.

Intraorally, the esthetic components are comprised of the teeth and dento-gingival complex. Restoratively driven implant placement dictates taking teeth size and proportion into account. For example, the average mesio-distal

dimension of a maxillary central incisor is 8.45 mm, while the lateral is only 6.44 mm. When assessing teeth, the shape or relative dimensions must also be considered. In 1999 Snow described and published what they determined to be the "Golden Percentages" of esthetics in relation maxillary anterior tooth size. In this ratio, the centrals take up 25% of the width respectively followed by the lateral incisors with 15% and the canines with 10%. This equates to a proportion of 1.618 : 1.618. The authors suggest that this proportion be used as a striating point, but not a definitive methodology due to anatomical and soft tissue variations that inherently exist. Assessment of the maxillary anterior teeth can also be made with respect to the axial alignment. Rufenacht (1990) described that the general mesial inclination is more pronounced from the central incisors to the canines. He went on to elaborate and describe the contact points of these teeth as descending from the incisal to cervical third as we move laterally towards the canines. The last component of tooth related esthetics is the gingival zenith, or rather, the most apical point of gingival tissue. The gingival zenith was noted to be 1 mm distal to the tooth midline on central incisors, 0.4 mm distal on lateral incisors, and coincident with the midline on the canines.

The dento-gingival complex is comprised of the periodontium (and its subsequent biotype), the gingival line, and the dimension of the supracrestal tissue. Generally speaking, there are two gingival biotypes: thick/flat and thin/scalloped. A thick gingival biotype is related to square teeth and bulbous convexities in the cervical third of the tooth. It often correlates to a gingival margin at the cementoenamel junction (CEJ) and has thicker and more fibrotic tissue, thicker bone, increased quality and quantity of keratinized attached gingiva, and greater contact areas between adjacent teeth. The thin/scalloped biotype is associated with a triangular tooth form has delicate soft tissue, presence of scalloped osseous form with dehiscence or fenestration, reduced keratinized tissue, and often lack of interproximal tissue fill (Olsson and Lindhe 1991; Weisgold 1977). Biotype will dictate response to bacteria and treatment. For example, a thick biotype is more resilient and therefore prone to pocket formation. In the same scenario with a thin biotype, recession is the most common outcome (Müller et al. 2000). Additionally, tissue biotype dictates the phenomenon known as creeping attachment. Thick biotypes demonstrated significantly more creeping attachment than thin biotypes (Pontoriero et al. 2001).

The gingival line, or junction between hard and soft tissue, is considered to be the key to esthetic harmony. This scallop is created by the confluence of the periodontium and teeth. The level of the gingival line on the central incisors is ideally the same as the canines, with the laterals being 1 mm coronal. It must harmonize bilaterally with the smile line, the facial midline, and axial inclination of the teeth (Smukler and Chaibi 1997). Schluger (1949) stated that the form of the underlying bone dictated soft tissue results and that the difference between the levels and shapes of osseous tissue and the soft tissue caused recurrent pocketing and recurrent periodontal disease. In contrast, Doza De Bastos (1977) found that the degree and configuration of osseous scalloping is determined by the surface topography of the tooth. Gingival form is dictated both by the osseous configuration and the surface anatomy of the tooth. In health, bone and tissue are adjacent to one another and consistent with each other in form. In periodontal disease, the hard and soft tissues are no longer consistent with or adjacent to each other, creating disharmony and a poor esthetic result. Overall, the contour or shape of the gingiva varies considerably and depends on the shape of the teeth, their alignment in the arch, the location and size of the area of proximal contact, and the dimension of the facial and lingual gingival embrasures.

The final component of the dento-gingival complex is the interdental papilla. The lateral borders and tip of the interdental papilla are formed by the free gingiva from adjacent teeth. The center portion is formed by attached gingiva. Filling of the interproximal contact space was noted in 98% of sites with 5 mm or less measured from the peak of bone to the contact point. If this distance was greater than 5 mm, a black triangle was evident (Tarnow et al. 1992). Incorporation of a customized temporary abutment and immediate fixed provisional facilitates the maintenance of the gingival architecture for optimal aesthetics and eliminates the need for a removable prosthesis during healing.

The indirect component associated with esthetics is the bony housing for the implants. In other words, the available height of bone, soft tissue volume, and three-dimensional position of the anticipated implant restoration are among the numerous concerns that must be addressed prior to the initiation of treatment (Saadoun et al. 1999). Insufficient bone can preclude proper implant positioning while inadequately treated soft tissue will not exhibit a gingival appearance similar to that of the adjacent teeth. If hard and soft tissue discrepancies are not corrected by regenerative techniques, the replaced tooth appears long or overbulked gingivally. In order to create hard and soft tissue harmony, an understanding of the biological variables and periodontal implications is necessary.

The Prosthetic Space

Careful consideration must be taken in implant placement for any given prosthetic space. From a mesio-distal stance, an implant must be placed at least 1.5 mm away from an adjacent tooth, and 3 mm from an implant to prevent interproximal bone loss and subsequent loss of soft tissue and esthetics (Kois and Jan 2001). In the bucco-lingual dimension, the average maxillary anterior bony wall thickness following extraction was approximately 0.8 mm, with 87% of cases having less than 1 mm thickness (Huynh-Ba et al. 2010). The proper bucco-lingual positioning of the implant simplifies the restorative procedure, resulting in a proper emergence profile and facilitating oral hygiene. In order to achieve this result, the centerline of the implant must often be located near the center of the tooth it replaces. Alterations to this concept are made in response to gingival biotype and overbite. Prevention of any buccal recession is achieved by ensuring at least 1 mm of buccal wall remains after implant placement. It was noted that as bone thickness approached 1.8–2 mm, bone loss decreased, and in some cases bone gain was seen (Kitagawa et al. 2005).

Temporization

Observations in temporization have been made that the response of peri-implant soft tissue to crown-abutment contour modifications will depend on the location of that contour change. Two areas of interest have been noted: the critical space and subcritical space.

Critical Space

The critical space describes the portion of the crown/abutment/implant which lies immediately apical to the gingival margin. This space wraps circumferentially around the restoration and was found to be significant within 1 mm range in the apico-coronal direction. Interproximal critical spaces will dictate the final shape of the crown ranging from triangular to square. Additionally, the location of the critical space is not permanent. In cases of recession, the critical space will shift apically. From a clinical perspective, the final design of the critical space around all aspects of the restoration should correlate to the desired gingival architecture and anatomy of the implant-supported crown being fabricated.

Subcritical Space

The subcritical space is located apically to the critical space. This is under the caveat that there is sufficient "running room," or distance from the implant neck to the gingival margin. This space, if of high enough magnitude, allows for the proper cervical contouring of the restoration. Any alterations to the subcritical contours should not have a clinical effect on the gingival margin. If an implant is placed too shallow for example, an insufficient amount of running room will be present, and no subcritical space will exist. Design of the subcritical space may be convex, flat, or even concave to dictate soft tissue filling and growth. Alterations can be made in circumferentially, helping to manage both interproximal and facial tissue.

Buccal Contour

The buccal contour is important in determining the zenith and facial gingival margin level. These alterations will ultimately have an impact on the clinical crown length. Additional changes to the critical and subcritical space of a temporary may also control and/or change the location of the gingival zenith. The convexity of the facial critical contour has an effect on the gingival margin scallop.

Final Restoration

Fabrication of the final restoration relies on the practitioner's clinical skill as well as their ability to select the correct abutment, and restorative materials. Implants should be placed so that the abutment ultimately resembles or mimics the preparation of a natural tooth. In order to achieve this, surgical guides can assist in angulation. If too much angulation (in a palatal, buccal, mesial, or distal direction) exists, esthetics and even function can be compromised (Davarpanah et al. 2001).

Abutment Options

Abutment options for implant crowns include stock and custom abutments. Stock abutments compromise the cheaper and faster option. They are premade and come in standard sizes that are either straight or angled. In general, stock abutments are not used in the aesthetic zone because tissue may not accurately form to the shape of the abutment. Some studies indicate a greater risk of peri-implantitis when using stock abutments. Custom abutments on the other hand, have better subgingival contour for esthetics. This allows the practitioner to control the position of the margin, and even compensate for poor implant angulation to some degree (Sullivan and Sherwood 1993).

Cemented Versus Screw Retained

Cement retained restorations: Often more esthetic, carry the ideal occlusal load, and are more flexible with implant angulation. Some disadvantages of cement retained restorations include the need for cement, and issues with crown retention as a result. Insufficient cement may result in poor retention of the implant crown, while excess cement becomes a foreign object to the immune system and elicits an inflammatory response which will lead to peri-implantitis and ultimately failure if not treated appropriately. Screw retained restorations have their own set of pros and cons. Advantages of a screw retained restoration include: use with limited inter-occlusal distance, no cement needed, and retrievability. Cons include the challenge in creating a screw access location, and if the implant is poorly angled it will alter screw placement and can have a significant effect on esthetics.

Restorative Materials

Restorative options for single or multiple unit implant crowns have taken great strides in recent years. Options include porcelain fused to metal (PFM), E.max, layered zironcia, full contour zirconia, gold, and composites. PFMs have been the standard especially in posterior regions due to their durability and strength; however, they can be esthetically challenging at the margins of the restoration (Schoenbaum et al. 2013) have shown success to restore implants and have a strength that is similar to zirconia in many cases. The downside of E.max is ensuring that the resin cements are not used in excess. Resin cements are known to be of low viscosity and translucency, additionally they bond well to titanium. Consideration of an alternative cement is indicated in many E.max cases for this reason (Kitagawa et al. 2005). Layered zirconia is another option to restore implant crowns. This material requires greater occlusal clearance (Tan et al. 2012). Careful consideration in esthetics should be taken for all the restorative materials and increasing the opaqueness as necessary dependent on the material selected for the abutment to ensure it isn't visible through the crown. Overall, a number of materials may be used for the fabrication of an implant supported prosthesis. Practitioner and lab technician skill are important factors in the decision-making process.

Additionally, the amount of restorative space present may dictate or contraindicate the use of a particular material and favor another. In the esthetic zone, special care should be taken to match the color of adjacent teeth, and ensure the restoration is opaque enough to prevent any visibility of the abutment.

This chapter has provided an in-depth review of the prosthetic considerations during implant restoration. With the advent of technological advances, the number of materials and tools available to fabricate the most aesthetic and functional restorations will remain a dynamic field of study.

References

Beyer, J.W. and Lindauer, S.J. (1998). Evaluation of dental midline position. *Semin. Orthod.* 4 (3): 146–152.

Davarpanah, M., Martinez, H., Celletti, R., and Tecucianu, J.F. (2001). Three stage approach to aesthetic implant restoration: emergence profile concept. *Pract. Proced. Aesthet. Dent.* 13: 761–767.

Doza De Bastos, C. (1977). *Correlation of Gingivo and Osseous Contour of the Surface Anatamy of Teeth: A Comparative Study in Animals*. Master's thesis, 26–37. Boston: Boston University Schooi of Graduate Dentistry.

Huynh-Ba, G., Pjetursson, B.E., Sanz, M., and Cecchinato, D. (2010). Analysis of the socket bone wall dimensions in upper maxilla in relation to immediate implant placement. *Clin. Oral Implants Res.* 21: 37–42.

Kitagawa, T., Tanimoto, Y., Odaki, M. et al. (2005). Influence of implant/abutment joint designs on abutment screw loosening in a dental implant system. *J. Biomed. Mater. Res. B Appl. Biomater.* 75 (2): 457–463.

Kois, J. and Jan, J. (2001). Predictable peri-implant gingival aesthetics: surgical and prosthodontic rationales. *Pract. Proced. Aesthet. Dent.* 13 (9): 691–698.

Müller, H.P., Schaller, N., Eger, T., and Heinecke, A. (2000). Thickness of masticatory mucosa. *J. Clin. Periodontol.* 27: 431–436.

Olsson, M. and Lindhe, J. (1991). Periodontal characteristics in individuals with varying form of the upper central incisors. *J. Clin. Periodontol.* 18 (1): 78–82.

Pontoriero, R. and Carnevale, G. (2001 Jul). Surgical crown lengthening: a 12-month clinical wound healing study. *J. Periodontol.* 72 (7): 841–848.

Rufenacht, C.R. (1990). *Fundamentals of Esthetics*. USA: Quintessence Publishing, Main.

Saadoun, A.P., LeGall, M., and Touati, B. (1999). Selection and ideal tridimensional implant position for soft tissue aesthetics. *Pract. Period. Aesthet. Dent.* 11 (9): 1063–1067.

Schluger, S. (1949). Osseous resection; a basic principle in periodontal surgery. *Oral. Surg. Oral. Med. Oral. Pathol.* 2 (3): 316–325.

Schoenbaum, T.R., Chang, Y.Y., and Klokkevold, P.R. (2013). Screw-access marking: a technique to simplify retrieval of cement-retained implant prostheses. *Compend. Contin. Educ. Dent.* 34 (3): 230–236.

Smukler, H. and Chaibi, M. (1997). Periodontal and dental considerations in clinical crown extension: a rational basis for treatment. *Int. J. Periodontics Restorative Dent.* 17: 464–477.

Snow, S.R. (1999). Esthetic smile analysis of maxillary anterior tooth width: the golden percentage. *J. Esthet. Dent.* 11 (4): 177–184.

Sullivan, S. and Sherwood, R.L. (1993). Considerations for successful single tooth implant restorations. *J. Esthet. Restor. Dent.* 5 (3): 119–126.

Tan, J.P., Sederstrom, D., Polansky, J.R. et al. (2012). The use of slow heating and slow cooling regimens to strengthen porcelain fused to zirconia. *J. Prosthet. Dent.* 107 (3): 163–169.

Tarnow, D.P., Magner, A.W., and Fletcher, P. (1992). The effect of the distance from the contact point to the crest of bone on the presence or absence of the interproximal dental papilla. *J. Periodontol.* 63 (12): 995–996.

Tjan, A.H., Miller, G.D., and The, J.G. (1984). Some esthetic factors in a smile. *J. Prosthet. Dent.* 51 (1): 24–28.

Weisgold, A.S. (1977). Contours of the full crown restoration. *Alpha Omegan* 70: 77–89.

Zaidel, D.W. and Cohen, J.A. (2005). The face, beauty, and symmetry: perceiving asymmetry in beautiful faces. *Int. J. Neurosci.* 115 (8): 1165–1173.

17

Digital Workflow in Surgery

Edgard El Chaar

Department of Periodontics, University of Pennsylvania, Dental medicine, Philadelphia, PA, USA

Introduction to Digital Dentistry

Digital dentistry is gaining more popularity in the last five years and more clinicians are integrating it into their clinical practice. A rise in the lectures on the matter in domestic and international symposium has been noticeable as well more and more publications have populated the literature. Eventually, it will be integrated in the curriculum of dental education.

The digital workflow or digital dentistry is a big umbrella that has benefits all over the restorative and surgical disciplines. It has two folds, one capturing a dental image instead of taking a conventional impression, which eliminates the error in elastomeric impression material setting and error in stone setting, all of which can result in an accurate outcome with the digital impression called intra-oral scanning (IOS) (Ender et al. 2016, 2019), to volumetric data acquisition using cone beam computerized tomography (CBCT).

For the purpose of surgical implementation, the two collected data can be combined together in a planning software (computer-aided design (CAD)) and will be able to produce through a process called (computer-aided manufacturing (CAM)) static computer aided implant dentistry. This terminology is important to differentiate it from the navigational implant surgery, which correlates the planned placement in a live feedback of the drill position in the three-dimensional (3D) image of the patient.

Terminology

Images collected from a CBCT can be exported into a universal language called digital imaging and communication in medicine (DICOM). The image captured by an IOS can be saved in a universal file format called (STL). It's widely believed to be an abbreviation of the word **St**ereo Lithography, though sometimes it is also referred to as "Standard Triangle Language" or "Standard Tessellation Language."

The STL format doesn't export colored images. To achieve that, there is another universal format called OBJ which allows exporting it in color. Each scanner and CBCT have their own format language, that's why it is important to be able to export them in a universal format that can be imported in a system of choice of a clinician or to be transferred to another colleague if the patient decides to seek another place for treatment.

Description of STL

The main purpose of the STL file format is to encode the surface geometry of a 3D object. It encodes this information using a simple concept called "tessellation."

Tessellation is the process of tiling a surface with one or more geometric shapes eliminating overlaps or gaps, such as a tiled floor or wall. Tessellation can involve simple geometric shapes or very complicated (and imaginative) shapes.

The basic idea was to tessellate the two-dimensional (2D) outer surface of 3D models using tiny triangles also called "facets" and store information about the facets in a file.

For example, if you have a simple 3D cube, this can be covered by 12 triangles. In a cube, there are two triangles per face. Since the cube has six faces, it adds up to 12 triangles.

If you have a 3D model of a sphere, then it can be covered by many small triangles.

The Albert Consulting Group for 3D Systems realized that if they could store the information about these tiny triangles in a file, then this file could completely describe the surface of an arbitrary 3D model. This formed the basic idea behind the STL file format.

In a nutshell, an STL file stores information about 3D models. This format describes only the surface geometry of a three-dimensional object without any representation of color, texture, or other common model attributes. This format allows the image to be 3D printed, models to be generated and crowns to be milled.

Description of 3D Volume

Today, the CBCT is a very common tool available in most of the dental practices. It provides lower radiations in order of 92–118 μSv. As discussed in the previous chapters, it provides an abundant information on anatomical landmarks and different images, sagittal, axial, and coronal. In relation to our needs, it provides the bone and the teeth known as high density tissue. One of the setbacks in the images collected, we can get artifacts in the shape of streaks originating from restorations and crowns. This can be an impediment since the guides and prosthetic work-up will depend on the clarity of the teeth image. To limit artifacts: reduction of the field of view (FOV), Placing cotton rolls between the arches and the mucobuccal fold during the acquisition may decrease the beam hardening artifact. Patient-related artifacts are typically due to motion during the acquisition of the data volume, such as pronounced respiration, eye motion, or tremors. Movement artifact ranges from blurring to double contours of bony outlines.

2D images are made of several pixels represented as squares, with height and width. The smaller the pixel, the better the quality of the picture. The same concept applies to a 3D data volume. A voxel is the smallest 3D element of the volume, and is typically represented as a cube or a box, with height, width, and depth. Each 3D voxel represents a specific X-ray absorption. The voxel size on CBCT images is isotropic, which means that all the sides are the same dimension with uniform resolution in all directions. This is considered an advantage of the CBCT because if a certain structure needs to be measured, the measurement will be exact in all the three orthogonal planes. There are different voxel sizes depending on the capabilities of each unit. Voxel size needs to be smaller than the desired anatomical structure for adequate representation. For example, the first sign of periapical inflammatory lesion is discontinuity of the lamina dura; thus, if visualization changes to the periapical area (lamina dura and PDL space) is desired, a CBCT less than 0.2 mm needs to be acquired. Structures smaller than the voxel size will not be visualized in the scan (example, small cracks in the enamel). As previously mentioned, soft tissue structures (mucosa, gingiva, cartilage, nerves, blood vessels) cannot be evaluated in a CBCT study.

During the *reconstruction phase*, the set of 150–600 basis images will be sent to a dedicated software that will then create a 3D volume reconstruction of the data volume which is called rendering. To render a 2D projection of the 3D data set, one needs to define the opacity and color of every voxel. This is usually defined using an RGBA (for red, green, blue, alpha) transfer function that defines the RGBA value for every possible voxel value. We are focused on teeth and the bone which each will have a value. This will allow the clinicians to do a segmentation of the rendering in certain planning software's making the image clearer from the artifacts or un-needed structures.

Applications of Interactive Software

Intra-Oral Scanners (IOS)

There are different IOS in the market. The older version required powder in order to capture the image not anymore in the new models. The principle is to stitch multiple images to make them continuous. Based on the literature, not much of difference between all of them other than the rapidity in capturing the images based on the stitching and the software that allows it to happen but yet a recent publication showed there is a difference between some (Nedelcu et al. 2018). The IOS have shown similar accuracy to conventional impressions (Ender et al. 2016) and some suggested can be used as a replacement for conventional impressions when restoring up to ten units without extended edentulous spans. In a Prosthetic case, a body scan is needed to capture the position of the implant and with the IOS you can even capture the emergence profile that was created without resorting to multiple steps done during the conventional way (Elian et al. 2007). There is a system that allows the use of the healing abutment as a scan body with a proprietary software to decoded called encode. Regardless, for prosthetic or to create a surgical guide, the IOS is an important phase to collect and to be able to export freely an STL file and from there it will be imported to a planning software. Our focus will be on a virtual Implant planning software for edentulous sites either single or multiple in one or different quadrant but not for full reconstruction in edentulous site.

Virtual Implant Software Planning

In order to achieve that, the following will need to happen regardless of the system maybe in a different set of order:

1. Import of the DICOM, cleaning of the 3D rendering via segmentation if the software is capable.

2. Importing the digital impression and matching it with the radiographical in a process called stitching or registration depending on the system in use.
3. You plan the implant following the 3D implant placement set rules (Grunder et al. 2005; Hämmerle et al. 2015).
4. Depending on the system, you can either use a feature of digital wax-up from a pre-set library and adjusted to the appropriate size or import a digital scan of the waxed-up site.
5. Once the positioning is satisfactory, you will follow the steps of the particular software to design a surgical guide and export it in STL format.

At this point, this exported file will be imported in a 3D printer resin based allowing the surgical guide to be manufactured. This constitutes the CAM part of the digital process. The virtual planning software (CAD) will generate a surgical protocol which will be discussed next.

Drilling Surgical Guide

A drilling surgical guide allows the transfer of the virtually planned treatment to surgery which is called in the literature "static computer aided Implant dentistry" (Vercruyssen et al. 2015). Depending on the system used, a specific part, drilling burs, and surgical protocol will be generated by the planning software. All the drilling guides will have in common the following:

1. A sleeve: a tube of titanium that inserts in the site of each implant. Depending on the systems, you can have a pilot drill sleeve, or a fully guided sleeve which will correspond to the diameter of the implant. Sometimes, the diameter for the fully guided can be too wide for the space and will be an impediment for it to be printed. The clinician might have to revert to less of a fully guided preparation and placement.
2. If you are going for fully guided preparation of the osteotomy, a key that correspond to each bur will be provided.
3. Set of burs with stoppers that will be held by the key of different length for each step of the osteotomy.
4. Lastly, a fixture mount with stopper in case of guided implant placement.
5. The planning software will generate through an algorithm, will calculate the appropriate length of the bur taking into consideration, the distance from its stopper over the key, the length of the sleeve, the distance of the sleeve from the bone and the necessary depth of osteotomy. A surgical protocol will be generated, stating the length of the bur, the key to use and the fixture mount appropriate key and depth marking. Tissue

punchers will be selected as well in case of flapless approach.

Although in theory, the guide should be perfectly correct, the clinician should always check to make sure the osteotomy is in the right direction and position (Wismeijer et al. 2018). A recent systematic review (Tahmaseb et al. 2018) reviewed 2238 implants in 471 patients that had been placed using static guides. The meta-analysis of the accuracy (20 clinical) revealed a total mean error of 1.2 mm (1.04–1.44 mm) at the entry point, 1.4 mm (1.28–1.58 mm) at the apical point and deviation of 3.5°(3.0–3.96°). There was a significant difference in accuracy in favor of partial edentulous comparing to full edentulous cases. They recommended a safety margin of at least 2 mm to be respected.

The deviation between CBCT and surface scan model resulting from inaccurate registration is transferred to the surgical field and results in a deviation between the planned and actual implant position (Flügge et al. 2017). Furthermore, the registration accuracy in commercial virtual implant planning software is significantly influenced by the preprocessing of imported data, by the user and by the number of restorations resulting in clinically non-acceptable deviations encoded in drilling guides. The authors advocate the manual segmentation of 3D models by the user proved better than the automatic segmentation especially in patients with multiple restorations. Further to that, the printing of the guide using additive manufacturing (3D printing), which uses a polymerizing resin and selective laser melting, can be subject to inaccuracies (Galante et al. 2019).

Use of Guided Surgery in Immediate Implant Placement

The benefits of placing an immediate implant in the anterior esthetic area are numerous and the challenges are plenty: from the positioning of the implant to achieve a prosthetically driven placement leading to a screw retained prosthesis, to preserving the gingival scallop and reducing gingival margin recession, to immediately temporizing the patient that helps both latter's and improve patient comfort.

The digital planning leading to a digital surgical guide can provide a more precise 3D implant position when it comes to buccal-lingual and mesio-distal placement. The depth control is bit tricky which will require more the clinician experience.

If we follow the fully guided implant placement, we can even design a temporary digitally that has built-in the position of the abutment.

Descriptively, once the IOS is taken with the site to be extracted and imported in either the planning software if it can provide the digital extraction or to free online software called meshmixer. Once the tooth is extracted and super-imposed over the DICOM, the planning proceed as the normal process but with the criteria of immediate implant which is the apical stabilization of 3 to 4 mm. Another added benefit is the visualization of the free gingival margin and being able to measure the 3 mm depth needed at time of immediate implant placement.

The process can then be synergized with a prosthetic software of the clinician choosing. It will allow for chairside provisionalization, among other features. By using these steps, the clinician will end up with a design that requires the clinician or technician to further shape digitally the submarginal contour, especially from the mesiobuccal line angle to the distobuccal line angle especially for the maxillary central. Once the design is established, it can be routed to make a digital model with a soft-tissue design depicting the implant position or straight with the temporary or skipping the model design with the soft tissue and just produce the temporary only. When the project is finalized, all three models if that route is chosen, designed temporary, soft tissue, and the model with the analog location, can be exported into STL format for three-dimensional printing. The designed temporary with the proper shade and adapted to a prosthetic abutment appropriates to the chosen implant system using the printed model with the printed soft tissue. We can also verify the fit of the surgical guide over the model and its lining up with the lab analog.

If the implant stability is not satisfactory to the clinician, the printed tooth can be trimmed to a 3D custom abutment or even designed as such from the beginning.

The goal of provisionalization at the time of immediate implant placement is also based on the concept that the buccal emergence profile can support the soft tissue from collapsing. This is discussed more in Chapter 18, but recently, El Chaar et al. introduced a mathematical concept to calculate the emergence profile based on the depth of the implant and the buccal gap that is created by the immediate implant placement (El Chaar et al. 2020). This can be integrated in both implant planning software with the prosthetic synergy and will make it defined better cutting down on the prosthetic time of the surgical phase.

Full Arch Guided Surgery

The digital surgical workflow was also included in the planning of a full arch case. This will consist on planning the placement of the implants either parallel or with angled posterior ones. In order to do that, we can create a leveling of all the implants with a cutting plane, allowing a straight leveling between the posterior and anterior implant and also based on the prosthetic distance needed between the implants interface and the incisal of the future prosthetic.

Once these established, the clinician or the lab technician can build the reduction guide, that will be the base, and stabilized with pins, the leveling can be finalized and then the implant surgical guide can be attached over it to place the implants. Once the implants are placed, the latter guide is removed and the temporary milled or printed bridge is stacked over the reduction guide and connected to the multi-unit abutments. This will allow the patient to walk out with immediate temporary load. I do call this temporary a surgical temporary that would need to be replaced or embellished when the healing is finished. (Figures 17.1–17.7)

Aid in Ridge Deficiency Diagnosis

We, as clinicians are dealing with more and more extensive and complicated cases that require more presurgical preparation. When the CBCT is taken, and uploaded to the planning implant software, some of them will allow you to manipulate the rendering image, clean it. That allows the clinician to segment the area that they need and then export it as an .stl image which in turn will be printed (Figure 17.8). Once the clinician has it in their hand, they can decide which procedure will be more beneficial to the situation in question, an autogenous bloc/monocortical

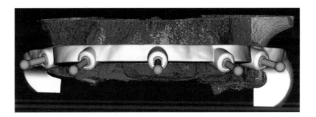

Figure 17.1 Planning of the reduction guide based on the cutting plane with the planned stabilization pins

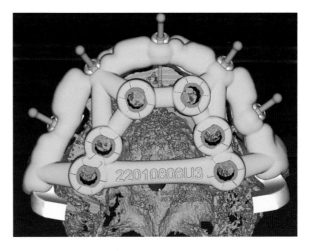

Figure 17.2 The stackable guide for implant placement sitting over the reduction guide.

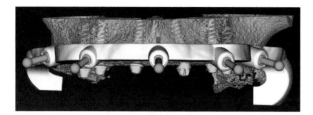

Figure 17.3 Buccal view of the reduced bone with the implant placed along with the multiunit abutments.

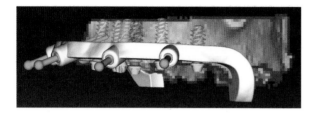

Figure 17.4 Side view of the reduced bone with the implant placed along with the multiunit abutments.

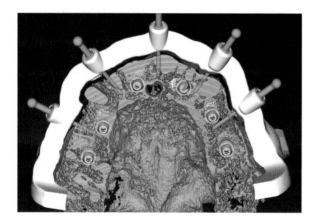

Figure 17.5 Occlusal view of the reduced bone with the implant placed along with the multiunit abutments.

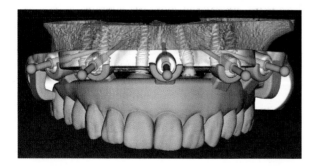

Figure 17.6 Buccal view of the temporary prosthesis sitting over the reduction guide which became the base of all the phases of treatment.

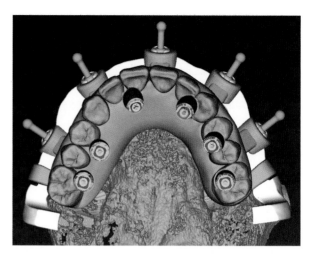

Figure 17.7 Side view of the temporary prosthesis sitting over the reduction guide which became the base of all the phases of treatment.

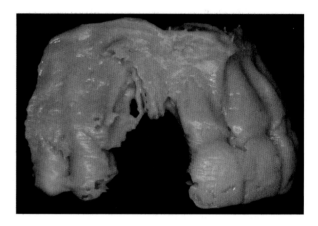

Figure 17.8 Printed image of the rendering allowing the clinician to assess the amount of bone destruction and here in particular there is still an implant that need to be removed.

plates, a titanium mesh, or just resorbable/nonresorbable membrane with or without tenting screws. There is also a free online software called slicer that can allow you to do the segmentation of the rendering. Both 3D preparation and treatment has been described by El Chaar et al. (2019) that can help you the reader to understand more in depth that critical phase.

As a conclusion, technologies in data acquisition in CBCT will keep improving both in reducing radiation and accuracies despite the dental restorations allowing the clinician to more accurately register the data from the IOS which in its turn will keep improving both in speed and stitching of the images even in the fully edentulous. The future is bright and this technology will be more adopted by the clinicians and it will become more affordable compared to the navigational and the robotic guided implant dentistry.

References

El Chaar, E., Urtula, A.B., Georgantza, A. et al. (2019). Treatment of atrophic ridges with titanium mesh: A retrospective study using 100% mineralized allograft and comparing dental stone versus 3D-printed models. *Int. J. Periodontics Restor. Dent.* 39 (4): 491–500.

El Chaar, E., White, C., Salama, T. et al. (2020). Clinical methodology quantifying the emergence profile contour for immediate provisionalization: A proposed mathematical model emergence profile in immediate provisionalization. *J. Oral. Implantol.* 47 (3): 191–198.

Elian, N., Tabourian, G., Jalbout, Z.N. et al. (2007). Accurate transfer of peri-implant soft tissue emergence profile from the provisional crown to the final prosthesis using an emergence profile cast. *J. Esthet. Restor. Dent.* 19 (6): 306–314.

Ender, A., Attin, T., and Mehl, A. (2016). In vivo precision of conventional and digital methods of obtaining complete-arch dental impressions. *J. Prosthet. Dent.* 115 (3): 313–320.

Ender, A., Zimmermann, M., and Mehl, A. (2019). Accuracy of complete-and partial-arch impressions of actual intraoral scanning systems in vitro. *Int. J. Comput. Dent.* 22 (1): 11–19.

Flügge, T., Derksen, W., Te Poel, J. et al. (2017). Registration of cone beam computed tomography data and intraoral surface scans–A prerequisite for guided implant surgery with CAD/CAM drilling guides. *Clin. Oral Implants Res.* 28 (9): 1113–1118.

Galante, R., Figueiredo-Pina, C.G., and Serro, A.P. (2019). Additive manufacturing of ceramics for dental applications: a review. *Dent. Mater.* 35 (6): 825–846.

Grunder, U., Gracis, S., and Capelli, M. (2005). Influence of the 3-D bone-to-implant relationship on esthetics. *Int J Periodontics Restorative Dent* 25 (2): 113–119.

Hämmerle, C.H., Cordaro, L., van Assche, N. et al. (2015). Digital technologies to support planning, treatment, and fabrication processes and outcome assessments in implant dentistry. Summary and consensus statements. The 4th EAO consensus conference 2015. *Clin. Oral Implants Res.* 26: 97–101.

Nedelcu, R., Olsson, P., Nyström, I. et al. (2018). Accuracy and precision of 3 intraoral scanners and accuracy of conventional impressions: a novel in vivo analysis method. *J. Dent.* 1 (69): 110–118.

Tahmaseb, A., Wu, V., Wismeijer, D. et al. (2018). The accuracy of static computer-aided implant surgery: a systematic review and meta-analysis. *Clin. Oral Implants Res.* 29: 416–435.

Vercruyssen, M., Laleman, I., Jacobs, R., and Quirynen, M. (2015). Computer-supported implant planning and guided surgery: a narrative review. *Clin. Oral Implants Res.* 26 (Suppl. 11): 69–76.

Wismeijer, D., Joda, T., Flügge, T. et al. (2018). Group 5 ITI consensus report: digital technologies. *Clin. Oral Implants Res.* 29: 436–442.

Further Reading

Benic, G.I., Elmasry, M., and Hammerle, C.H.F. (2015). Novel digital imaging methods to assess the outcome of implant therapy: a narrative review. *Clin. Oral Implants Res.* 26 (Suppl. 11): 86–96.

Buser, D., Martin, W., and Belser, U.C. (2004). Optimizing esthetics for implant restorations in the anterior maxilla: anatomic and surgical considerations. *Int. J. Oral Maxillofac. Implants* 19 (7).

Patzelt, S.B.M. and Kohal, R.J. (2015). CAD/CAM–fabricated implant-supported restorations: a systematic review. *Clin. Oral Implants Res.* 26 (Suppl. 11): 77–85.

18

Socket Management

Aikaterini Georgantza

Ashman Department of Periodontology and Implant Dentistry, New York University College of Dentistry, New York, NY, USA

Anatomical Features of the Alveolar Process

The Alveolar Process

The bone that supports teeth in the maxilla and mandible may be divided into two parts: the alveolar process and the basal bone, which are continuous with no distinct border dividing them. The alveolar process of the jaw develops along with the eruption of the teeth and is composed of the alveolar bone proper and the supporting bone. The volume and the shape of the alveolar process are determined by the form of the teeth, their axis of eruption, and eventual inclination (Schroeder 1985).

The Alveolar Bone Proper

Compact bone that composes the alveolus (tooth socket). Also known as cribriform plate or lamina dura, the fibers of periodontal ligament insert into it (American Academy of Periodontology, 2001). The function of the alveolar bone proper is to form the attachment apparatus of the tooth in conjunction with the root cementum and the periodontal ligament.

Alveolus and Extraction Socket

Alveolus is the socket in the bone into which a tooth is attached by means of the periodontal ligament. (American Academy of Periodontology, 2001). The extraction socket is a term used to describe the tissues remaining after tooth removal. The outer walls of the extraction socket consist mainly of cortical bone with the buccal bone plate being usually thinner (<1 mm in the anterior region) than the lingual or palatal wall.

The Alveolar Ridge

When the alveolar process heals following loss of teeth, the remaining bone is referred to as the alveolar ridge and is the result of bone formation within the socket and bone resorption externally.

Classification of Remaining Bone

Lekholm and Zarb (1985) classified the "quality" of the bone in the healed edentulous ridges into four categories according to which classes 1 and 2 are characterized by thick cortical plates and small volume of bone marrow. Sites that belong to classes 3 and class 4 present with thin walls of cortical bone surrounding large amount of cancellous bone (spongiosa), including trabeculae of lamellar bone and marrow.

Alterations of the Alveolar Process Following Tooth Extraction

Biological Events and Histologic Ridge Alterations

The healing of an extraction socket was studied in specimens obtained from humans (Amler et al. 1960, 1969; Evian et al. 1982) and in animal models (Cardaropoli et al. 2003; Araújo and Lindhe 2005).

In the study by Amler (1969), the socket healing was monitored in volunteers, after tooth extraction and soft tissue biopsies were harvested from the extraction sites after varying intervals; from 48 hours to 32 days. From his observations, Amler concluded that a blood clot formed within the socket soon after the removal of a tooth. Within two to three days the clot was gradually replaced with granulation tissue and subsequently with young connective tissue and osteoid with signs of mineralization after three weeks. After six weeks of healing, there was pronounced bone formation in the socket and trabeculae of newly formed bone.

The limitations of this study are the following: (i) The tissue sampled was not demineralized prior to sectioning as a result only events of that preceded hard tissue formation could have been analyzed. (ii) The study was of short duration and did not include the important later phase of socket healing that involves the process of modeling and remodeling. (iii) The biopsy was restricted to the superficial region of the wound and the marginal portions of the socket. Thus, the tissue composition of the fully healed extraction site was not documented in the study.

Cardaropoli et al. (2003) published the results of a long-term experimental study in dogs, which described in more detail the various phases of socket healing including processes of both modeling and remodeling.

Overview of the Histologic Sequence of Healing

The healing of an extraction socket is characterized by a sequence of histologic events taking place in four clear stages:

- **Blood clotting**: The blood clot acts as a physical matrix that directs cellular movements, contains growth factors, and enhances the activity of inflammatory cells.
- **Wound cleansing**: When neutrophils and macrophages that migrate into the wound clean the site from bacteria and damaged tissue before formation of new tissue can start.
- **Tissue formation**: A new tissue, i.e. granulation tissue gradually, replaces the blood clot. The granulation tissue contains macrophages, a large number of fibroblast-like cells, and newly formed blood vessels. A provisional connective tissue is established through a combination of fibroplasia (intense synthesis of matrix components exhibited by the mesenchymal cells) and angiogenesis (formation of new vessels).
- **Tissue modeling and remodeling**: Within few weeks the entire socket is filled with woven bone which is replaced gradually with lamellar bone and marrow.

Dimensional Ridge Alterations

Knowledge of healing events following tooth extraction is essential for prosthetically driven treatment planning.

Studies measuring the mean apico-coronal and bucco-lingual change in ridge dimensions following tooth extraction:

Pietrokovski and Massler (1967), Schropp et al. (2003), Araújo and Lindhe (2005).

In the study by Pietrokovski and Massler (1967), the authors had access to 149 dental cast models (72 maxillary and 77 mandibular) in which one tooth was missing (and not replaced) on one side of the jaw. The outer contours of the buccal and lingual/palatal portions of the ridge at a tooth site and at the contralateral edentulous site were determined by the use of a profile stylus and an imaging technique. A pilot study was also carried out to test the accuracy of the technique and the degree of symmetry of normal and edentulous ridges. The authors reported the following findings:

1. From the pilot study the human dental arches found to be symmetrical but not identical with a small and not significant difference.
2. The buccal plate of the maxillary and mandibular arch was resorbed to a greater extend shifting the position of the edentulous ridge toward the palatal/lingual site and shortening the total arch length.
3. The amount of tissue resorption was significantly greater in the edentulous molar region than in the incisor and premolar region of both jaws.

Schropp et al. introduced subtraction radiography as a new method for assessing morphologic changes and remodeling processes of extraction sites during the healing period. This prospective clinical trial demonstrated that major changes of an extraction site take place during the 12 months following atraumatic tooth extraction. The width of the alveolar ridge was reduced by 50% during the observation period and two thirds of this reduction occurred within the first three months after tooth extraction. Regarding the soft tissue height, only slight changes, less than 1 mm, took place in both jaws during the 12 months of healing (Schropp et al. 2003).

Araújo and Lindhe (2005) described alterations in the edentulous ridge profile following tooth extraction in an experimental study in a dog model. Over eight weeks of healing, the margin of the buccal wall shifted apically by approximately 2 mm. According to the authors, bone loss during socket healing is greater along the buccal than the lingual wall for several reasons. First, the crestal portion of the buccal bone wall is primarily compromised of bundle bone, especially in the anterior region. Bundle bone is a tooth-dependent tissue that completely resorbs after tooth extraction. On the contrary, bundle bone typically comprises a smaller proportion of the lingual or palatal socket wall. Also, the lingual bone wall of the socket is thicker than the buccal wall.

Clinical Implications for Ridge Preservation and Implant Treatment

Adequate dimensions of the alveolar ridge promote implant placement in the proper three-dimensional position and provide proper mechanical support for the implant and soft tissues. Numerous experimental and clinical studies have shown that resorption of the alveolar process is an inevitable consequence after tooth extraction.

Many factors have been suggested to influence post-extraction ridge reduction. These include:

- Pre-existing pathological processes
- Thin bone and soft tissue phenotype
- Number of missing teeth
- Traumatic tooth extraction

Preventing or reducing this resorption is desirable for long-term success in implant dentistry since ideally the implant must be circumferentially surrounded by healthy bone and a wide band of keratinized mucosa.

Atraumatic Tooth Extraction

Tooth extraction is the first step in treatment and even though it has been considered a simple and straight-forward procedure, it is an invasive procedure. It disrupts vascular structures and damages soft tissues and associated periodontal ligament. It should be performed as minimally traumatic as possible, with care to avoid additional bone resorption. Flapless tooth extraction is important and has been shown to reduce the amount of bone loss in the early healing phase four to eight weeks post extraction compared with full-thickness flap elevation (Fickl et al. 2008).

Indications for Ridge Preservation

Ridge preservation may be defined as a procedure that aims to preserve the ridge volume existing at the time of extraction. General indications:

- Maintenance of the existing soft and hard tissue envelope
- Maintenance of a stable ridge volume for optimizing functional and esthetic outcomes
- Simplification of treatment procedures subsequent to the ridge preservation (Hämmerle et al. 2012).

It is also indicated when an immediate or early implant placement is not feasible due to:

Patient-Specific Indications

- Adolescent people (too young for implant placement)
- Pregnancy
- Medical reasons
- Financial reasons

Site-Specific Indications

- Extended apical bone defects where primary stability may be compromised
- Extended soft tissue deficiency
- Multi-rooted sites

Contraindications for Ridge Preservation

- General contraindication against oral surgical interventions
- Infection at the extraction site, which cannot be taken care of during the ridge preservation surgery
- Patients radiated in the area planned for ridge preservation
- Patients taking bisphosphonates
- Implant placement anticipated within six to eight weeks of extraction
- Thick periodontal phenotypes with expected sufficient amount of bone after extraction and healing

Ridge Preservation Procedures

Several procedures have the potential to modulate the degree of the inevitable ridge changes.

Maintenance of the Root and the Socket Shield Technique

Historically, the first therapeutic attempts to prevent alveolar ridge resorption were performed by root retention, with primary goal of maximizing the stability of removable prostheses (Osburn 1974). Later in 1994, Langer introduced the spontaneous *in situ* gingival augmentation technique to increase the quantity of gingival tissue around a tooth scheduled for extraction.

Salama et al. in 2007 described the advantages of the "Root Submergence technique" for pontic site development in esthetic implant dentistry. Hürzeler et al. published in 2010 the "Socket-shield" technique, according to which the retaining of the buccal aspect of the root during implant placement did not appear to interfere with osseointegration and could be beneficial in preserving the buccal bone plate.

Forced Eruption

Forced eruption has been used as a site development for future implant placement.

Socket Grafting

Over the past two decades, multiple studies have been conducted to evaluate the efficacy of different socket grafting approaches (Avila-Ortiz et al. 2014). In these studies a large variety of biomaterials have been employed and tested, including autologous bone, bone substitutes (allografts, xenografts, and alloplasts), autologous blood-derived products, and bioactive agents (Darby et al. 2009).

Socket Grafting Technique: Clinical Recommendations

- Minimally traumatic tooth extraction
- Socket debridement
- Raising of a flap and placement of biomaterials (biomaterial for ridge contouring and/or barrier membrane)

- Primary wound closure when possible (soft tissue punch, connective tissue graft, barrier membrane, soft tissue replacement matrix, pedicle flap)
- Suturing
- Antibiotics

Materials Used for Socket Grafting The materials used for ridge preservation are those that have been used for guided bone regeneration (GBR) and guided tissue regeneration (GTR) and reflect what is available commercially. Demineralized freeze-dried bone allograft (DFDBA) and deproteinized bovine bone mineral (DBBM) have been used extensively. Other graft materials include autologous bone, calcium sulfate (CMC/CaS), solvent-preserved cancellous allograft, and biocoral (Darby et al. 2009).

Membranes placed were most commonly expanded polytetrafluoroethylene (e-PTFE) membranes or collagen membranes. In addition, a polylactic/polyglycolic membrane was assessed by Lekovic et al. (1998) and Simon et al. (2000). Other membranes investigated were those manufactured from titanium or acellular dermal matrix graft (ADMG). Finally sponges made of polylactic/polyglycolic acid (PL/PG) or collagen have been placed in extraction sockets to preserve the ridge. The collagen sponges acted as a carrier for either recombinant human bone morphogenetic protein 2 (rhBMP-2) or synthetic cell-binding peptide p-15 (Darby et al. 2009).

The Osteology Consensus Conference in 2012 concluded that the majority of studies and systematic reviews did not reveal significant differences between various biomaterials and treatment approaches (Hammerle et al. 2012).

However, bone grafting materials that will be resorbed and replaced with the host's bone are preferable. An ideal material would be one that resorbs at the same rate as new bone formation occurs. If a bone graft material resorbs too rapidly, it will permit shrinkage or contraction to occur before the space can be filled with new bone. Conversely, an implant that resorbs too slowly may delay bone formation (Seibert 1993).

Healing and Implant Placement After placing the biomaterial in the extraction socket and subsequently covering the area with a membrane and a flap or only with a soft tissue substitute material, the area should be left to heal for four to six months prior to implant placement. The healing period depends on the size of the extraction socket. It is recommended that a molar socket be allowed to heal for six months, and a lateral incisor socket for four months. In general, ridge preservation procedures are accompanied by varying degrees of bone formation and residual graft material in the extraction socket. This depends on the materials and techniques used. Ridge preservation procedures do not prevent 100% of the ridge alteration that takes place following tooth extraction. Thus, even if enough bone is preserved for implant placement, some flattening of the ridge should be expected. In maxillary anterior regions, additional procedures such as contour augmentation or soft tissue grafting may be required at the time of implant placement to compensate for this deficiency.

Socket Grafting Complications Occasionally complications may result from a ridge preservation procedure. These are mostly related to healing and bacterial contamination of the wound. The most common complications include:

- Infection
- Soft tissue dehiscence
- Gingival graft necrosis
- Membrane exposure
- Exposure and loss of graft material

Management of Socket at the Esthetic Zone

Extraction Socket Classifications

Extraction socket classifications and treatment protocols are designed to help guide clinicians through diagnosis and therapy. There have been various proposed systems to classify extraction sockets.

Elian and coworkers presented a simplified socket classification and repair technique according to which there are three types of sockets:

- **Type I Socket**: The facial soft tissue and buccal plate of bone are at normal levels in relation to the cementoenamel junction of the pre-extracted tooth and remain intact post-extraction.
- **Type II Socket**: Facial soft tissue is present but the buccal plate is partially missing following extraction of the tooth.
- **Type III Socket**: The facial soft tissue and the buccal plate of bone are both markedly reduced after tooth extraction.

A simple, noninvasive approach to the grafting and management of sockets when soft tissue was present but buccal plate was compromised following tooth extraction was also introduced (Elian et al. 2007).

El Chaar et al. in 2016 proposed a classification of extraction sockets for single rooted teeth based on the biologic principles of wound healing and guided by the topography of the extraction socket. The treatment protocol for each socket type is directed by the anatomy of the remaining bone, the soft tissue biotype, and the location of the socket in the maxilla or the mandible.

Timing of Implant Placement

Several classifications have been proposed for the timing of implant placement following tooth extraction with various time intervals. In 2004, Hämmerle et al. proposed a classification of four categories (Type I–IV), which was later modified by Chen and Buser (2008) adding a descriptive terminology in the 3rd volume of the ITI Treatment Guide series (Figure 18.1).

Immediate Implant Placement

Diagnosis and Indications In the esthetic sites, immediate implant placement may be considered in single-tooth sites when the anatomical situation is ideal. Specifically when the buccal plate of the socket is fully intact, the tissue biotype is thick with a thick facial bone wall (≥1 mm) and primary stability can be achieved. However, additional procedures may be required even in these favorable conditions in order to prevent mucosal recession. Such procedures may include adjunctive connective tissue grafts and flap advancement.

Outline of favorable clinical conditions for immediate implant placement:

- In the esthetic zone, sites with a low esthetic risk and low esthetic demands:
  - Thick tissue biotype
  - Intact thick buccal bone wall
- Intact bone walls and favorable apical topography
- Single-rooted sites
- Absence of acute purulent infection

When the clinical conditions are favorable, then an immediate implant placement is planned with pre-operative three-dimensional radiographic images cone beam computed tomography (CBCT).

Immediate Implant Placement Surgical Technique

- **Minimally traumatic tooth extraction**: Flapless tooth extraction is important to avoid additional bone resorption from the bony surface related to the elevation of the mucoperiosteal flap (Wood et al. 1972).
- **Socket debridement and inspection**: Immediately after tooth extraction all granulomatous tissue is removed with curettes and the socket is examined to confirm that all bone walls are intact.
- **Implant osteotomy**: The implant osteotomy is prepared utilizing a surgical template to ensure ideal implant position. Verification for proper three-dimensional implant placement. A gap of 2 mm is maintained between the implant shoulder and the internal aspect of the facial wall. This marginal gap is grafted with particles of cortical allograft.
- **Suturing**: A horizontal mattress suture is placed.
- **Interim tooth replacement**: Removable dental prosthesis or vacuum-formed overlay bridge (Essix) are provided for patients as interim tooth replacements. Care is taken to relieve the prosthesis to avoid contact with the implants and underlying mucosa.
- **Post-operative care**: Patients are instructed to rinse twice daily with chlorhexidine digluconate and to refrain from removing plaque by mechanical means at the surgical sites for two weeks.
- **Suture removal**: Sutures are removed two weeks post-operatively and patients are asked to commence plaque removal at the exposed healing caps with a soft-bristle toothbrush.
- **Final restorative treatment**: Patients are referred for restorative treatment three to four months after implant surgery and are recalled for examination and instruction in home care following connection of the implant crowns.
- **Annual recalls scheduled**.

Complications

- **General complications related intraoral surgical procedures**: Infection, pain, swelling, wound dehiscence, and exposure of the graft.
- **Midfacial recession**: Soft tissue recession may be expected following immediate implant placement and

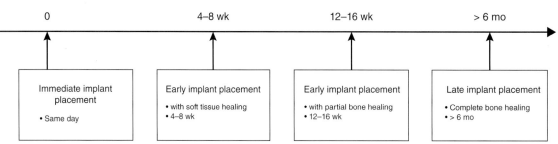

Implant placement post extraction

Treatment options

Figure 18.1 The four treatment options for post-extraction implant placement as defined by the ITI in two ITI Consensus Conferences (2003 and 2008). Source: Chen and Buser (2008)/Quintessence Publishing Co, Inc.

a wide range regarding the amount of recessions is reported in the literature. Several factors for the development of mucosal recession have been identified such as smoking, presence of a thin buccal bone plate (i.e. <1 mm thick), presence of a thin soft tissue biotype, and a facial implant position.

esthetic Maximization The esthetic implications of immediate implants, especially for single anterior teeth in the esthetic zone are of increasing significance. The peri-implant mucosal tissues often immediately collapse after tooth extraction, socket debridement, and implant placement making it challenging to preserve the original soft tissue architecture.

Temporization Versus Shell Several studies have reported high success rates following a provisional restoration of a single endosseous implant placed immediately following tooth extraction in the maxillary anterior area.

Generally, an immediate implant provisional restoration should be screw retained to avoid problems associated with inadequate cement removal. The provisional restoration can be either fabricated chairside, processed by the prosthodontist, conventionally or computer-guided.

Kan and Rungcharassaeng (2000) proposed a surgical and prosthodontic rationale for immediate implant placement and provisionalization of maxillary anterior single implants. According to the author's technique, an acrylic resin provisional shell of the to-be-extracted tooth was fabricated prior to implant surgery. After the placement of the implant, a metal temporary abutment was placed onto the implant and autopolymerizing acrylic resin was applied to the temporary abutment to capture the cervical gingival emergence of the extracted tooth. The customized metal temporary abutment was then prepared extraorally and hand tightened onto the implant, and the relined provisional shell was provisionally cemented. The provisional restoration was adjusted to clear all contacts in centric occlusion and during eccentric movements.

Chu et al. (2014) developed a prefabricated polymethyl methacrylate (PMMA) shell device to replicate the shape and dimensions of the extracted root at the cervical area and properly support the subgingival mucosal tissues. Additionally the shell device can restore the pre-extraction state of the tooth cervical region and act as a prosthetic socket-sealing device for bone graft containment.

Contour of the Temporary Restoration The concept of "contour" was originally adapted from tooth-supported restorations and needed to be redefined for the implant dentistry. Ideally, the implant abutment should mimic a full crown preparation. Su et al. (2010) defined two distinct zones within the implant abutment and crown and

introduced the *critical* and *subcritical contour* terms. The *critical contour* is the area of the implant abutment and crown located immediately apical to the gingival margin. The facial profile of the critical contour is important in determining the zenith and labial margin level. The *subcritical contour* is located apical to the critical contour, provided that sufficient "running room" is present (if the implant placement is too shallow, this contour will not exist). Alterations of both critical and subcritical contour can be used to enhance peri-implant soft tissue esthetics.

Digital Guided Surgery Computed tomography (CT)-guided implant surgery was first introduced in the early 2000s. Guided implant surgery involves a reverse engineering workflow, first establishing the ideal position and morphology of the planned restoration, and then virtually planning the ideal position of the dental implant(s) according to that restoration. Surgical guides are then produced to aid the surgeon in placing the implants accurately, according to the virtual plan (Orentlicher et al. 2017).

Placement of implants using guided surgery can be performed fully guided or using pilot guides. Fully guided placement involves osteotomies and implant placement, using implant-specific guided surgery instrumentation, to final depth and angulation, through the surgical guide. While with the use of pilot guides, the final implant placement is done freehand using conventional instrumentation.

Immediate Implant Placement in Posterior Sites Due to the wider socket dimensions in multi-rooted tooth sites, there might be a decreased amount of implant surface in direct contact with the adjacent bone walls. This might impede the achievement of optimal primary stability (Lang et al. 2012).

Molar sites present situations with limited indications due to anatomical reasons and when immediate implants are placed in these sites, soft and hard tissue augmentation is frequently necessary.

Premolars represent the sites with the most favorable indication due to the normally favorable anatomical situation and generally low esthetic demands (Hämmerle et al. 2012).

Surgical Technique for IIP in Posterior Sites Proposed protocol for immediate implant placement in posterior jaws by El Chaar and Castano (2017).

- After careful patient selection and evaluation of the preoperative anatomy of the extraction site by CBCT, an atraumatic extraction is performed.
- Osteotomy preparation for single rooted tooth: Engage the lingual aspect of the extraction socket. Drill 3–4 mm

past the apex of the extracted tooth to form a primary stability rectangle.

- Place the implant at a minimum of 2 mm away from the lingual aspect of the facial socket wall.
- Osteotomy preparation for multi-rooted tooth: Engage the center of the furcational dome. Drill 3–4 mm past the apices of the extracted tooth.
- Optimal position of the implant's prosthetic platform is 3–5 mm below the free gingival margin.
- Graft residual peri-implant voids with composite cortical-cancellous (70 : 30) allograft.
- Cover the graft with bovine pericardium membrane.
- If there is inadequate bone volume for implant placement then graft the maxillary sinus with cancellous, cortical, or composite particulate allograft ≥4 mm vertical subantral space required.
- Determine the optimal implant loading time. Immediate loading when ≥40 Ncm of implant insertion torque. Delayed when <40 Ncm of implant insertion torque.
- Suturing.

Complications
- Lack of primary stability
- Infection
- Early implant failure
- Related to simultaneous crestal sinus elevation (sinus membrane perforation)

Early Implant Placement with Soft Tissue Healing (4–8 Weeks)
Indications When the buccal bone wall of the socket is damaged, early placement is preferred, even in cases where tissue biotype is thick. Other favorable clinical conditions for early implant placement are as follows:

- In the esthetic zone, sites with low to high esthetic risk:
  - High lip line
  - Presence of a buccal bone defect
  - Thin buccal bone wall (≤1 mm)
  - Thin tissue biotype
  - Multiple-tooth gaps
- Local infection at the extraction site
- Large apical bone defects where initial stability may be compromised

Surgical Technique
- At implant surgery, four to eight weeks post extraction a palatal incision is carried out in this area, with the blade cutting along the inner surface of the palatal bone wall deep into the former socket.

- With the help of a fine tissue elevator, the soft tissues of the former socket are mobilized as part of the mucoperiosteal flap to the facial aspect, offering a thick flap with excellent vascularity.
- The osteotomy is prepared utilizing a surgical template to ensure ideal implant positioning.
- Assessment for additional grafting.
- Assessment of primary stability for implant loading time.
- Suturing to ensure tension free primary closure.

Early Implant Placement with Partial Bone Healing (12–16 Weeks)

Indications
- Multi-rooted sites
- Local infection involving the tooth
- Large apical bone defects where primary stability with immediate and early soft tissue healing placement approach is compromised

Late Implant Placement Complete Bone Healing (>6 months)

Indications It represents the original protocol for implant placement and was considered the standard of care in the 1980s. Although this approach is rarely used today, there are some clinical conditions where it is indicated. These are the following:

- In growing adolescent patients
- In situations where increased time for bone healing and modeling is desired, e.g. large cystic lesions, sinus floor
- Medical or other patient-related factors that may require treatment after extraction to be significantly delayed

Surgical Technique
- Mid-crestal incision (avoid vertical incisions)
- Flap reflection
- Osteotomy preparation with a surgical template and according to the manufacturer
- Placement of the implant in the ideal three-dimensional position
- Assessment for additional grafting
- Assessment of the primary stability for implant loading time
- Suturing to ensure tension free primary closure

Complications
- Loss of primary stability
- Early implant failure
- Infection

References

Amler, M. H. The time sequence of tissue regeneration in human extraction wounds. *Oral Surg. Oral Med. Oral Pathol.*, 1969 196927, 309–318.

Amler, M., Johnson, P., and Salman, I. (1960). Histological and histochemical investigation of human alveolar socket healing in undisturbed extraction wounds. *J. Am. Dent. A* 61: 32–44.

American Academy of Periodontology (2001). *Glossary of Periodontal Terms*, 4e. Chicago, IL: American Academy of Periodontology.

Araújo, M.G. and Lindhe, J. (2005). Dimensional ridge alterations following tooth extraction. An experimental study in the dog. *J. Clin. Periodontol.* 32 (2): 212–218.

Avila-Ortiz, G., Rodriguez, J.C., Rudek, I. et al. (2014). Effectiveness of three alveolar ridge preservation techniques: A pilot randomized control trial. *Int. J. Periodontics Restorative Dent.* 34: 509–521. https://doi.org/10.11607/prd.1838.

Cardaropoli, G., Araújo, M., and Lindhe, J. (2003). Dynamics of bone tissue formation in tooth extraction sites. An experimental study in dogs. *J. Clin. Periodontol.* 30: 809–818.

Chen, S.T. and Buser, D. (2008). ITI Treatment Guide Vol 3: Implants in extraction sockets. In: *Implants in Post-Extraction Sites: A Literature Update* (ed. D. Buser, U. Belser and D. Wismeijer), 9–16. Berlin: Quintessence Publishing Co, Ltd.

Chu, S.J., Hochman, M.N., Hui-Ping Tan-Chu, J. et al. (2014). A novel prosthetic device and method for guided tissue preservation of immediate postextraction socket implants. *Int. J. Periodontics Restorative Dent.* 34 (9): 885–890.

Darby, I., Chen, S.T., and Buser, D. (2009). Ridge preservation techniques for implant therapy. *The Int. J. Oral Maxilloac. Implants* 24 (Supplement): 260–271.

El Chaar, E. and Castano, A. (2017). A retrospective survival study of trabecular tantalum implants immediately placed in posterior extraction sockets using a flapless technique. *J. Oral Implantol.* 115–124.

El Chaar, E., Oshman, S., and Fallah Abed, P. (2016). Single-rooted extractions sockets: classification and treatment protocol. *Compend. Contin. Educ. Dent.* 537–541.

Elian, N., Cho, S.C., Froum, S. et al. (2007). A simplified socket classification and repair technique. *Pract. Proced. Aesthet. Dent.* 19 (2): 99–104.

Evian, C., Rosenberg, E., Coslet, J., and Corn, H. (1982). The osteogenic activity of bone removed from healing extraction sockets in humans. *J. Periodontol.* 19.

Fickl, S., Zuhr, O., Wachtel, H. et al. (2008). Tissue alterations after tooth extraction with and without surgical trauma: a volumetric study in the beagle dog. *J. Clin. Periodontol.* 35: 356–363.

Hämmerle CHF, Araújo MG, Simion M, On Behalf of the Osteology Consensus Group 2011. Evidence-based knowledge on the biology and treatment of extraction sockets. *Clin. Oral Implants Res.* 23(Suppl. 5), 2012, 80–82 doi: https://doi.org/10.1111/j.1600-0501.2011.02370.x

Hürzeler, M.B., Zuhr, O., Schupbach, P. et al. (2010). The socket-shield technique: a proof-of-principle report. *J. Clin. Periodontol.* 37: 855–862. https://doi.org/10.1111/j.1600-051X.2010.01595.

Kan, J.Y. and Rungcharassaeng, K. (2000). Immediate placement and provisionalization of maxillary anterior single implants: a surgical and prosthodontic rationale. *Pract. Periodont. Aesthet. Dent.* 12 (9): 817–824.

Lang, N.P., Pun, B.L., Lau, I.K.Y. et al. (2012). A systematic review on survival and success rates of implants placed immediately into fresh extraction sockets after at least one year. *Clin. Oral Implants Res.* 23 (Suppl. 5): 39–66.

Langer, B. (1994). Spontaneous in situ gingival augmentation. *Int. J. Periodontics Restorative Dent.* 14 (6): 524–535.

Lekholm, U. and Zarb, G.A. (1985). Patient selection and preparation. Chapter 12. In: *Tissue-Integrated Prostheses. Osseointegration in Clinical Dentistry* (ed. P.-I. Branemark, G.A. Zarb and T. Albrektsson), 199–209. Chicago, Ill: Quintessence Publishing Co Inc.

Lekovic, V., Camargo, P.M., Klokkevold, P. et al. (1998). Preservation of alveolar bone in extraction sockets using bioabsorbable membranes. *J. Periodontol.* 69: 1044–1049.

Orentlicher, G., Horowitz, A., Goldwaser, B., and Abboud, M. (2017). Ten myths of guided implant surgery. *Compend. Contin. Dent.* 38 (8): 552–557.

Osburn, R.C. (1974). Preservation of the alveolar ridge: a simplified technique for retaining teeth beneath removable appliances. *J. Indiana State Dent. Assoc.* 53 (1): 8–11.

Pietrokovski, J. and Massler, M. (1967). Alveolar ridge resorption following tooth extraction. *J. Prosthet. Dent.* 17: 21–27.

Salama, M., Ishikawa, I., Salama, H. et al. (2007). Advantages of the root submergence technique for pontic site development in esthetic implant therapy. *Int. J. Periodontics Restorative Dent.* 27: 521–527.

Schroeder, H.E. (1985). *The Periodontium*. Berlin Heidelberg: Springer-Verlag.

Schropp, L., Wenzel, A., Kostopoulos, L., and Karring, T. (2003). Bone healing and soft tissue contour changes following single-tooth extraction: a clinical and radiographic 12-month prospective study. *Int. J. Periodontics Restorative Dent.* 23 (4): 313–324.

Seibert, J.S. (1993). Treatment of moderate localized alveolar ridge defects. *Prev. Dent. Clin. North Am.* 37.

Simon, B., von Hagen, S., Deasy, M.J. et al. (2000). Changes in alveolar bone height and width following ridge augmentation using bone graft and membranes. *J. Periodontol.* 71: 1774–1791.

Su, H., Gonzalez-Martin, O., Weisgold, A., and Lee, E. (2010). Considerations of implant abutment and crown contour: critical contour and subcritical contour. *Int. J. Periodontics Restorative Dent.* 30: 335–334.

Wood, D.L., Hoag, P.M., Donnenfeld, O.W., and Rosenfeld, L.D. (1972). Alveolar crest reduction following full and partial thickness flaps. *J. Periodontol.* 43: 141–144.

Further Reading

Hammerle, C.H., Chen, S.T., and Wilson, T.G. Jr., (2004). Consensus statements and recommended clinical procedures regarding the placement of implants in extraction sockets. *Int. J. Oral Maxillofac. Implants* 19 (Suppl): 26–28.

19

Deficient Ridges Augmentation

Edgard El Chaar[2], Aikaterini Georgantza[1], and Wayne Kye[1]

[1] Ashman Department of Periodontology and Implant Dentistry, New York University College of Dentistry, New York, NY, USA
[2] Department of Periodontics, University of Pennsylvania, Dental Medicine, Philadelphia, PA, USA

Crestal Sinus Elevation

Background

Earliest description of a transalveolar approach to the sinus floor elevation procedure dates to Tatum (1986). It was later modified by Summers (1994), and since then, numerous iterations have been reported. This chapter will highlight the BAOSFE (bone-added osteotome sinus floor elevation) technique originally described by Summers.

Indications

A transalveolar (aka crestal, transcrestal, vertical, internal) sinus floor elevation is indicated when an implant is planned in the posterior region of the maxilla and there is inadequate residual bone height (RBH) for an adequately sized implant. It provides a conservative alternative to the lateral window (Caldwell-Luc) approach in that flap reflection is minimal, access is limited to the implant osteotomy, and predictable installation of the implant can usually be obtained concurrent to the procedure (versus a staged approach often encountered with the Caldwell-Luc technique). Localized elevation of the sinus floor limits unnecessary manipulation of the Schneiderian membrane, thereby mitigating the risk of sinus complications including tears, perforations, and post-operative infections. Additionally, when compared with the lateral window technique, there is a decrease in post-surgical morbidity, healing period prior to implant loading, chair time, materials, and overall financial costs to the patient and practitioner alike.

The multi-center retrospective study by Rosen et al. (1999) reported greater than 95% success rate for implants placed with the BAOSFE technique when the RBH was ≥5 mm. However, when the RBH was ≤4 mm RBH, successful osseointegration decreased to 85.7%. A recent systematic review by Shi et al. (2016), corroborated the results of Del Fabbro's systematic review, where the cumulative survival rates were significantly lower when the RBH was <5 mm. These results strongly suggest that the transalveolar sinus elevation is most predictable with an RBH ≥5 mm. The decision whether the implant placement would be concurrent to the sinus floor elevation or delayed after subsequent healing would be primarily dependent upon the primary stability of the implant.

Compared with a lateral window approach, the crestal sinus approach is seen to be as successful, if not more. In Del Fabbro's (2012) systematic review, the researchers found a 97.2% survival rate with follow-up of six years for the crestal approach compared with 93.7% for lateral window approach. However, as with any procedure, there are some risks and drawbacks. Anatomical variations in patients including the presence of septae at the implant sites, or pneumatization of the sinus following tooth loss are contraindications for the procedure. The technique is "blind" as there is no direct visualization of the sinus floor elevation. This may potentially increase the risk of perforations and complicate its management. Unlike the lateral window approach, the transalveolar sinus approach are usually limited to one to two implant sites and have a mean bone gain of 3.8 mm (Toffler 2004).

The specific type of sinus floor elevation depends on criteria including, but not limited to RBH, marginal bone width sinus anatomy, presence of intact Schneiderian membrane, extent of sites needing rehabilitation, clinician training and experience, and patient-related factors (medical history, preference, etc.). Practitioners need to consider alternative treatment options and develop patient catered care for each individual's needs as well as the surgeon's technical ability. These may include the lateral window approach, the use of osseodensification burs or the placement of short implants.

Armamentarium

In additional to the traditional implant surgical set-up, a number of additional instruments and materials should be at the practitioner's disposable for the transalveolar approach:

- **Drill stops** to allow the surgeon to limit the osteotomy to 1 mm short of the sinus floor
- **Ball-tipped probe or blunt depth gauge** to confirm the presence of bone or feel the exposed membrane
- **Offset osteotomes and mallet** to both infracture the sinus floor and pack the grafting material into the sinus cavity
- **Biomaterials**, such as bone replacement grafts and barriers, to augment the recipient site, to provide a buffer prior to grafting within the osteotomy, or to repair any tears or perforations

Surgical Technique

In the past, traditional intraoral radiographs and panoramic images have been sufficient to diagnose and treatment plan for a transcrestal sinus floor elevation of limited sites. However, with developments in radiographic technology, cone beam computed tomography would yield the ideal and recommended images to visualize sinus pneumatization, anatomy including septae, rule out any sinus pathology, and confirm residual ridge height.

Upon successful and profound anesthesia, appropriate incisions are made and a full-thickness mucoperiosteal flap is elevated to provide adequate visibility and access to the underlying ridge. Initiate osteotomy according to manufacturer's recommended protocol under copious sterile irrigation. Osteotomy depth should be approximately 1 mm crestal/occlusal to sinus floor. For example, if the RBH is 6 mm from the alveolar crest to the sinus floor, the depth of the osteotomy should NOT exceed 5 mm. Depth of prepared osteotomy should be verified with ball-tipped probe. Drill stops would be advantageous to ensure the tip of the drill does not extend further than planned. Continue widening your osteotomy to the final width. In most cases, this will be about 0.5 mm narrower than the final width of the proposed implant fixture. This ensures a wider surface area for the graft and osteotome and minimizes sinus perforations. Add a small amount of hydrated BRG (one scoop of a Miller or Lucas curette). BRG should be filled to no more than $\frac{1}{2}$ the depth of the osteotomy. Using the example of a 5 mm osteotomy depth, graft about 2.5 mm in height.

Next, select the widest osteotome possible to passively fit into your prepared osteotomy. Ensuring proper angulation and finger rests, gently tap the osteotome with the mallet. You should feel a decrease in resistance (or the "break"). Summers (1998) stated that the concave tip of the osteotome traps the BRG and fluids as the instrument is inserted, which in turn, creates a hydraulic force which exerts pressure in all directions ("Pascal's law"). The BRG within the osteotomy appears to serve as a buffer/cushion for the sinus floor infracture. Important point is to ensure that the osteotome NEVER exceed the initially measured RBH. In this way, you are providing a safety check so that perforation of the sinus secondary to the osteotome extending into the sinus cavity is taken out of the equation. The Valsalva maneuver should be performed to test for any sinus perforations by gently holding the patient's nostrils and asking to blow through the nose. If air is noted from the osteotomy, it's a probably indication that there is a sinus perforation and the grafting should be aborted.

Continue the process of grafting, aligning osteotome and gently tapping for about 10 times prior to exposing a radiograph. Ten times is an arbitrary number but adequate to have enough crestal sinus elevation that would be apparent and visible on the radiograph. A "dome" of the BRG should be noted. Generally, 0.5–1 cc of BRG would suffice for a single site. If an implant is to be placed simultaneously, complete your last osteotome crestal tap similarly and do NOT extend the osteotome to the final proposed depth. The final installation of the fixture ensures further displacement of the BRG within the sinus cavity.

If it is determined that this will be a staged transalveolar sinus augmentation, then the procedure should be completed with BRG placed all the way to the most crestal portion of the osteotomy. A barrier may be considered to cover the grafted site. Usually, a four to six month healing period appears to be adequate in time to ensure that proper healing and consolidation of the crestal sinus graft has occurred. At the time of fixture placement, adequate RBH should be present. If further crestal augmentation is necessary, an additional crestal sinus augmentation may be performed with a concurrent implant placement.

Complications

Tan et al. (2008) reported the most commonly reported complication was perforation of the sinus membrane, which varied from 0–21.4%, with a mean of 3.8%. Post-operative infection was observed less than 1% of the time. Attempts can be made to repair the perforation and/or tear with a variety of materials (i.e. resorbable collagen membrane, wound dressings). If the perforation/tear is irreparable or too severe, the procedure should be aborted. Infrequently, complications such as benign paroxysmal positional vertigo and detached retina have been reported.

Follow-Up

Post-surgical medications may include an analgesic or NSAID, an antibiotic, an anti-bacterial rinse and a nasal decongestant. A routine post-surgical appointment should be performed within 7–14 days of the procedure. Results from a three-year multicenter randomized controlled trial demonstrated that short implants (5–6 mm) have demonstrated similar success rates compared with longer implants (10 mm) placed in osteotome-mediated sites (Gastaldi et al. 2017).

Lateral Sinus Floor Elevation

Background

The introduction of sinus floor augmentation, which has facilitated the placement of longer implants in the posterior maxilla, has led to an improvement of overall prognosis of maxillary implants. The first paper concerning the treatment of patients with endosseous implants associated with maxillary sinus elevations operations was published in 1980 by Boyne and James. The maxillary sinus was accessed via antrostomy in order to create a "bone window" on the lateral wall which was then delicately pushed and turned inside the antrum. The material used for the graft was generally autogenous bone harvested from the iliac crest and blade implants were inserted in a subsequent operation, some months after the sinus elevation procedure. Since then, this procedure has become a very predictable and well documented one that is an integral part of dental implant treatment.

Indications

Insufficient residual alveolar bone height in the posterior maxilla of equal or less than 5 mm may result from alveolar bone resorption following tooth loss, bone loss due to periodontal disease, pneumatization of the maxillary sinus, or a combination of the above.

Wallace and Froum (2003) found the overall of implant survival rate was 91.8% after reviewing 3220 implants placed and Del Fabbro (2004) found it to be 91.49% after reviewing 6913 implants placed in 2046 subjects. More recently, Del Fabbro (2013), found an overall implant survival after a minimum of three years loading was 93.7% and 97.2% for the lateral window and transalveolar approaches, respectively. Of importance is the fact that 80% of failures occurred within the first year and 93.1% of the failures occurred within three years.

Grafting Materials

Grafting materials range from autogenous bone to allograft to xenograft, to synthetic bone used with or without membrane over the lateral osteotomy. The important points to cover are the vitality of grafted material, survivability of the implants in these grafts, and the amount of remodeling of the grafted material.

In relation to bone vitality, Tarnow et al. (2000) showed that the use of the membrane has affected the vitality of bone from 11.9% vital bone without using membranes versus 25.5% when using membranes in 12 bilateral cases. Further to that, they found a higher survival rate of 100% with membrane versus 92.6% without membrane in 55 placed dental implants over five years.

Later, Froum et al. in (2006) conducted a histomorphometric bi-lateral study comparing xenograft versus allograft in a 13 bilateral sinus lifts found twice more vital bone with the allograft sinuses and ¼ less residual material as well.

In relation to survivability of the implants in grafted sinuses and of importance, Del Fabbro (2004) correlated the grafting material to the survival rate of dental implant placed in a grafted sinus as follows:

1. 87.7% when autogenous bone was used alone.
2. 94.88% when combining autogenous with various bone substitutes
3. 95.98% when various bone substitute were used alone

which brings us to the amount of residual bone graft. Mordenfeld in a 30 maxillary sinus lifts using a Mixture of Xenograft (DPBB) 80% and 20% autogenous bone did a histomorphometric analysis at 6 months and 11 years and found no statistically significant differences between the length and area of the particles after 11 years compared with those measured after 6 months in the same patients or to pristine particles from the manufacturer.

Later, Danesh-Sani et al. (2017), in a systematic review evaluating histomorphometric variables, the amount of new bone (NB), residual graft (RG) particles, and soft tissue (ST), related to various grafting materials assess the effect of graft healing time on different histomorphometric outcomes. They found: Autogenous bone (AB) resulted in the highest amount of NB and lowest amount of RG compared with other grafting materials. Based on this meta-analysis, a significant difference was noticed in the amount of NB formation in grafts with a healing time of >4.5 month when compared with the grafts with less healing time. However, when comparing biopsies taken at 4.5–9 month of healing (average = 6.22 month) to the ones taken at ≥9–13.5 month (average = 10.36 month), no significant difference was noticed in the amount of NB formation of various grafts except allografts that resulted in a significantly higher percentage of NB at 9.5 month of healing. Based on histomorphometric analysis, AB results in the highest amount of NB formation in comparison with the other grafting materials. Bone substitute materials (allografts, alloplastic materials, and xenografts) seem to be good alternatives to autogenous bone and can be considered as grafting materials to avoid disadvantages related to AB, including morbidity rate, limited availability, and high volumetric change. Combining AB with alloplastic materials and xenografts brings no significant advantages regarding NB formation.

Anatomical Considerations

The maxillary sinuses are bilateral bony cavities in the maxilla, containing an air space volume of approximately 15 cc each, lined by pseudostratified columnar epithelium. The maxillary sinus is located in the body of the maxilla and is the largest of the pneumatic paranasal chambers.

It has the shape of a pyramid:

- Apex: extends into zygomatic process of maxilla
- Base or medial wall makes part of lateral wall of the nasal cavity
- 4 walls:
  a. anterior similar to the maxilla anterior wall
  b. posterior corresponds to the infratemporal surface of maxilla
  c. inferior or floor corresponds to alveolar process
  d. superior or roof is the orbital surface of the maxilla
     The majority of maxillary sinuses have their floors at varying distances below the level of the floor of the nasal fossa. The maxillary sinus communicates with the nasal fossa through *the ostium maxillare, which is the Ostium of maxillary sinus* using the middle nasal concha.
     The ostium also communicates with the ethmoidale cells thru infundibulum ethmoidale.

A healthy sinus is self-maintained by postural drainage and actions of the cilicated epithelial lining, which propels bacteria toward the ostium. It also produces mucous with lysozyrnes and immnoglobulins. The rich vascularity of the sinus membrane helps to maintain it in a healthy state by facilitating lymphocyte and immunoglobulin access to the membrane and the sinus cavity. The healthy sinus contains its own flora, of which Haemophilus is the most common species.

Other than the descriptive anatomy of the sinus, there are two important landmarks:

A. Vascularizations
   Vascularization of the lateral maxilla is supplied by branches of the posterior superior alveolar artery (PSAA) and the infraorbital artery (IOA) that form an anastomosis in the bony lateral antral wall, which also supplies the Schneiderian membrane. Both arteries had an average diameter of 1.6 mm.

Solar et al. (1999), in 18 maxillary specimens, they found the PSSA divide itself in two intra-osseous anastomosis connecting with the IOA, the Internal intra-osseous anastomosis (IA) and the external intra-osseous anastomosis (EA) that lounges in the external wall. The mean distance between the alveolar ridge and the external intraosseous-anastomosis was 23 mm.

The blood supply of the graft periphery is provided by the Schneiderian membrane, intraosseous vascular bundles, and the center of the graft from the endosseous anastomosis; thus the bony window should be as small as possible.

B. Septae
Bornstein is a study that included 294 maxillary sinuses in 212 patients (126 women and 86 men) with a mean age of 53.8 years. Sinus septa were present in 141 patients (66.5%) and in 166 of 294 sinuses (56.5%). The most common orientation of the septa was coronal (61.8%), 7.6% were oriented axially, and 3.6% were aligned sagittally. Most septa were located on the floor of the maxillary sinus (58.6%), commonly (60.7%) in the region of the first and second molars.

Another important fact that he found in his study that can be of great relevance, is the maxillary sinuses were diagnosed in 36.4% of cases as healthy and without thickening of the sinus membrane. Sex was a significant variable in the health of the maxillary sinus; 57.7% of the sinuses in women and 72.3% in men were diagnosed as pathologic.

Armamentarium

- Presurgical cone beam computed tomography (CBCT) scans to disclose sinus pathology and difficult anatomy
- Round diamond burs
- Specially designed hand instruments for lateral sinus elevation
- Piezoelectric surgery with sinus specific inserts
- Materials to control bleeding (electrocautery, local with 1 : 50 000 epinephrine, bone wax)
- Biomaterials, such as bone replacement grafts and barrier membranes, to graft the sinus cavity, or to repair any tears or perforations of the sinus membrane

Surgical Technique

Upon successful and profound anesthesia, mid-crestal and anterior releasing incisions are made. A full-thickness mucoperiosteal flap is elevated to provide adequate visibility and access to the underlying ridge. After the flap reflection the window at the lateral wall of the sinus is designed with a round diamond bur. This can be done with a piezoelectric insert too, which minimizes the risk of sinus membrane perforation. Then the sinus membrane is carefully elevated with the specially designed hand and/or piezoelectric instruments. Care must be taken to ensure that the membrane is elevated all the way to the medial wall. The bone graft material is then placed and carefully packed in the sinus cavity while the membrane is held up with a hand instrument. A resorbable membrane can be placed in the sinus to prevent or manage a small perforation and on top of the window.

Factors Influencing Lateral Sinus Augmentation Success and Implant Survival Rate

- Type of grafting material (autogenous, allograft, xenograft, alloplast)
- Type of implants (rough versus smooth surface)
- Loading conditions (immediate versus delayed)
- Residual bone quality and quantity
- Use or non-use of barrier membrane over the lateral window
- Smoking habits
- Skill of the surgeon

Complications

The maxillary sinus elevation procedure is today considered to be the most predictable of the pre-prosthetic surgical techniques with success rates, as determined by the secondary outcome measure of implant survival, in the high 90th percentile (Aghaloo and Moy 2007; Del Fabbro et al. 2013). However, each surgical step of the sinus elevation surgery, if not performed properly, may lead to complications. These complications may occur intraoperatively or postoperatively.

A. Intraoperative complications
  ○ Bleeding
  ○ Sinus (Schneiderian) membrane perforation: Perforation of the Schneiderian membrane is the most frequent intra-operative complication associated with this procedure. Krenmair et al. (2007) reported a prevalence rate for perforation of 58.3%. In an interesting retrospective study, Froum et al. (2013)) found the augmented sinuses that exhibited perforation of the Schneiderian membrane and were repaired showed statistically greater vital bone percentages compared with the non-perforated sinus group. They postulated that if perforations are repaired properly during surgery, do not appear to be an adverse complication in terms of vital bone production or implant survival.
  Vlassis and Fugazzotto (1999) introduced a classification system for sinus membrane perforations

encountered during a sinus augmentation procedure. Five of the perforations are discussed, as are the therapeutic options for their repair. Classes I and II perforations are most easily repaired, while Class IV is the most difficult to successfully treat. In addition, the effect of the sinus membrane perforation on the course of proposed therapy is discussed. When classified and managed appropriately, sinus membrane perforations are not an absolute indication for aborting the augmentation procedure which is in progress.
  There are two anatomical that contribute to increasing the odds of sinus perforations. One is the Palato-nasal Recess on medial wall of the maxillary sinus (Chan et al. 2013), and the second is the angle that is formed between the lateral wall and the medial wall at the level of the sinus floor, leading both of them to higher risk of perforations.
  ○ Tears in the buccal flap and injury to the infraorbital nerve that generally result from poor surgical technique
B. **Postoperative complications**
  ○ Infection
  ○ Postoperative sinusitis
  ○ Loss of graft material through the window
  ○ Migration of implants into sinus or sinus graft

Prevention of Complications

- Obtain preoperative CBCT scan for accurate diagnosis and treatment planning
- Prescribe antibiotics
- Use piezoelectric surgery for lateral osteotomy and initial membrane elevation to avoid trauma to the vessels and minimize the risk of perforating the sinus membrane
- Have materials on hand to control intraoperative bleeding (electrocautery, local with 1:50 000 epinephrine, bone wax)
- Elevate the membrane from lateral to medial wall, maintain contact of the instrument with the bone at all times

Follow-up

Post-surgical medications may include an analgesic or NSAID, an antibiotic, an anti-bacterial rinse, and a nasal decongestant. A routine post-surgical appointment should be performed within 7–14 days of the procedure.

Ridge Augmentation

Fundamentals of Ridge Augmentation

Correcting ridge deficiency has always been a goal in modern dentistry. Many classifications for the shape of the defects with treatment modalities have been described. Before we dive in reviewing these classifications, one has to cover the principles of bone regeneration.

Developmentally, the alveolar bone of the maxilla and mandible is formed through a process called *intramembranous* bone formation. It is also seen in the cranial vault and in the mid shaft of long bones. In contrast, bone formation in the remaining part of the skeleton occurs via a process called *endochondral* bone formation.

Chronically one will focus on the paper by Seibert and Nyman of 1990 (Seibert and Nyman 1990) done on beagle dogs. Ridge defects were created bi-laterally. One side had the sites treated with membrane and implanted material under the membranes to create a space did generate active NB and in the control side, two sites were treated with a membrane with no implantable graft and one site with implantable graft with no membrane, in both control scenarios no NB was formed.

The second paper, by Schenk et al. (1994) found the following:

1. The placement of barrier membranes promotes bone regeneration in alveolar ridge lesions by:
   physical support of the overlying soft tissue
   creation of a space filled with a blood clot into which osteogenic cells can migrate, and protection of the granulation tissue and the delicate vascular network during the organization of the hematoma;
   exclusion of competing non-osteogenic cells
   possible local accumulation of growth factors and other bone-promoting substances.
2. Bone regeneration in membrane-protected defects closely follows the pattern of bone development and growth:
   a. The first stage corresponds to intramembranous (direct) ossification and results in the formation of primary spongiosa.
   b. In the second stage, this scaffold is reinforced by parallel-fibered and lamellar bone.
   c. The third stage is characterized by cancellous and cortical bone remodeling.
3. A prolonged healing period may be required in larger defects (the study was done up to four months).
4. The metal reinforced membranes reliably preserved their original form throughout the healing period, whereas the standard e-PTFE membranes partially collapsed.

Those two papers lead us to three cardinal points in ridge augmentation: space creation, space maintenance, and stabilization are key for a successful regeneration.

Surgical Techniques

Various therapeutic approaches can be considered in ridge augmentation, autogenous block bone grafting (Cordaro et al. 2002), inter-positional autografts (Jensen 2006), distraction osteogenesis (Garcia-Garcia et al. 2003) and guided bone regeneration with membranes (Simion et al. 2001; Ronda et al. 2014), or titanium meshes (Louis et al. 2008; El Chaar et al. 2019).

Ridge Classifications

Classification systems are generally used to establish guidelines for treatment of a particular clinical situation. The available classification systems of ridge volume represent valuable guidelines for evaluating alveolar ridge defects. However, certain limitations that restrict their applicability in daily clinical practice can be found. For example, Seibert's classification (Cordaro et al. 2002) represents the three broad categories of ridge defects, but a division of those defects into subcategories is lacking. Each of the three classifications can be further subdivided into categories based on the size of the defect. Such division may prove useful in selecting treatment modalities and predicting treatment outcomes. Furthermore, Seibert's classification was originally used to address treatment of ridge defects in preparation for receiving a pontic. As such, presented treatment options were all ST augmentation procedures used to enhance the esthetic appearance of fixed partial dentures. For that reason, dividing defect types into different size categories may again prove valuable for predicting the degree of success of the various treatment modalities available for the treatment of both soft and hard tissue defects.

Seibert
Class I: buccolingual loss of tissue with normal apico-coronal ridge height
Class II: apico-coronal loss of tissue with normal buccolingual ridge width
Class III: combination-type defects (loss of both height and width)

Misch and Judy (1987) (Jensen 2006) wrote a classification

A: abundant bone
B: barely sufficient bone
C: compromised bone with sub-classification (C-h: compromised height; C-w: compromised width)

Lekholm and Zarb (1985) (Garcia-Garcia et al. 2003) in their classification they defined the following:

A: virtually intact alveolar ridge

B: minor resorption of alveolar ridge

C: advanced resorption of alveolar ridge to base of dental arch

D: initial resorption of base of dental arch

E: extreme resorption of base of dental arch

Allen et al. (1985) (Simion et al. 2001)

A: apicocoronal loss of tissue

B: buccolingual loss of tissue

C: combination

In this classification, numeric measurements of severity have been introduced as follows:

Mild: <3 mm; Medium: 3–6 mm; Severe: >6 mm

HVC System classification (Ronda et al. 2014):

This system is a modification of Seibert's classification that attempts to address some of its limitations. The three broad categories are still present, with the use of simpler terminology, referring to Classes I, II, and III defects as Horizontal (H), Vertical (V), and Combination (C) defects, respectively.

Each category is further subdivided into:

- small (s, ≤3 mm)
- medium (m, 4–6 mm)
- large (l, ≥7 mm) subcategories

Both soft and hard tissue defects are considered in this classification scheme, with treatment options suggested based on the type and size of the defect and the planned restorative treatment plan.

In this classification, they gave a treatment options based on HVC classification as described as follows:

Defect class	Soft tissue augmentation	Hard tissue augmentation
H-s	Pouch procedure Roll procedure	Ridge expansion procedures
H-m	Tunnel procedure	Advanced flap + GBR
H-l	Advanced flap + CTG	Advanced flap + monocortical block bone grafts (MBG)

Defect class	Soft tissue augmentation	Hard tissue augmentation
V-s	Advanced flap + CTG	Orthodontic extrusion
V-m	Interpositional graft	Advanced flap + GBR/MBG
V-l	Onlay soft tissue graft	Distraction osteogenesis

Defect class	Soft tissue augmentation	Hard tissue augmentation
C-s	Advanced flap + CTG	Advanced flap + GBR
C-m	Advanced flap + CTG	Advanced flap + GBR OR
C-l	Advanced flap + CTG	Large extraoral block grafts (tibia, rib, calvaria)

Expectations of Ridge Augmentation

We will divide this part in two:

Horizontal Ridge Augmentation

Buser et al. (1996) (Wang and Shammari 2002) using autogenous bone blocks covered with expanded polytetrafluoroethylene membranes reported a mean crest width gain of 3.53 mm to 7.1 mm average of *5.3 mm*.

The sites were *mainly in the maxilla*.

Fifty-eight sites were augmented, including 41 sites *located in the anterior maxilla*.

Von Arx and Buser (2006) (Buser et al. 1996), using xenograft with resorbable collagen membrane, a mean initial crest width measured 3.06 mm. At re-entry, the mean width of the ridge was 7.66 mm, *with a calculated mean gain of horizontal bone thickness of 4.6 mm* (range 2–7 mm). Only minor surface resorption of 0.36 mm was observed from augmentation to re-entry.

Vertical Ridge Augmentation

Simion et al. (1998) made a comparative study between implant positioned to the desired height and in one side grafted with demineralized freeze-dried bone allograft Group A and the other side autogenous bone chips Group B with titanium-reinforced expanded polytetrafluoroethylene membranes were used to cover the implants and complete membrane fixation was established. The clinical measurements from Group A demonstrated a mean vertical bone gain of 3.1 mm and in Group B a mean vertical bone gain of 5.02 mm. Both the clinical and histologic results indicate a beneficial effect of the addition of demineralized freeze-dried bone allograft or autogenous bone particles to vertical ridge augmentation procedures in humans. In a long-term retrospective study of implants placed in vertically augmented bone, Simion et al. (2001) concluded that

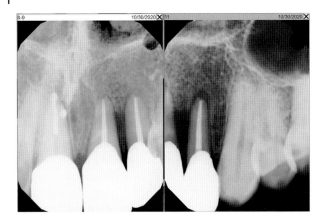

Figure 19.1 Radiograph showing the amount of bone loss that this 43-year-old male presented with. He had a ski accident a year before and subsequently he was treated by two endodontic treatments on #9 and 10.

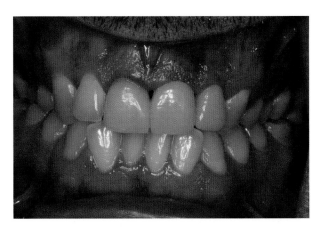

Figure 19.4 Patient was temporized at first with a bridge going from #8.

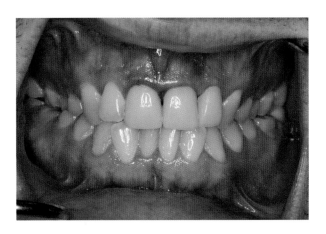

Figure 19.2 He received three crowns including #8.

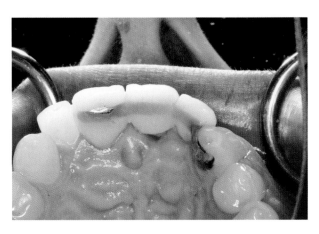

Figure 19.5 The temporary bridge was bonded on the lingual of #11.

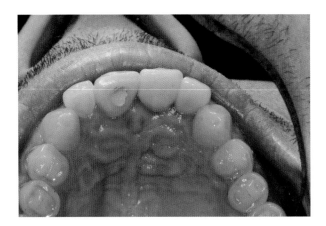

Figure 19.3 #8 later ended up re-treated endodontically 6 months after the crown inserted.

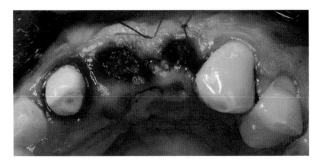

Figure 19.6 #9 and 10 were extracted and a resorbable collagen plug were placed in each socket to enhance soft tissue healing.

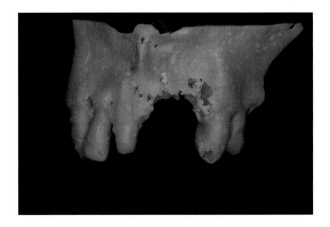

Figure 19.7 The bony defect was 3 D printed. This is the buccal view buccal.

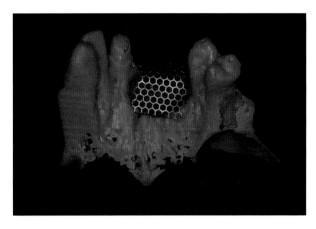

Figure 19.10 Occlusal view of the titanium mesh medical grade fitted.

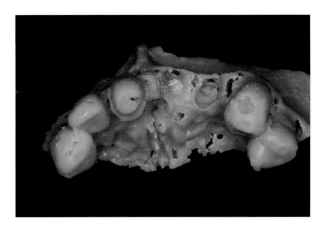

Figure 19.8 Occlusal view of the 3 D printed model.

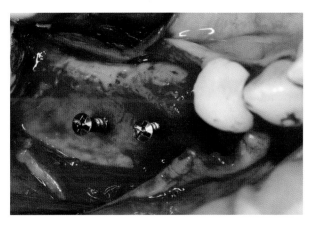

Figure 19.11 Creating a space can be also created using tenting screws as shown here from a different case.

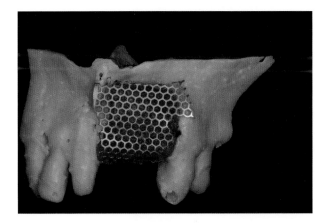

Figure 19.9 A was shaped to fit over the volume needed that was built using wax. Buccal view.

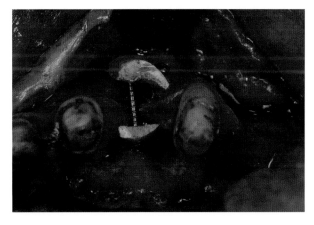

Figure 19.12 Creating a space can be also created using autogenous blocks as shown here from a different case.

vertically augmented bone with GBR techniques responds to implant placement like native, non-regenerated bone.

Urban et al. (2019) in a systematic review and meta-analysis found that Clinical vertical bone gain and complications rate varied among the different procedures, with a weighted mean gain of 8.04 mm and complications rate of 47.3% for distraction osteogenesis, 4.18 mm and 12.1% for guided bone regeneration (GBR), and 3.46 mm and 23.9% for bone blocks. In comparative studies, GBR achieved a significant greater bone gain when compared with bone blocks.

In regard to the use of titanium mesh mainly medical grade ones, a semi rigid allows the rigidity needed to shape the space and make it resist to the bending forces of the chewing forces in the oral cavity. Louis et al. (2008) (Louis et al. 2008) found a mean augmented height of 13.7 mm and the success of the bone grafting was 97.72%.

El Chaar et al. (2019) used titanium mesh with 100% allograft, group 1 the titanium mesh was prepared from stone models and ingroup 2 from 3D printed models. They found the following:

Group 1: horizontal gain 6.91 mm; and vertical gain of 5.76 mm
Group 2: horizontal gain 5.94 mm and vertical of 6.99 mm

Fundamentals of Successful Surgical Technique

Since the three cardinal points of a successful ridge augmentation are space creation, space maintenance/containment and stabilization, the clinicians need to prepare the site properly that will start with the incisions, flap management, decortication, stable semi-rigid of the space maintainer, stabilization of the graft, and finally passivation of the flap (El Chaar et al. 2019; Ronda and Stacchi 2011; Ronda and Stacchi 2015; Abed et al. 2020).

The careful management of the ST is key to the success: Obtaining and maintaining primary closure of the flap during healing is necessary to prevent contamination and infection of the membrane, an event that always compromises the augmentation procedure (Ronda and Stacchi 2015; Abed et al. 2020; Simion et al. 1994). Maintaining closure of the flap over non-resorbable membranes is even more because expanded polytetrafluoroethylene separates the flap from the underlying periosteal vascularization, depriving it of an important blood supply (Ronda and Stacchi 2015; Abed et al. 2020; Simion et al. 1994).

Clinical Case of Ridge Augmentation

A 43 year old male presented for a treatment of his two maxillary left incisors #9 and 10. He had a ski accident a year

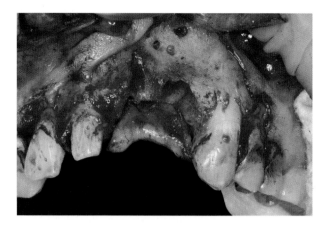

Figure 19.13 Upon flap reflection, we confirmed the defect was similar to what we saw from the 3 D printing. Buccal view.

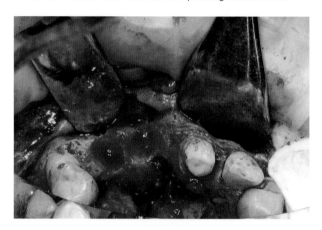

Figure 19.14 Occlusal view, confirming the defect as similar to the 3 D printed one.

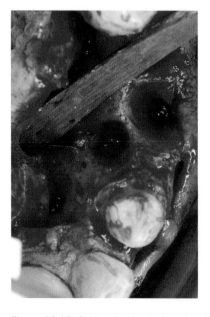

Figure 19.15 Occlusal-palatal view showing the cleaned up naso-palatine orifice.

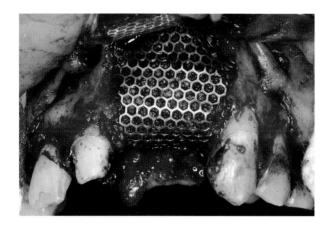

Figure 19.16 The titanium mesh was secured after the allograft layered cancellous cortical was placed by titanium screws. Buccal view.

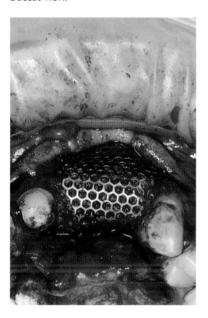

Figure 19.17 Occlusal view of the secured titanium mesh.

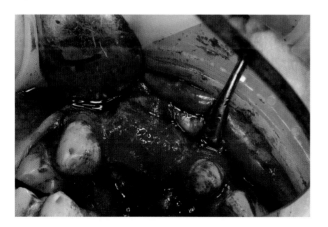

Figure 19.18 In 8 months, the titanium mesh was removed. We can appreciate the volume gained. Occlusal view.

before and subsequently he was treated by two endodontic treatment on #9 and 10 and three crowns including #8. The latter ended up treated endodontically 6 months after the crown inserted. (Figures 19.1–19.3). Patient was temporized (Figures 19.4, 19.5) and #9 and 10 extracted and a resorbable collagen plugs were placed to enhance soft tissue healing (Figure 19.6). The bony defect was 3 D printed (Figures 19.7, 19.8). One of the pillar of a successful ridge augmentation is space creation, in this case we decided to use titanium mesh medical grade that we shaped to fit to the volume that is needed to build (Figures 19.9, 19.10).

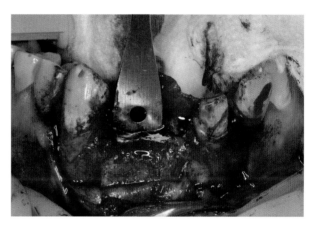

Figure 19.19 Buccal view of the rebuilt bone.

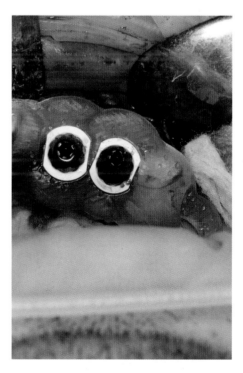

Figure 19.20 Two implants placed in a guided manner.

Creating a space can be also created using tenting screws (Figure 19.11), or autogenous blocks (Figure 19.12).

Once flap was reflected, we confirmed the defect was similar to what we saw from the 3 D printing (Figures 19.13, 19.14). The titanium mesh was secured after the allograft layered cancellous cortical was placed (Figures 19.15, 19.16). In 8 months, the titanium mesh was removed (Figures 19.17, 19.18) and two implants placed in a guided manner (Figures 19.19, 19.20).

(This figures were provided by Dr. El Chaar).

References

Abed, P.F., El Chaar, E., Boltchi, F., and Bassir, S.H. (2020). The novel periosteal flap stretch echnique: a predictable method to achieve and maintain primary closure in augmentative procedures. *J. Int. Acad. Periodontol.* 22 (1): 11–20. PubMed PMID: 31896103.

Aghaloo, T. and Moy, P.K. (2007). Which hard tissue augmentation techniques are the most successful in furnishing bony support for implant placement? *Int. J. Oral Maxillofac. Implants* 22 (Suppl): 49–70.

Allen, E.P., Gainza, C.S., Farthing, G.G., and Newbold, D.A. (1985). Improved technique for localized ridge augmentation: a report of 21 cases. *J. Periodontol.* 56: 195–199.

Buser, D., Dula, K., Hirt, H.P., and Schenk, R.K. (1996). Lateral ridge augmentation using autografts and barrier membranes: a clinical study with 40 partially edentulous patients. *Int. J. Oral Maxillofac. Surg.* 54: 420–432.

Chan, H.L., Monje, A., Suarez, F. et al. (2013). Palatonasal recess on medial wall of the maxillary sinus and clinical implications for sinus augmentation via lateral window approach. *J. Periodontol.* 84 (8): 1087–1093.

Cordaro, L., Amadé, D.S., and Cordaro, M. (2002). Clinical results of alveolar ridge augmentation with mandibular block bone grafts in partially edentulous patients prior to implant placement. *Clin. Oral Implants Res.* 13: 103–111.

Danesh-Sani, S., Engebretson, S.P., and Janal, M. (2017). Histomorphometric results of different grafting materials and effect of healing time on bone maturation after sinus floor augmentation: a systematic review and meta-analysis. *J. Periodontal Res.* 52 (3): 301–312.

Del Fabbro, M., Testori, T., Francetti, L., and Weinstein, R. (2004). Systematic review of survival rates for implants placed in the grafted maxillary sinus. *Int. J. Periodontics Restorative Dent.* 24 (6).

El Chaar, E., Urtula, B., Georgantza, A. et al. (2019). Treatment of atrophic ridges with titanium mesh: a retrospective study using 100% mineralized allograft and comparing dental stone versus 3D-printed models. *Int. J. Periodontics Restorative Dent.* 39: 491–500. https://doi .org/10.11607/prd.3733.

Del Fabbro, M. et al. (2013). Long-term implant survival in the grafted maxillary sinus: a systematic review. *Int. J. Periodontics Restorative Dent.* 33: 773–783.

Froum, S.J., Wallace, S.S., Elian, N. et al. (2006). Comparison of mineralized cancellous bone allograft (Puros) and anorganic bovine bone matrix (Bio-Oss) for sinus augmentation: histomorphometry at 26 to 32 weeks after grafting. *Int. J. Periodontics Restorative Dent.* 26 (6).

Froum, S.J., Khouly, I., Favero, G., and Cho, S.C. (2013). Effect of maxillary sinus membrane perforation on vital bone formation and implant survival: a retrospective study. *J. Periodontol.* 84: 1094–1099.

Gastaldi, G., Felice, P., Pistilli, R. et al. (2017). Short implants as an alternative to crestal sinus lift: a 3-year multicenter randomized controlled trial. *Eur. J. Oral Implantol.* 10 (4): 391–400.

Jensen, O.T. (2006). Alveolar segmental "sandwich" osteotomies for posterior edentulous mandibular sites for dental implants. *J. Oral Maxillofac. Surg.* 64: 471–475.

Krenmair, G., Krainhofner, M., Schmid-Schwap, M., and Piehslinger, E. (2007). Maxillary sinus lift for single implant-restorations: a clinical study. *Int. J. Oral Maxillofac. Implants* 22: 351–358.

Lekholm, U. and Zarb, G. (1985). Patient selection and preparation. In: *Tissue-Integrated Prostheses: Osseointegration in Clinical Dentistry* (ed. P.-I. Branemark), 199–209. Chicago: Quintessence.

Louis, P.J., Gutta, R., Said-Al-Naief, N., and Bartolucci, A.A. (2008). Reconstruction of the maxilla and mandible with particulate bone graft and titanium mesh for implant placement. *J. Oral Maxillofac. Surg.* 66: 235–245.

Misch, C.E. and Judy, K.W. (1987). Classification of partially edentulous arches for implant dentistry. *Int. J. Oral Implantol.* 4: 7–13.

Ronda, M. and Stacchi, C. (2011). Management of a coronally advanced lingual flap in regenerative osseous surgery: a case series introducing a novel technique. *Int. J. Periodontics Restorative Dent.* 31 (5): 505.

Ronda, M. and Stacchi, C. (2015). A novel approach for the coronal advancement of the buccal flap. *Int. J. Periodontics Restorative Dent.* 35 (6): 795–801.

Ronda, M., Rebaudi, A., Torelli, L., and Stacchi, C. (2014). Expanded vs. dense polytetrafluoroethylene membranes in vertical ridge augmentation around dental implants:

a prospective randomized controlled clinical trial. *Clin. Oral Implants Res.* 25: 859–866.

Rosen, P.S., Summers, R.B., Mellado, J.R. et al. (1999). The bone-added osteotome sinus floor elevation technique: multicenter retrospective report of consecutively treated patients. *Int. J. Oral Maxillofac. Implants* 14: 853–858.

Schenk, R.K., Buser, D., Hardwick, W.R., and Dahlin, C. (1994). Healing pattern of bone regeneration in membrane-protected defects: a histologic study in the canine mandible. *Int. J. Oral Maxillofac. Implants* 9 (1).

Seibert, J. and Nyman, S. (1990). Localized ridge augmentation in dogs: a pilot study using membranes and hydroxylapatite. *J. Periodontol.* 61: 157.

Shi, J.Y., Gu, Y.X., Zhuang, L.F. et al. (2016). Survival of implants using the osteotome technique with or without grafting in the posterior maxilla: a systematic review. *Int. J. Oral Maxillofac. Implants* 31: 1077–1088.

Simion, M., Baldoni, M., Rossi, P., and Zaffe, D. (1994). A comparative study of the effectiveness of e-PTFE membranes with and without early exposure during the healing period. *Int. J. Periodontics Restorative Dent.* 14: 166–180.

Simion, M., Jovanovic, S.A., Trisi, P. et al. (1998). Vertical ridge augmentation around dental implants using a membrane technique and autogenous bone or allografts in humans. *Int. J. Periodontics Restorative Dent.* 18 (1).

Simion, M., Jovanovic, S.A., Tinti, C., and Benfenati, S.P. (2001). Long-term evaluation of osseointegrated implants inserted at the time or after vertical ridge augmentation: A retrospective study on 123 implants with 1–5 year follow-up. *Clin. Oral Implants Res.* 12 (1): 35–45.

Solar, P., Geyerhofer, U., Traxler, H. et al. (1999). Blood supply to the maxillary sinus relevant to sinus floor elevation procedures. *Clin. Oral Implants Res.* 10 (1): 34–44.

Summers, R.B. (1994). A new concept in maxillary implant surgery: the osteotome technique. *Compendium* 15 (2): 152–158.

Summers, R.B. (1998). Sinus floor elevation with osteotomes. *J. Esthet. Dent.* 10 (3): 164–171.

Tan, W.C., Lang, N.P., Zwahlen, M. et al. (2008). A systematic review of the success of sinus floor elevation and survival of implant inserted in combination with sinus floor elevation Part II: transalveolar technique. *J. Clin. Periodontol.* 35 (Suppl 8): 241–254.

Tarnow, D.P., Wallace, S.S., Froum, S.J. et al. (2000). Histologic and clinical comparison of bilateral sinus floor elevations with and without barrier membrane placement in 12 patients: part 3 of an ongoing prospective study. *Int. J. Periodontics Restorative Dent.* 20 (2).

Tatum, O.H. (1986). Maxillary and sinus implant reconstruction. *Dent. Clin. North Am.* 30: 207–229.

Toffler, M. (2004). Osteotome-mediated sinus floor elevation: a clinical report. *Int. J. Oral Maxillofac. Implants* 19: 266–273.

Urban, I.A., Montero, E., Monje, A., and Sanz-Sánchez, I. (2019). Effectiveness of vertical ridge augmentation interventions: a systematic review and meta-analysis. *J. Clin. Periodontol.* 46: 319–339.

Vlassis, J.M. and Fugazzotto, P.A. (1999). A classification system for sinus membrane perforations during augmentation procedures with options for repair. *J. Periodontol.* 70 (6): 692–699.

Von Arx, T. and Buser, D. (2006). Horizontal ridge augmentation using autogenous block grafts and the guided bone regeneration technique with collagen membranes: a clinical study with 42 patients. *Clin. Oral Implants Res.* 17: 359–366.

Wallace, S.S. and Froum, S.J. (2003). The influence of sinus angmentation on the implant stability. The systematic rebus. *Ann. Periodontol.* 8: 328–343.

Wang, H. and Shammari, K. (2002). HVC ridge deficiency classification. *Int. J. Periodontics. Restorative Dent.* 22: 335–343.

Further Reading

Bornstein, M.M., Seiffert, C., Maestre-Ferrín, L. et al. (2016). An analysis of frequency, morphology, and locations of maxillary sinus septa using cone beam computed tomography. *Int. J. Oral Maxillofac. Implants* 31 (2).

Calin, C., Petre, A., and Drafta, S. (2014). Osteotome-mediated sinus floor elevation: a systematic review and meta-analysis. *Int. J. Oral Maxillofac. Implants* 29: 558–576.

Del Fabbro, M., Corbella, S., Weinstein, T. et al. (2012). Implant survival rates after osteotome-mediated maxillary sinus augmentation: a systematic review. *Clin. Implant Dent. Relat. Res.* 14 (Suppl 1): e159–e168.

Emmerich, D., Att, W., and Stappert, C. (2005). Sinus floor elevation using osteotomes: a systematic review and meta-analysis. *J. Periodontol.* 76: 1237–1251.

Esposito, M., Cannizzaro, G., Barausse, C. et al. (2014). Cosci versus Summers technique for crestal sinus lift:

3-year results from a randomized controlled trial. *Eur. J. Oral Implantol.* 7 (2): 129–137.

Garcia-Garcia, A., Somoza-Martin, M., Gandara-Vila, P. et al. (2003). Alveolar distraction before insertion of dental implants in the posterior mandible. *Br. J. Oral Maxillofac. Surg.* 41: 376–379.

Lundgren, S., Cricchio, G., Hallman, M. et al. (2000). Sinus floor elevation procedures to enable implant placement and integration: techniques, biological aspects and clinical outcomes. *Periodontology* 2017 (73): 103–120.

Machtei, E.E. (2001). The effect of membrane exposure on the outcome of regenerative procedures in humans: a meta-analysis. *J. Periodontol.* 72: 512–516.

Mordenfeld, A., Hallman, M., Johansson, C.B., and Albrektsson, T. (2010). Histological and histomorphometrical analyses of biopsies harvested 11 years after maxillary sinus floor augmentation with deproteinized bovine and autogenous bone. *Clin. Oral Implants Res.* 21: 961–970.

Pjetursson, B.E. and Lang, N.P. (2000). Sinus floor elevation utilizing the transalveolar approach. *Periodontology* 2014 (66): 59–71.

Seibert, J.S. (1983). Reconstruction of deformed, partially edentulous ridges, using full thickness onlay grafts. Part I. Techniques and wound healing. *Compend. Contin. Educ. Dent.* 4: 437.

20

Soft Tissue Assessment and Enhancement in Implant Dentistry
Edgard El Chaar

Department of Periodontics, University of Pennsylvania, Dental Medicine, Philadelphia, PA, USA

Introduction

With the advent in Implant surface technology, the need of having keratinized tissue (KT) became an important point in the long run in order to have a sustainable healthy dental implant. In the world work shop in periodontics (Berglundh et al. 2018), it has been stated that a minimum of 2 mm appears to be the magical number to achieve this goal. Before a dental implant is placed and from the moment of treatment planning, the clinician has to assess both the hard and soft tissues. The parameters to place a dental implant have been set and well established as the 3D implant placement (Buser et al. 2004) in relation to the amount of bone facial to the placed implant and its relation to the adjacent teeth especially in partially edentulous patients. Now we will need to add to the agreed-on amount of KT. That is now known as the phenotype would it be around natural tooth, a site to be extracted or a site for implant placement. Clinicians today must balance biology, functionality, and esthetics when treatment planning and executing implants.

In most of the instances, these procedures will be used to correct an esthetic or functional failure of placed implants. Failures that compromise the health of an implant fixture are inflammatory in nature and include peri-implantitis and peri-implant mucositis. While the result of these pathologic changes is often unesthetic, the underlying cause of the disease must first be addressed before steps can be made to restore the esthetics. When an implant is healthy but the result of the surgical and prosthetic placement is unsatisfactory to both the patient and clinician, immediate steps can be taken to achieve a more desirable esthetic result. As with all dental treatment, the disease process and pathology must be eliminated or controlled before steps can be taken to repair the damage that it has caused. It is best to take measures to prevent both

infectious and esthetic implant failures through proper planning and surgical execution.

Some common esthetic failures are loss of interdental papilla "black triangles," midfacial gingival recession, a non-harmonious gingival margin, buccal concavities, and translucency of the implant body or prosthetic margins. There are steps that can be taken to avoid these failures during the planning and surgical execution of implant placement including augmentation prior to implant placement, flap design during placement, and soft tissue management during second stage. The fundamental point is to assess the hard and soft tissue prior to implant placement in order to determine if there is a need for augmentation prior to the placement. Bone height and thickness are major determinants of soft tissue contours, which will affect the implant placement subsequently will dictate the tooth morphology, which will determine the contact point from the crest of bone and finally this will lead to the tissue quality and quantity important for the long term success of the dental implant.

This chapter will discuss manipulation and/or augmentation of existing soft tissue, rather than prosthetic gingiva, in combination with implant-supported crowns, to achieve an ideal esthetic result.

Techniques to Create Contour, Thickness, and Increase Keratinized Tissue

A-Flap Management

Over the years we all have been faced with the concept of flapless versus flap and many designs have been promoted for the latter. The clinician has to always remember that we are replacing a lost dental organ which is our ultimate goal. By setting that goal we need to start thinking from it backwards which I often quote as "set your goal and walk your way back." Would it be an anterior or posterior tooth, it has a specific shape at its coronal level. A central maxillary incisor is triangular, canine is oval, transitioning from the premolars to the molars it becomes a rectangle; yet the coronal part of the implant is a circle regardless of that implant diameter. All of that takes place at the flap level.

Gomez-Roman (2001) showed that even if there is adequate crestal bone height prior to implant placement, the flap design can affect the amount of crestal bone resorption following placement. By preserving the proximal tissue of the adjacent teeth "limited flap design" a 0.29 mm bone was noted versus a 0.79 mm versus "widely mobilized flap procedure," which includes the proximal tissue. Another advantage of preserving that tissue is giving the clinician a visual marker to keep the 1.5 mm from adjacent teeth during the placement (Buser et al. 2004; Esposito et al. 1993).

For years, I personally used and taught my residents and colleagues to use the H design, in which you evaluate the position of the adequate amount of KT and you initiate your crestal incision followed by two cross arches on the buccal and lingual, extending up to mucogingival line (MGL) on the buccal side and enough on the lingual to allow exposure of the crestal bone. On the buccal side, it can extend passed MGL in case an apically repositioning is needed. Although it covers all the criteria cited earlier, suturing the flap and controlling the level of it either coronal or apical becomes a challenge since we have a raised flap on the lingual and we need to suture together the buccal and lingual component. To avoid this hurdle, I designed a flap that I call the U shape, where the crestal incision is made depending on the adequate KT that the clinician judged is necessary coupled with two buccal only crestal incisions extending up to MGL. The lingual portion at the crestal level is elevated without being mobilized. The major advantage of this design is the clinician can control the positioning of the flap either coronal or apical depending on the esthetic assessment done during the treatment planning, namely, the Pink Esthetic score, assessment of papilla height, and pink and white esthetic score in gingival display (Figures 20.1–20.5).

As a side technical important note, to position the flap coronally you position the flap at the level needed and you place the first suture coronally on both sides. It is important that the two cross arch incisions on the buccal are parallel and not widened at the apical part to avoid shrinkage of the coronal part of the flap. If so, it will difficult to have enough width to cover the buccal aspect. For the apical position, it's the opposite, you place the flap in the desired place and you suture first the apical part followed by the coronal.

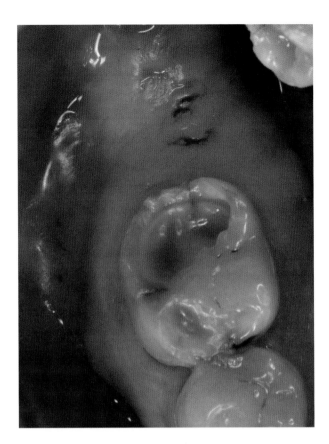

Figure 20.1 Occlusal view showing the mucogingival line buccal more coronal with less than 1 mm keratinized tissue buccal.

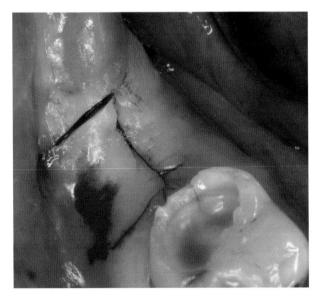

Figure 20.2 The U shape incision to the buccal with parallel vertical incisions.

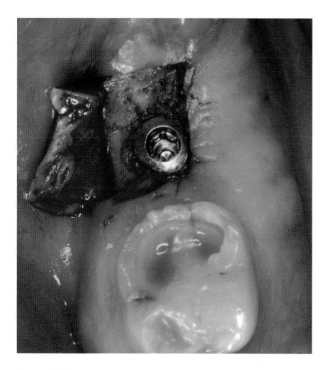

Figure 20.3 Full thickness flap elevated, exposing the implant.

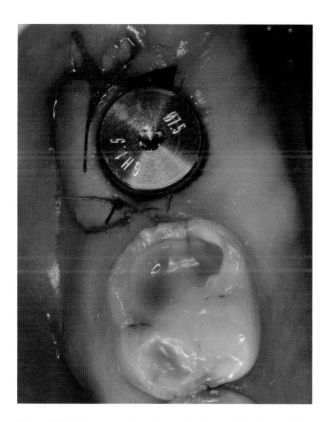

Figure 20.4 Flap sutured at the needed coronal level matching the adjacent margins.

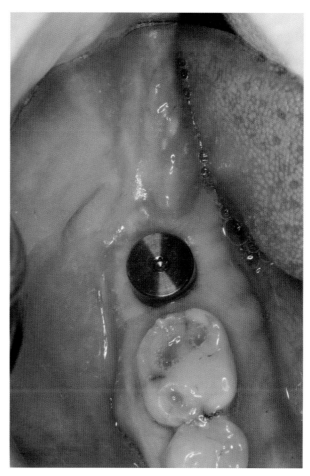

Figure 20.5 Six weeks healing revealing a good band of keratinized tissue with buccal contour continuous with the adjacent teeth and coronal levels of tissue similar to the adjacent as well.

Roll Technique

A roll flap procedure was developed by Abrams in 1980 as a means of correcting small Seibert class I ridge defects that result in a buccal concavity. This technique is useful in correcting a ridge defect at a future site for a pontic, or a small buccal concavity present in the area where an implant has been placed. If there is an implant present in the site, this technique can be used in combination with the uncovery procedure. This technique employs a pedicle connective tissue graft that is harvested from the palate and then folded under into a pouch created on the buccal. The augmentation provided by the pedicle is meant to match the root eminences of the adjacent teeth therefore if the edentulous span is greater than one tooth multiple pedicle grafts may prepared.

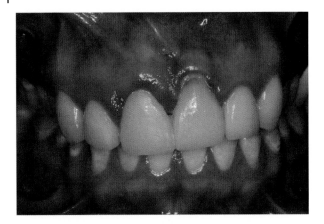

Figure 20.6 Buccal view showing the soft tissue buccal discrepancy.

The roll technique presented here is a **modification** to the roll technique introduced by Scharf and Tarnow in 1992 (Scharf and Tarnow 1992) and will be illustrated in the series of figures (Figures 20.6–20.11). The main modifications, no vertical incisions on both sides and the shape of the harvested connective tissue is trapezoidal not rectangular as designed by Schaarf and Tarnow. It begins with making three measurements. First measure from the crest of the ridge or the anticipated gingival margin of the future crown to the most apical extent of the concavity, second measure the apical width 1 mm from mesial side of each adjacent apex of the adjacent teeth, and third measure the interproximal distance between the adjacent teeth coronally accounting for the papillary like tissue to be left on the side of each tooth. Those lines of measurements will form a trapezoid shape. These measurements will determine the size of the pedicle that needs to be harvested from the palatal area. The buccal limit of the donor site is the mid-crest of the pontic site preparation or above

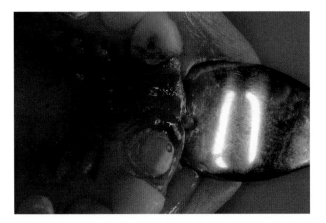

Figure 20.8 The trapezoidal shaped incisions were made on the palate to accommodate the needed tissue on the buccal, full thickness of that tissue were made after de-epithelizing the surface.

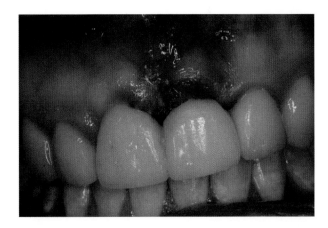

Figure 20.9 Tissue was rolled under the pouch made buccal and part of it was kept coronal to match the adjacent tooth. A narrow healing abutment was placed to support the tissue.

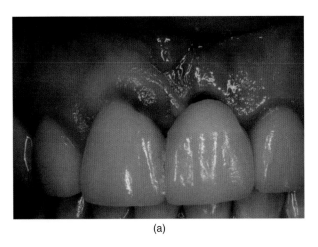

(a)

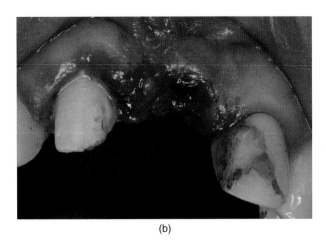

(b)

Figure 20.7 (a) The implant was disconnected to let the tissue grow over it and bury it (b).

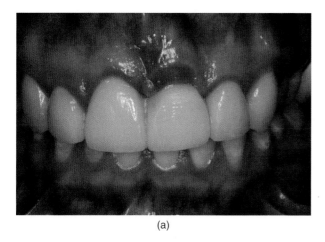

(a)

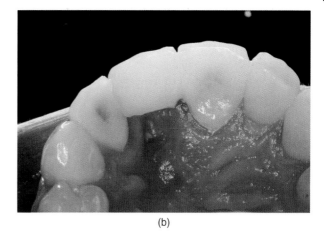

(b)

Figure 20.10 Eight weeks healing of the rolled tissue (a) buccal view and (b) palatal showing the fill of the donor site and the placed healing abutment.

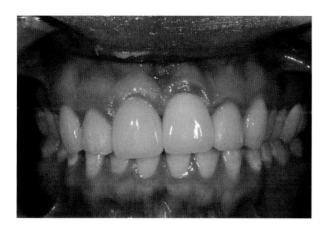

Figure 20.11 Final prosthesis in place with marginal tissue matching the adjacent tooth.

the middle of the cover screw for implants. Delineate the donor site with incisions extending to the underlying bone in all areas except the crestal limit, which will serve as the base of the pedicle. Once the site is delineated de-epithelialize that area and sharply elevate the connective tissue pedicle to full thickness leaving exposed bone on the palate. Some authors suggested dissecting the pedicle graft leaving behind periosteum, but doing so risks severing the supra-periosteal capillary bed that may lead to flap necrosis and jeopardize the end result. Full thickness elevation also reduces risk of perforation of the pedicle flap, allows for a thicker graft, and maintains the supra-periosteal blood supply to the graft. Once the pedicle is elevated to the buccal transition area, create a full thickness pouch in the area of the defect on the buccal following the planned trapezoidal architecture. After elevation of the pouch, roll the pedicle graft into the area of the buccal defect. At this time the pedicle may be trimmed and adjusted to fit. Once the graft is in place, place two

stabilizing sutures coronally on either side of the trapezoid. At this point, the healing abutment can be placed and any periosteum or any osseous structure over the implant cover screw should be removed.

Autograft Subepithelial Connective Tissue (CTG), a Free Gingival Graft (FGG), or Allograft Dermis

Used in lack of KT surrounding implant fixture or in case there is not enough tissue present to be displaced apically, or rolled buccally, one may employ a free gingival graft (FGG), connective tissue autograft (CTG), or allograft dermis. Connective tissue grafts can be used to increase tissue thickness and/or to increase attached KT in areas of esthetic concern. An FGG can also be used to increase a zone of KT but will heal with a more blanched looking tissue and it is not advised in areas of esthetic concern. Alternatively, and for the same reason, an allograft dermis can be used to increase KT. The main advantage of using a connective tissue graft is the color match with the surrounding tissue compared with the FGG. These techniques are easiest to perform at time of the second stage surgery or implant placement but can be done with a prosthesis in place if necessary but will require a more diligent and refined execution.

Free Gingival Graft (FGG)

This technique is mainly used to increase the amount of KT while preserving the marginal gingiva. A sub-marginal incision is made down to the bone in case of implant that is already exposed or sub marginal to the existent KT in a healed ridge. The extent of the incision depends on the extent of the area to be treated. At the margins of this area extend the incisions curved apically. A full-thickness flap was reflected.

In case when implants are not uncovered, an incision is made at the MGL and a full-thickness flap was reflected to expose the previously placed implant.

In both instances, the flap is apically positioned and stabilized with tacks to establish the new vestibule. Once the flap is secured, measure the recipient area to determine the amount of tissue that needs to be harvested from the palate. Next, harvest a full thickness graft from the palate to place in the area of deficient tissue. The donor tissue should be taken at least 2 mm from the palatal gingival margin as tissue contractions occurs during healing and recession may occur as a result of the wound edge being too close to teeth. The shape of the donor tissue is outlined with a scalpel at a right angle to the palate at the desired depth, which can be gauged by the bevel on a #15C scalpel blade (approximately 1 mm). The blade is then turned parallel to the palate and a graft of the desired uniform thickness is removed by sharp dissection from the palate. The donor tissue is transferred to the recipient site to check the fit and modified if needed. Suturing techniques vary widely, but stabilization of the graft is the most important principle and can be accomplished using stabilizing structures adjacent to the surgical site. Reducing graft mobility and dead spaces between tissues will improve the graft success and after an average of eight weeks the donor and recipient sites are healed. This technique does give a high discomfort at the palate site reported by most patients regardless of which kind of cover is used over the donor site and does not provide a high esthetic result due to the color mismatch.

Connective Tissue Grafts (CTG)

Following the development and use of FGG, Langer and Calagna in 1980 described the subepithelial connective tissue graft for root coverage and ridge augmentation as the second major type of free soft tissue autograft (Langer and Calagna 1980). The esthetics advantages, healing period, and superior color match of CTG versus FGG make CTG the most widely used soft tissue autograft technique used in periodontal plastic surgery (Langer and Calagna 1982). A connective tissue graft used under a pedicle flap yields to a mean root coverage of 89.3% around natural teeth (Langer and Langer 1993). When the palatal masticatory mucosa is used as autogenous donor material for a connective tissue graft, it is important to control the thickness of the graft harvested. Harvesting a thick graft aids in vascularity and ease of manipulation of the donor tissue but delays the healing period, while use of a thin graft decreases the healing time but often results in graft shrinkage or early necrosis (Mörmann et al. 1981; Sullivan and Atkins 1968). Histologic analysis of the mucosa by Yu et al. showed that the thickness of the lamina propria decreased toward the posterior palatal area and mid-palatal suture, while that of

the submucosa increased (Yu et al. 2014). Yu's results suggest that the most appropriate donor site for it is the region 3 mm below the cementoenamel junction (CEJ) between the distal surface of the canine and the midline surface of the first molar. When harvesting from this area also keep in mind the anatomical landmarks of the palate. The greater and lesser palatine vessels and nerves lie in a bony groove, the greater palatine groove, which traverses the palate anteriorly at the junction of the horizontal and vertical palate. It is important to avoid the nerves and vessels located along this neurovascular line. The location of this line relative to the CEJ varies with palatal vault depth. In shallow palatal vaults the average distance between the neurovascular line and the CEJ is 7 mm, whereas in high vaults the maximum average distance is 17 mm. In an average vault there is about a distance of 12 mm from the neurovascular line to the CEJ (Reiser et al. 1996; Rose 2004). Major problems can occur when the surgeon violates the neurovascular area such as paresthesia and excessive bleeding. Paresthesia of the anterior palate is more noticeable to the patient during speech due to the phonetic impact of an absence of feeling in this area. This paresthesia is generally temporary and often dissipates over the span of 6–12 months due to regeneration of nerve fibers. Bleeding can be a major problem in the palate but most bleeding can be controlled by pressure, increasing the number of sutures, and the use of chemical or electrical coagulants. Taking to account an incision starts 23 mm from the free gingival margin and ended 2 mm prior to the neurovascular line then the maximum width of donor tissue needed will vary from 3 to 9 mm harvesting a graft from an individual with a shallow palatal vault may not be adequate and doing so could risk in neurovascular damage. In these cases, a clinician should consider allogenic grafting as the best treatment option.

A CTG can be used in two different manners. One is to increase the bulk of tissue in the area of a small concavity or thin mucosa and the other is to increase the zone of KT. If the intention is to increase the zone of KT, one should employ a free connective tissue graft while if tissue thickness needs to be increased a classical connective tissue graft procedure should be applied. These two connective tissues grafting techniques will be presented separately.

A Free Connective Tissue Graft A Free Connective Tissue Graft is performed in the same manner as an FGG at the recipient site and the harvesting from the palate is performed by dissecting the connective tissue rather than harvesting a full thickness graft. When harvesting connective tissue from the palate begin by doing a single horizontal incision 2 mm apical to the gingival margins especially at the first molar without vertical incisions than elevate a full thickness envelope flap from which connective tissue is dissected out and the remaining flap

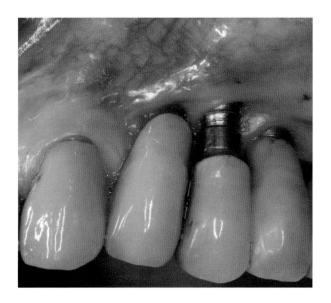

Figure 20.12 The focus on this case is implant in position #11, where there is an aberrant frenum with loss of keratinized tissue and recession on the abutment buccally.

epithelium cover is left attached to the remaining palatal tissue. Once the graft has been removed, the remaining flap will be sutured to the adjacent immobile palatal tissue.

The recipient site will be denuded in a full thickness manner by making a horizontal incision which is a submarginal one of the intended zone of width augmentation (Figures 20.12 and 20.13). The mobilized mucosa needs to

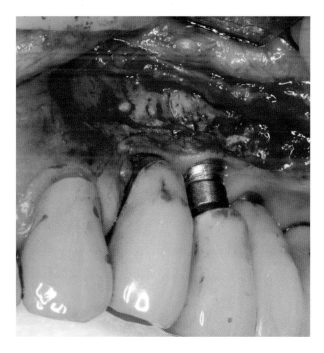

Figure 20.13 A full thickness bed is made in the area of the recipient site and the apically repositioned mucosa was tacked apically.

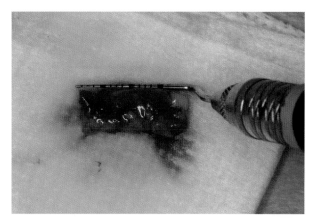

Figure 20.14 A thick Connective tissue graft was harvested from the palate for placement over the defect.

be stabilized apically, which I recommend to tack it using titanium tacks one on each corner and one in the middle (Figure 20.13). At this point the harvested connective tissue (Figure 20.14) is placed over the prepared site and sutured coronally with interrupted sutures (Figure 20.15). The advantage of using a free connective tissue graft is the color match avoiding this very bulky keloid white tissue that results from using an FGG (Figure 20.16).

Covered Connective Tissue Graft A conventional connective tissue graft is useful in areas where one needs to increase the thickness of the buccal tissue around an implant or in areas where it is necessary to improve the quality of the tissue. In a covered connective tissue graft, the flap created at the donor site is placed over the graft and positioned

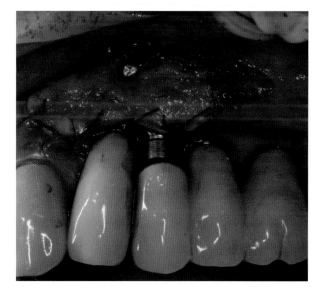

Figure 20.15 The free connective tissue was secured coronally to the recipient site and one was used to affix it to on the apical side.

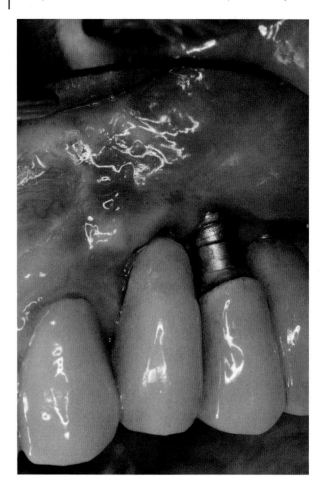

Figure 20.16 A six month healing showing the gained keratinized tissue that blends in color with the adjacent tissue.

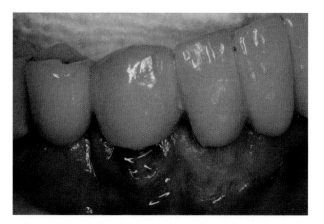

Figure 20.17 Purulent exudate and a lack of keratinized tissue with recession on the buccal of implant in positions #27–28 to be treated with implant decontamination and connective tissue graft.

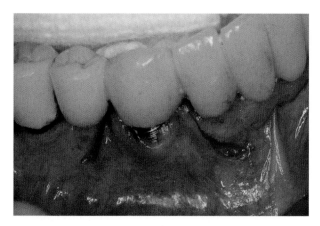

Figure 20.18 The procedure began with debridement and elevation of a full thickness flap.

coronally, called coronally advanced flap (CAF). The CAF increases the graft survival by increasing the blood supply necessary as well as the thickness (El Chaar et al. 2016; Goaslind et al. 1977). We will be describing the CAF with the connective tissue in a case of peri-implantitis treatment to make it more exciting (Figure 20.17).

1) Begin with preparation of the recipient bed: lay a full thickness envelope flap exposing the bone in the area which needs augmentation. Use intra-sulcular incisions on the coronal portion of the flap in areas of surrounding natural teeth and the same in the area of the implant. All interproximal papilla should be sliced (de-epithelized) exposing the underlying connective tissue and leaving the base intact and attached to the underlying bone. If any elements of the implant fixture are exposed following flap elevation, these areas should be disinfected following the clinician's chosen protocol (Figures 20.18–20.21).

2) As done in previous techniques, measure the area of the defect and harvest a connective tissue graft from the palate (Figure 20.22).

3) Place the CTG into the opened flap and suture it to the interproximal non-elevated tissue with interrupted sutures using a vicryl P-3 5.0 sutures. In this case, I placed mineralized cancellous allogaft in the interproximal two wall defects (Figure 20.21).

4) Stretch the elevated flap and cover the now stabilized graft. Affix the overlaying flap using single sling with 5.0 vicryl P3 sutures (Figure 20.23).

5) If the overlying tissue is mainly from mucosa, another step may be done following healing where the mucosa is split to expose the underlying matured tissue (Figure 20.24).

Allograft Dermis While autografts such as connective tissue and FGG have been considered the gold standard for soft tissue grafting, improvement in processing mechanisms and development of soft tissue allografts have made them a predicable alternative to autografts (Hirsch et al. 2005;

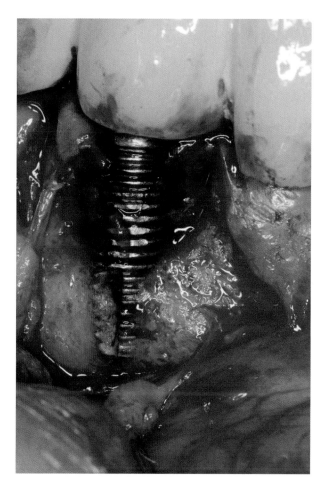

Figure 20.19 Once the flap was elevated it was confirmed that the implant was placed outside of the boney housing. Note the intra-bony defects present on both the mesial and lingual of the implant. The area was debrided and prepped for implantoplasty.

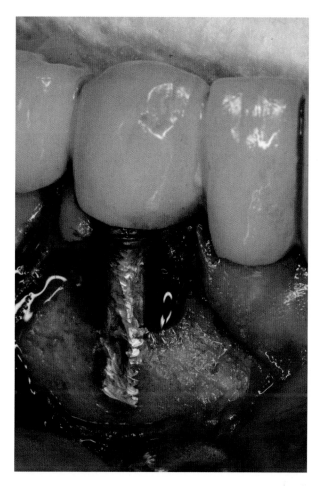

Figure 20.20 High-speed handpiece and irrigation was used to preform implantoplasty on all exposed areas of the implant. Following implantoplasty the implant surface was treated with phosphoric etch solution and then thoroughly irrigated with saline.

Paolantonio et al. 2002). There are many different acellular dermises available on the market, each type differs in processing and sterilization techniques but all serve a sterile acellular collagen matrix, which acts a scaffold for ingrowth of surrounding tissue (Hirsch et al. 2005; Schlee and Esposito 2011). The current processing technique involves complete removal of the epithelium by uncoupling the bond with the dermis, ensuring no damage to the dermal structure and maintaining the basement membrane. This process renders the dermal matrix free from cellular components, while the graft still contains blood vessel channels, collagen, elastin, and proteoglycans. The acellular dermal matrix (ADM) allograft is in the thin to medium range of graft thickness (0.75–1.4 mm) (Schlee and Esposito 2011).

The use of ADM is technique sensitive in case of KT augmentation around implants. Allograft dermis doesn't provide a predictable outcome used as a free graft due

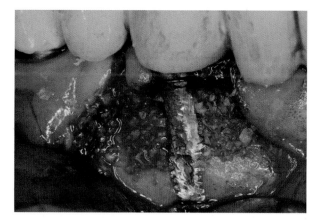

Figure 20.21 A cancellous mineralized allograft bone graft was placed in the intrabony defect on the mesial and distal Note the wicking of the blood into the area between the bone particles and the creation of an overall red tone to the otherwise white graft material.

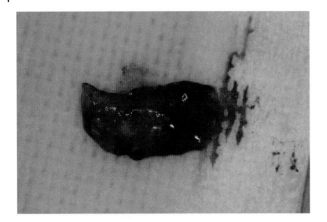

Figure 20.22 A thick connective tissue graft was harvested from the palate for placement over the defect.

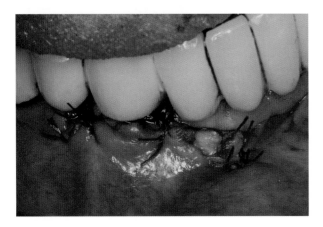

Figure 20.23 The flap is elevated over the donor tissue and both the flap and graft are sutured into place.

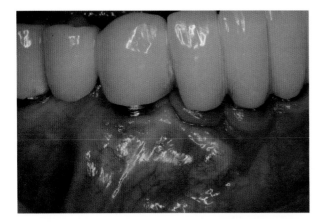

Figure 20.24 A eight year follow up shows thick firm pink healthy tissue surrounding the implant.

to rate of necrosis and delay in vascularization when not covered by a flap, yet studies demonstrated ADM was a compatible graft material to increase KT around implant (Park 2006; Wei et al. 2000; Yan et al. 2006).

In order to increase its predictability, we introduced a new procedure based mainly on stabilizing the Dermis to the recipient site using tacks (Yan et al. 2006). The surgical step of this technique is described as following:

(1) An incision following the mucogingival junction is made.
(2) A full-thickness flap was reflected to expose the previous placed implant.
(3) The flap was apically positioned and stabilized with tacks to establish a new vestibule.
(4) Tacks were used to stabilize the ADM as well. No sutures were used.

In this article (Yan et al. 2006), we compared an FGG where the flap was sutured apically (control) and the contralateral flap where the ADM was used stabilized with tacks. We can see the dramatic effect that immobilization has made compared with the contralateral side where sutures were used. The basement membrane side of the ADM facing the oral cavity did slough partially due to lack of complete vascularization but was repopulated by epithelium at four to six weeks. The tacks covered by tissue can be maintained submerged if no irritation was reported. Otherwise, it can be easily removed with topical anesthetic. We believe that the stabilization of the ADM with tacks increase the chance of plasmatic fluid phase in the first three to four days to populate the dermis and allow the neo-vascularization to take place, which is essential in any graft survivability. Secondly, stabilizing the flap of the recipient site with tacks apically, allows also in both cases of FGG as described previously and, in this case, to inhibit the disengagement of this flap from the sutures and the creeping coronally of the flap, which limits the chance of the graft to mature.

Tunnel Technique The tunnel technique allows for placement of a connective tissue graft or an allograft dermis without reflection of a conventional flap. A tunnel flap is in essence an alteration of a pedicle flap as it maintains blood supply from the papillary and the mucogingival aspects. This increase in blood supply as compared with a conventional flap aids in graft stability and circulation (Rose 2004). A full-thickness dissection prepares the donor site to receive the connective tissue graft. This style of flap is difficult and time consuming when compared to a conventional flap. This technique of reflection should only be undertaken after many conventional flaps have been reflected and a working knowledge of the anatomy is learned. This technique has many advantages as it allows for increased blood supply, a more rapid healing but lack good stability of the graft (Allen 1994; Blanes and Allen 1999; Zabalequi et al. 1999).

Keep in mind, these techniques are mainly described for natural teeth.

In a tunnel technique, the recipient bed is a tunneled full thickness pouch spanning the area of the defect. Elevate the tissue with a tunnel technique in the area of the defect without opening the flap at the gingival crest. Ensure the instrument tip is resting underlying osseous structure and with a gentle back and forth pushing motion develop and dissect a full thickness pouch under the tissue. Extend the plane of dissection close to but not breaking the free gingival margin. Harvest the connective tissue graft from the palate as previously described or use an allograft dermis. In this case we are illustrating, thread the suture through the created pouch grab the allograft and pull it through the pouch. Once the graft is satisfactorily placed into the area, suture it into place through the flap while coronally elevating the flap using multiple interrupted sling suture. Particularly when using an Allograft dermis, the latter should be completely covered by the patient's tissue for successful results and the overlying flap needs to be of at least 1 mm in thickness (Cairo et al. 2016; Stefanini et al. 2018) (Figures 20.25–20.27).

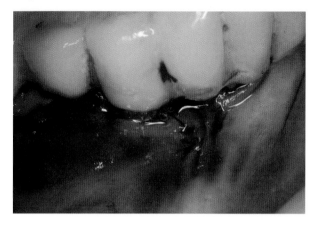

Figure 20.26 The Allograft Dermis is sutured in place and the vertical incisions are closed.

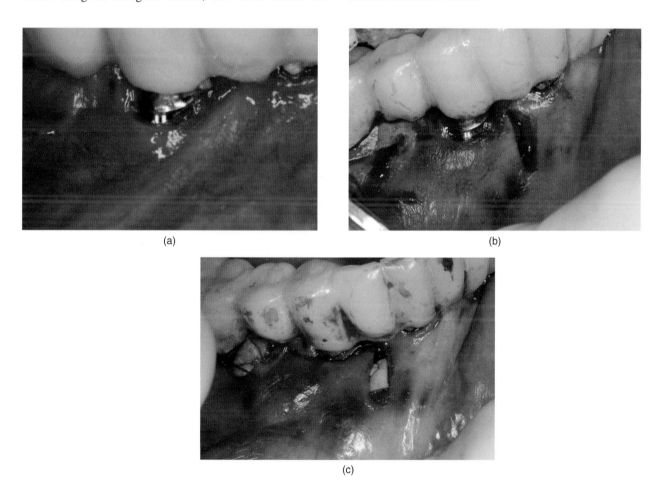

(a)

(b)

(c)

Figure 20.25 (a) There is thin tissue and a shallow vestibule in the area of this mandibular implant. A tunnel technique to place allograft dermis was used to thicken the tissue and deepen the vestibule. (b) Two vertical incisions are made and a full thickness tunnel flap is elevated. (c) The Allograft Dermis is suture on one end to aid in pulling the allograft dermis through the tunnel and pass it inside.

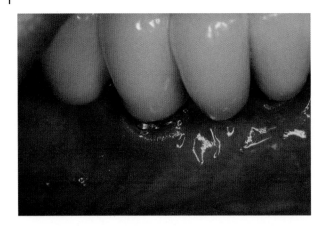

Figure 20.27 The area healed and providing a good vestibule for a good plaque control.

Techniques for Papilla Management

Second stage surgery or soft tissue augmentation in sites with multiple implants in a row presents a very specific challenge that is managing the inter-proximal implant tissue. When using the roll technique, apically repositioned flaps, free gingival, or connective tissue grafts during second stage around multiple implants the interproximal areas are left exposed to heal through secondary intention. This type of healing can lead to inter-implant crestal bone loss and the formation of flat or even inverted inter-implant papilla tissue. All of these outcomes are of extreme esthetic detriment and prevent adequate embrasure space fill following final restoration. Fortunately, there are techniques to manage soft tissue in a way to correct or minimize this set back.

Rotated Pediculated Marginal Tissue

Palacci (1995) described a technique to create papilla-like formation. The attached gingiva is displaced buccally beginning with a crestal incision in line with the palatal or lingual limits of the implant cover screws two vertical releasing incisions and a full thickness flap. The flap is elevated and pushed buccally, while the healing abutments are placed to hold the flap buccally. The excess buccal tissue is dissected into pedicles that are then rotated into the interproximal spaces. Dissection and rotation is done with semi-lunar incisions starting from the distal and rotation of the pedicle 90° in the palatal direction. The pedicles should be sutured without tension or engagement of the pedicles, an eight-shape figure suture is suggested to hold them in place (Palacci 1995). The down turn of this

suturing, it will not attach the peak of the rotated papilla to provide it with blood supply in the early phases of healing knowingly that the lingual flap is not the greatest in blood supply and scary in nature subsequent to the previous loss of the tooth.

Rotated Pediculated Lingual Marginal Tissue

El Chaar introduced a major modification to the Palacci technique takes advantage of the abundance of soft tissue on the palate while reducing risk of buccal gingival recession and the early necrosis of the rotated papilla, which can be caused by use of the buccal as a donor site. In this modification the attached gingiva is displaced buccally beginning using the U shape flap, described earlier, by having the crestal incision over the center of the cover screws. The elevated flap is displaced buccally and is secured at the level intended either coronal or apical. Contrary to the Palacci technique, the pedicle is created from the palatal tissue. That is laying over half of the cover screw and rotated forward rather than from the buccal. This is advantageous because no buccal KT is sacrificed. The rotated pediculated papilla like tissue is sutured to the buccal flap using a horizontal mattress suture. The sutures started from the buccal flap allowing the pediculated papilla to cover the interproximal bone covered and lay passively in the inter proximal space, which is a very important variant

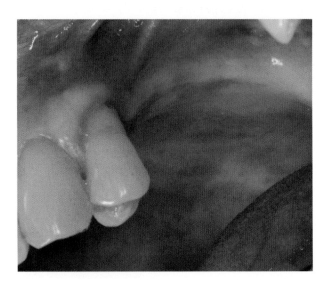

Figure 20.28 Maxillary posterior prior to placement of two adjacent implants and closure using the Rotated Pediculated Lingual marginal tissue El Chaar Technique. This technique can be used at time of single stage implant placement or during implant uncovery of adjacent implants. Note the inadequate keratinized tissue on the buccal.

to the Palacci technique securing more the rotated pedicle and accelerating the revascularization between the two joining tissues. This technique can be utilized anywhere including the anterior. In cases where the two sides right and left are both involved, one might end up having a two rotated papilla in the midline or inter-implant in positions #8 and 9. Before committing the two sides, one has to measure the inter-implant space. If the midline interproximal space is 3 mm than one side's (right or left) rotated pedicle should fill up the space. If that space exceeds the 4 mm, then the two pedicles from both sides right and left should be rotated to fill the up the space. If needed those two pedicles can be affixed together via a 6.0 polypropylene sutures (Figures 20.28–20.31).

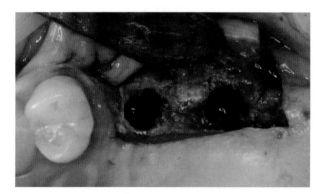

Figure 20.29 A U shape flap as described previously is made with full thickness flap elevation, two TLX Straumann were placed in a previously grafted maxillary sinus.

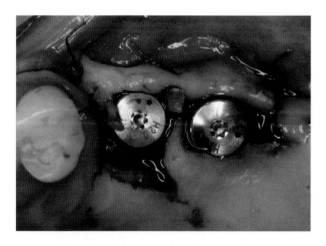

Figure 20.30 After the healing abutment were placed and the flap secured at the coronal level, a pedicule is dissected out of the lingual tissue and rotated to the interproximal and sutured to the buccal flap with a horizontal mattress.

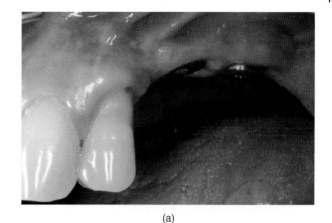

(a)

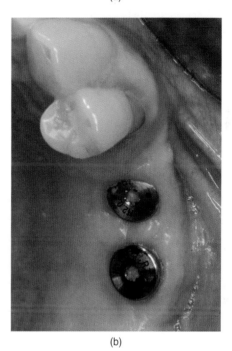

(b)

Figure 20.31 (a) Note the abundant keratinized soft tissue height and papilla like structure present between the two healing abutments most visible in the buccal view. (b) A palatal view showing the thickness achieved and the continuous contour with the adjacent teeth.

Techniques of Soft Tissue for Extraction Socket Grafting

It has been well established that after an extraction of a tooth, the alveolus undergoes a volumetric change (Schropp et al. 2003) and the thinner the phenotype, the more volumetric change will take place (Chappuis et al. 2013) by mean of losing buccal bone. This has a vast effect on the esthetic due to the flattening of the gingival scallop,

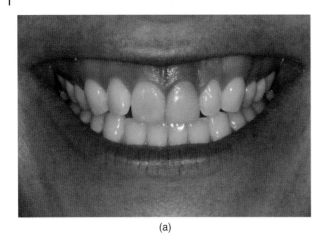

(a)

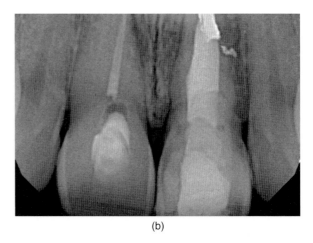

(b)

Figure 20.32 A 24 years old female presented with composite restored centrals with very pronounced gingival scallop (a) and fractured roots with a history of endodontically treated and re-implanted when she was 11 years old due to bike accident (b).

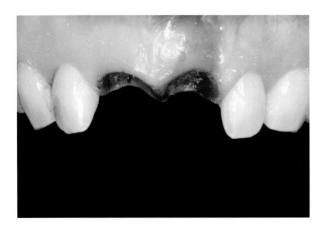

Figure 20.33 An atraumatic extraction was done.

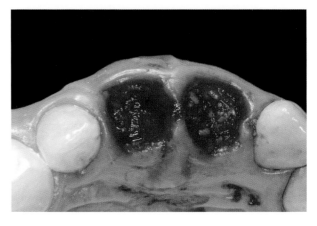

Figure 20.34 The socket was grafted with a layered cancellous, cortical mineralized allograft.

which is the critical part of the esthetic. This becomes more of an issue when we have loss of interproximal bone that will lead to proximal attachment loss on the adjacent teeth, mainly the papilla. El Chaar et al. 2016 (El Chaar and Oshman 2016) introduced a roadmap in which indicated the need of soft tissue coverage at the time of socket grafting in a single rooted maxillary tooth. In order to do so, without altering the gingival scallop, El Chaar introduced in 2012, an original technique for the posterior maxillary extraction teeth and a modification for the maxillary anterior teeth using a rotated pedicle graft form the palate to seal the socket which allows to preserve the gingival scallop intact at the time of hard tissue grafting (El Chaar 2010; El Chaar et al. 2017). In four to six months, the implant placement will be done flapless especially nowadays with the advent of digital dentistry increasing the accuracy and allowing for accurate temporization to maximize the esthetic outcome (El Chaar et al. 2020) (Figures 20.32–20.40).

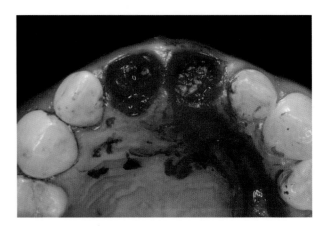

Figure 20.35 The harvesting of the connective tissue starts from the disto-lingual line angle of the canine leaving it pediculated anteriorly. The de-epithelization of the palatal tissue from that point to the lingual gingival margins of the extracted central on both sides will be done.

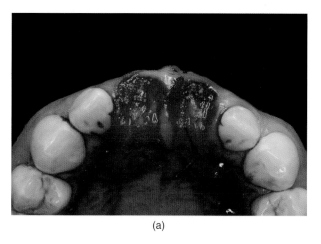

(a)

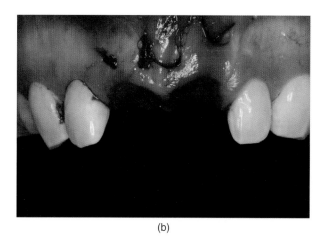

(b)

Figure 20.36 The pediculated rotated subepithelial connective tissue graft is rolled over the socket and laid inside of it in the coronal (a) part and secured by three horizontal mattresses from the buccal side (b).

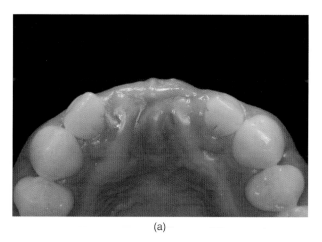

(a)

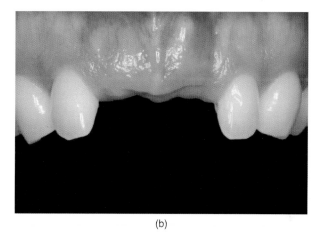

(b)

Figure 20.37 Six month healing buccal and palatal views of the site prior to implant placement.

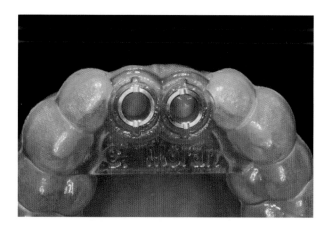

Figure 20.38 A 3D printed digital guide for the implant placement is inserted.

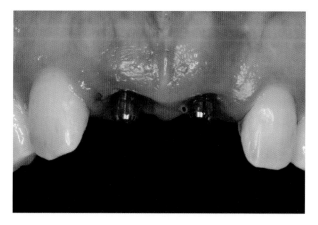

Figure 20.39 The two implants placed flaplessly to the needed depth.

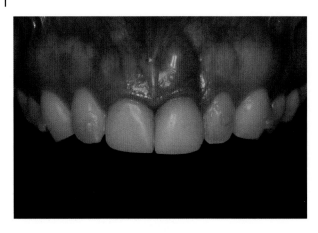

Figure 20.40 Facial view of the temporary in place four month post placement.

References

Allen, A.L. (1994). Use of the supraperiosteal envelope in soft tissue grafting for root coverage. I. Rationale and technique. *Int. J. Periodontics Restorative Dent.* 14: 217–227.

Berglundh, T., Armitage, G., Araujo, M.G. et al. (2018). Peri-implant diseases and conditions: consensus report of workgroup 4 of the 2017 world workshop on the classification of periodontal and peri-implant diseases and conditions. *J. Periodontol.* 89: S313–S318.

Blanes, R.J. and Allen, E.P. (1999). The bilateral pedicle flap-tunnel technique: a new approach to cover connective tissue grafts. *Int. J. Periodontics Restorative Dent.* 19 (5): 471–479.

Buser, D., Martin, W., and Belser, U.C. (2004). Optimizing esthetics for implant restorations in the anterior maxilla: anatomic and surgical considerations. *Int. J. Oral Maxillofac. Implants* 19 (7).

Cairo, F., Cortellini, P., Pilloni, A. et al. (2016). Clinical efficacy of coronally advanced flap with or without connective tissue graft for the treatment of multiple adjacent gingival recessions in the aesthetic area: a randomized controlled clinical trial. *J. Clin. Periodontol.* 43 (10): 849–856.

Chappuis, V., Engel, O., Reyes, M. et al. (2013). Ridge alterations post-extraction in the esthetic zone: a 3D analysis with CBCT. *J. Dent. Res.* 92 (12_suppl): 195S–201S.

El Chaar, E.S. (2010). Soft tissue closure of grafted extraction sockets in the posterior maxilla: the rotated pedicle palatal connective tissue flap technique. *Implant. Dent.* 19 (5): 370–377.

El Chaar, E. and Oshman, S. (2016). Single-rooted extraction sockets: classification and treatment protocol. *Compend. Contin. Educ. Dent. (Jamesburg, NJ: 1995)* 37 (8): 537–541.

El Chaar, E.S., Oshman, S., Danesh-Sani, S.A. et al. (2016). Increasing contact between soft tissue graft and blood supply. *J. Cosmet. Dent.* 32 (3).

El Chaar, E., Oshman, S., Cicero, G. et al. (2017). Soft tissue closure of grafted extraction sockets in the anterior maxilla: a modified palatal pedicle connective tissue flap technique. *Int. J. Periodontics Restorative Dent.* 37 (1).

El Chaar, E., White, C., Salama, T. et al. (2020). Clinical methodology quantifying the emergence profile contour for immediate provisionalization: a proposed mathematical model emergence profile in immediate provisionnalization. *J. Oral Implantol.* 47: 191–198.

Esposito, M., Ekestubbe, A., and Gröndahl, K. (1993). Radiological evaluation of marginal bone loss at tooth surfaces facing single Brånemark implants. *Clin. Oral Implants Res.* 4 (3): 151–157.

Goaslind, G., Roberston, P., Mahan, C. et al. (1977). Thickness of facial gingiva. *J. Periodontol.* 48: 768–771.

Gomez-Roman, G. (2001). Influence of flap design on peri-implant interproximal crestal bone loss around single-tooth implants. *Int. J. Oral Maxillofac. Implants* 16: 61–67.

Hirsch, A., Goldstein, M., Goultschin, J., and Boyan, B.D. (2005). A 2 year follow-up of root coverage using subpedicle acellular dermal matrix allografts and subepithelial connective tissue allografts. *J. Periodontol.* 76: 1323–1328.

Langer, B. and Calagna, L. (1980). The subepithelial connective tissue graft. *J. Prosthet. Dent.* 44: 363.

Langer, B. and Calagna, L. (1982). The subepithelial connective tissue graft. A new approach to the enhancement of anterior cosmetics. *Int. J. Periodontics Restorative Dent.* 2: 22–33.

Langer, L. and Langer, B. (1993). The subepithelial connective tissue graft for treatment of gingival recession. *Dent. Clin. N. Am.* 37: 243–264.

Mörmann, W., Schaer, F., and Firestone, A.R. (1981). The relationship between success of free gingival grafts and transplant thickness. Revascularization and shrinkage: a one-year clinical study. *J. Periodontol.* 52: 74–80.

Palacci, P. (1995). Peri-implant soft tissue management: papilla regeneration technique. In: *Optimal Implant Positioning and Soft Tissue Management for the Brånemark System* (ed. P. Palacci), 59–70. Chicago: Quintessence.

Paolantonio, M., Dolci, M., Esposito, P. et al. (2002). Subpedicle acellular dermal matrix graft and autogenous connective tissue graft in the treatment of gingival recessions: a comparative 1-year clinical study. *J. Periodontol.* 73: 1299–1307.

Park, J.B. (2006). Increasing the width of keratinized mucosa around endosseous implant using acellular dermal matrix allograft. *Implant. Dent.* 15: 275–281.

Reiser, G., Bruno, J., Mahan, P., and Larkin, L. (1996). The subepithelial connective tissue graft palatal donor site: anatomic considerations for surgeons. *Int. J. Periodontics Restorative Dent.* 16: 131–137.

Rose, L.F. (2004). *Periodontics: Medicine, Surgery, and Implants.* Mosby.

Scharf, D.R. and Tarnow, D.P. (1992). Modified roll technique for localized alveolar ridge augmentation. *Int. J. Periodontics Restorative Dent.* 12: 415–425.

Schlee, M. and Esposito, M. (2011). Human dermis graft versus autogenous connective tissue grafts for thickening soft tissue and covering multiple ginigival recessions: 6 months results from a preference clinical trial. *Eur. J. Implantol.* 4 (2): 119–125.

Schropp, L., Wenzel, A., Kostopoulos, L., and Karring, T. (2003). Bone healing and soft tissue contour changes following single-tooth extraction: a clinical and radiographic 12-month prospective study. *Int. J. Periodontics Restorative Dent.* 23 (4).

Stefanini, M., Zucchelli, G., Marzadori, M., and de Sanctis, M. (2018). Coronally advanced flap with site-specific application of connective tissue graft for the treatment of multiple adjacent gingival recessions: a 3-year follow-up case series. *Int. J. Periodontics Restorative Dent.* 38 (1).

Sullivan, H.C. and Atkins, J.H. (1968). Free autogenous gingival grafts. I. Principles of successful grafting. *Periodontics* 6: 121–129.

Wei, P.C., Laurell, L., Geivelis, M. et al. (2000). Acellular dermal matrix allografts to achieve increased attached gingiva. Part 1. A clinical study. *J. Periodontol.* 71: 1297–1305.

Yan, J.J., Tsai, A.Y., Wong, M.Y., and Hou, L.T. (2006). Comparison of acellular dermal graft and palatal autograft in the reconstruction of keratinized gingiva around dental implants: a case report. *Int. J. Periodontics Restorative Dent.* 26: 287–292.

Yu, S.K., Lee, M.H., Kim, C.S. et al. (2014). Thickness of the palatal masticatory mucosa with reference to autogenous grafting: a cadaveric and histologic study. *Int. J. Periodontics Restorative Dent.* 34: 115–121.

Zabalequi, I., Sicilia, A., Cambra, J. et al. (1999). Treatment of multiple adjacent gingival recessions with the tunnel subepithelial connective tissue graft: a clinical report. *Int. J. Periodontics Restorative Dent.* 19: 199–206.

Further Reading

Shi, Y., Segelnick, S.L., and El Chaar, E.S. (2020). A modified technique of tacking acellular dermal matrix to increase keratinized mucosa around dental implants as an alternative to a free gingival graft: a case report. *Clin. Adv. Periodontics* 10 (4): 175–180.

Tal, H., Moses, O., Zohar, R. et al. (2002). Root coverage of advanced gingival recession: a comparative study between acellular dermal matrix allograft and sub-epithelial connective tissue grafts. *J. Periodontol.* 73: 1404–1411.

21

Peri-Implant Diseases

Edgard El Chaar[1] and Cecilia White[2]

[1] Department of Periodontics, University of Pennsylvania, Dental Medicine, Philadelphia, PA, USA
[2] Private practice, Princeton, NJ, USA

Introduction

The prevalence of inflammatory diseases of bacterial origin around dental implants has been very well reported in literature making it an essential component of clinical implant care (Lang and Berglundh 2011; Sanz and Chapple 2012; Shibli et al. 2008; Lindhe et al. 2008). Two clinical conditions are described: peri-implant mucositis and peri-implantitis, defined as the inflammation in the mucosa surrounding an implant without signs of loss of supporting bone (Lindhe et al. 2008; Zitzmann and Berglundh 2008).

Peri-implantitis: Inflammatory disease of the soft tissues surrounding an implant, accompanied by bone loss that exceeds normal physiologic remodeling (Zitzmann and Berglundh 2008; Sanz and Chapple 2012). It is accepted that mucositis precedes peri-implantitis (Jepsen et al. 2015) and if left untreated, peri-implant mucositis can lead to peri-implantitis (Jepsen et al. 2015; Costa et al. 2012).

The world workshop between the AAP and EFP in 2017 (Schwarz et al. 2018) concluded the following parameters related to peri-implantitis:

- Peri-implantitis is a pathological condition occurring in tissues around dental implants, characterized by inflammation in the peri-implant connective tissue and progressive loss of supporting bone.
- The histopathologic and clinical conditions leading to the conversion from peri-implant mucositis to peri-implantitis are not completely understood.
- The onset of peri-implantitis may occur early during follow-up and the disease progresses in a non-linear and accelerating pattern.
- Peri-implantitis sites exhibit clinical signs of inflammation and increased probing depths compared with baseline measurements.

- At the histologic level, compared with periodontitis sites, peri-implantitis sites often have larger inflammatory lesions.
- Surgical entry at peri-implantitis sites often reveals a circumferential pattern of bone loss.
- There is strong evidence that there is an increased risk of developing peri-implantitis in patients who have a history of chronic periodontitis, poor plaque control skills, and no regular maintenance care after implant therapy. Data identifying "smoking" and "diabetes" as potential risk factors/indicators for peri-implantitis are inconclusive.
- There is some limited evidence linking peri-implantitis to other factors such as: post-restorative presence of submucosal cement, lack of peri-implant keratinized mucosa, and positioning of implants that make it difficult to perform oral hygiene and maintenance.
- Evidence suggests that progressive crestal bone loss around implants in the absence of clinical signs of soft tissue inflammation is a rare event.

Prevalence

Multiple authors have studied the prevalence of peri-implantitis and peri-mucositis on implant level and patient level. Differences in inclusion criteria have led to a wide range of results. Recently, Derks et al. (2016) reviewed 588 patients and 2277 implants over nine years and found:

Patient level: Mucositis: 32% Peri-implantitis: 45% *Implant* level: Mucositis: 35.1% Peri-implantitis: 24.9%. Additionally, Pimentel et al. (2018) included 147 patients with 490 implants and found: Patient level: Mucositis: 80.9% Peri-implantitis: 19.1% Implant level: Mucositis: 85.3%, peri-implantitis: 9.2%.

Criteria for Diagnosis of Peri-implantitis: Case Definition

According to the 2017 World Workshop (Schwarz et al. 2018), a diagnosis of peri-implantitis will be based on the following:

1. Presence of peri-implant signs of inflammation: redness, swelling, line or drop of bleeding within 30 seconds following probing, and/or suppuration
2. Increasing probing depth as compared with probing depth values compared with measurements obtained at placement of the prosthetic superstructure
3. Radiographic evidence of bone loss following initial healing (one year following prosthetic superstructure delivery)
4. In the absence of previous radiographs, radiographic bone loss ≥3 mm, and/or PD ≥6 mm in combination with bleeding on probing (BOP)

Additionally, clinical and radiographic examinations are necessary to evaluate peri-implant health (Jepsen et al. 2015; Schwarz et al. 2018). Clinical evaluation of the peri-implant soft tissue should include assessment of the patient's oral hygiene and the presence or absence of bacterial biofilm and visual evaluation of dental implants should be completed at least once per year including probing with a light force (~0.25 N). Implant health is indicated by a peri-implant probing depth of ≤5mm and an absence of bleeding on probing. Radiographic analysis requires a baseline X-ray, preferably with the suprastructure in place, and the reference point of the implant platform will allow assessment of changes in the bone level over time.

Risk Factors

History of Periodontitis

In a study involving 80 patients with peri-implant mucositis followed for five years, Costa et al. (2012) found the overall incidence of peri-implantitis to be 31.2% and that periodontitis patients had significantly higher odds of developing peri-implantitis with an odd ratio ranging from 4.1 to 9 (Costa et al. 2012; Koldsland et al. 2011; Derks et al. 2016). Complete edentulism resulted in a significant reduction of bacteria related to periodontitis and peri-implantitis, with the exception of *Aggregatibacter actinomycetemcomitans*, which might indicate that key pathogens can survive without pockets (Quirynen and Van Assche 2011).

The specific diagnosis and severity of the periodontal condition can also influence the risk for peri-implantitis.

The risk ratio for failure in patients with aggressive periodontitis is significantly higher when compared with healthy patients and those with chronic periodontitis (Monje et al. 2014). Additionally, the more severe the diagnosis and those with greater probing depths were at a greater risk (Daubert et al. 2015; Pimentel et al. 2018).

Implant Maintenance

Implant success depends largely on good plaque control and regular maintenance. The incidence of peri-implantitis in non-maintained patients is 44% while the incidence in maintained patients is 18% (Costa et al. 2012). Tan et al. (2017) found periodontally susceptible patients following a strict periodontal maintenance program had similar peri-implant crestal bone loss as compared with periodontally non-susceptible subjects over six years of follow-up. This study highlights the benefits of a strict periodontal maintenance.

Number of Implants

The number of implants a patient has also affects their risk. Patients with ≥4 implants had a greater risk of developing peri-implantitis (Derks et al. 2016; Pimentel et al. 2018).

Clinician Experience

Implants are more successful when placed by surgical specialists as those implants placed and restored by general dentist have a greater risk with an odds ratio of 4.3 (Derks et al. 2016).

Implant Brand

Peri-implantitis risk also varied between manufacturers with Nobel: OR 3.8 Astra: OR: 3.6 Other: OR 5.6. (Derks et al. 2016).

Smoking

Smokers had greater risk for peri-implantitis and for implant failure (Pimentel et al. 2018; Chen et al. 2013; Johnson and Hill 2004). The mechanism for this may be: smoking negatively influences oral microbial profile, suppresses the immune system, and alters microvascular environment, leading to disrupted healing (Johnson and Hill 2004). Factors relating to the greater risk with smokers include an altered oral microbial profile, reduced tissue oxygenation caused by carbon monoxide, vasoconstrictive properties of nicotine, and its cytotoxic effects on fibroblasts and PMNs (Johnson and Hill 2004; Liddelow and Klineberg 2011).

Microbiota

The most studied risk factor for peri-implantitis has been the microbiota (Padial-Molina et al. 2016). Zitzmann et al. (2001) demonstrated that once plaque deposits are from implants, the signs of inflammation in the peri-implant tissue disappeared. There have been cases where the primary causative agent in peri-implantitis was non-bacterial, such as the presence of irritating excess cement under the implant crown or implant fracture. However, it has been shown that these causative agents create a different ecological environment that shifts the composition of the biofilm to a more pathogenic one that is harmful to the peri-implant tissues (Mombelli and Décaillet 2011; Wilson 2009). Therefore, the ensuing tissue destruction and bone loss is still caused by the bacteria in the plaque biofilm that has accumulated on the implant surface (Canullo et al. 2016).

Various studies have been conducted to study the composition of this microbiota. Similar bacteria to those found in periodontal disease, such as *Porphyromonas gingivalis*, *Prevotella intermedia*, *Fusobacterium nucleatum*, *Tannerella Forsythia*, and *Treponema. denticola* have been implicated (Mombelli and Décaillet 2011; Maximo et al. 2009). Additionally, a general shift from Gram-positive coccoid species in health to anaerobic Gram-negative rods in peri-implantitis was seen (Padial-Molina et al. 2016). Successful implants contained little amounts of cultivable bacteria and they had mostly Gram-positive coccoid bacteria. Bacteria around implants with peri-implantitis were found at high levels and mostly consisted of Gram-negative anaerobic rods. More specifically, there was an abundance of Fusobacterium and *P. intermedia* (Mombelli et al. 1987). Peri-implantitis biofilm represents a mixed infection, with a majority consisting of diverse anaerobic Gram-negative bacteria (Mombelli and Décaillet 2011).

Earlier literature cites periodontal pathogens as the culprits behind peri-implantitis. However, the methods of detection involve either bacterial cultures or DNA probe analysis. Both types of methods may be biased because they involve pre-selection of bacteria for detection. Newer techniques such as metagenomics and 16S rRNA sequencing are beginning to elucidate new bacterial species beyond periodontopathogens. These include *Streptococcus, Eubacterium, Filifactor alocis, Parvimonas micra, Staphylococcus*, and more (Padial-Molina et al. 2016; Tamura et al. 2013). There have also been a number of fungi and viruses detected at higher levels around implants with peri-implantitis (Schwarz et al. 2018).

Treatment

It has been generally accepted that peri-implantitis is caused by microbial infection. As a result, any treatment protocol for peri-implantitis must include decontamination of the exposed contaminated implant surface. This said, decontamination is a difficult task that is complicated by the basic structure of the implant. Most modern implants have a medium rough surface structure in order to increase the bone-implant contact area and facilitate osseointegration. This can complicate the management of infections deep inside the peri-implant pocket, as increased surface area and surface roughness may facilitate microbial colonization and enhance biofilm formation.

Recent evidence suggests that the surface roughness and chemical composition of the implant surface can have an impact on plaque accumulation and thus contribute to the difficulty in reducing the bacterial load to a level necessary for resolution of peri-implant inflammation (Teughels et al. 2006).

Nonsurgical Therapy

Non-surgical treatment should always be done prior to surgical intervention as it allows the clinician to gauge the healing response and to assess the patient's ability to perform effective oral hygiene.

Peri-implant Mucositis

Similar to gingivitis, symptoms of peri-implant mucositis can be reversed via improved oral hygiene or effective removal of excess cement or other foreign material. The treatment for peri-implant mucositis often involves mechanical debridement alone. Schenk et al. (1997) found improved results after three months with scaling with rubber cup polishing; Strooker et al. (1998) found similar results using a carbon fiber brush with rubber cup polishing; and Thöne-Mühling et al. (2010) used plastic curettes + ultrasonic scaling.

The use of 0.12% CHX was found to be similar compared with a placebo as an adjunct to non-surgical therapy in patients with peri-implant mucositis (Menezes et al. 2016). The effect of local antibiotics as a treatment for peri-implantitis is limited. One study concluded that antibiotics as an adjunct to mechanical therapy had no impact on bacterial counts after six months and limited clinical effect (Hallström et al. 2012).

Peri-implantitis

Unlike peri-implant mucositis, treatment for peri-implantitis must take into account the extension of the inflammation beyond the soft tissue leading to destruction of hard and soft tissue attachment around the implant body.

Mechanical Debridement Karring et al. (2005) studied the vector system carbon fiber tip versus manual carbon-fiber curette. Only minor changes in bleeding at six months were noted with no change or increase in PD. Renvert et al. (2009) used titanium curettes versus ultrasonic device designed for implants. Decreased BOP and PI at six months. No change in PD Muthukuru et al. (2012): In a review of the non-surgical management of peri-implantitis: The available evidence suggested that submucosal debridement with adjunctive local delivery of antibiotics, submucosal glycine powder air polishing, or Er:YAG laser treatment may reduce clinical signs of peri-implant mucosal inflammation to a greater extent relative to submucosal debridement using curettes with adjunctive irrigation with chlorhexidine.

Sahm et al. (2011) conducted a prospective randomized clinical trials (RCT) using an air-abrasive device or mechanical debridement with carbon curettes and local application of CHX. Statistical significant decrease in BOP using air-abrasive, limited improvements noted at three and six months for both modalities.

Antibiotic Therapy As far as antibiotic therapy, systemic antibiotics had limited effects on the reduction of persisting implant sites (Stein et al. 2018). Alternatively, local delivery has been used with success. Mombelli et al. (2001) found the use of tetracycline (actisite) led to PD reduction of 1.9 mm over 12 months while Renvert et al. (2006) in a 12 months follow-up, minocycline (arestin) led to PD reduction of 0.6 mm.

Photodynamic Treatment (PDT) The use of lasers and photodynamic therapy has been used with increasing frequency in recent years. Schwarz et al. (2006) found that Er:Yag laser has a bactericidal effect and studied implant surface decontamination prior to guided bone regeneration (GBR) in the treatment of peri-implantitis. Er:YAG laser yielded similar clinical outcomes compared with plastic curettes, cotton pellets, and saline solution (Schwarz et al. 2012).

Er:YAG and ER,CR:YSGG lasers were more advantageous in removing calcified deposits on microstructure surface of titanium implants without inducing damage, compared with mechanical therapy by cotton pellet or titanium curette (in-vitro study). *Er-YAG* is the laser best suited for implant surface detoxification in the treatment of peri-implantitis lesions (Ogita et al. 2015; Takagi et al. 2018).

Alternatively, Chambrone et al. (2018) found that Photodynamic treatment (PDT) showed similar improvements in PD and clinical attachment level (CAL) compared with conventional therapy for both periodontitis and peri-implantitis.

Surgical Treatment

Claffey et al. (2008), in a systematic review of the literature, divided their findings into human and animal studies.

In the animal studies they found: re-osseointegration can occur on previously contaminated surfaces. The surface characteristics are decisive for regeneration and re-osseointegration. No single chemical surface decontamination method appears to be distinctly superior (chemical decontamination consisted of: hydrogen peroxide, citric acid, sodium chloride, chloramines, tetracycline hydrochloride, and CHX). Open debridement with surface decontamination can achieve resolution.

In the human studies they found: in access surgery resolution occurred in 58% of the lesions. No single method of surface decontamination (chemical agents, air abrasives, and lasers) was found to be superior. The use of regenerative procedures such as bone graft techniques with or without the use of barrier membranes has been reported with various degrees of success. However, it must be stressed that such techniques do not address disease resolution but rather merely attempt to fill the osseous defect.

Renvert et al. (2009) in a systematic review of 25 animal studies found that: re-osseointegration is possible to obtain on a previously contaminated implant surface. Implant surface characteristics may influence the degree of re-osseointegration. Surface decontamination doesn't achieve substantial re-osseointegration on a previously contaminated implant surface. No method predictably accomplished complete resolution of the peri-implant defect.

The most widely used chemical decontaminant is hydrogen peroxide for two minutes due to availability, efficiency, and safety and must be rinsed thoroughly with sterile saline (Renvert and Polyzois 2000).

DeWaal et al. (2013) studied surface decontamination during flap surgery leads to greater suppression of anaerobic bacteria in the short term but does not lead to better clinical results. Aghazadeh et al. (2012) found that surgical debridement followed by placement of either bovine bone graft versus autogenous bone. They found significantly better clinical results with bovine for bone levels, BOP, suppuration.

What Is the Most Predictable or Superior Treatment Modality?

Subramani and Wismeijer (2012) found that both mechanical and chemical decontamination techniques should be applied alongside regenerative surgical procedures to obtain optimum re-osseointegration and successfully treat peri-implantitis (Strooker et al. 1998).

Mellado-Valero et al. (2013) found that there is sufficient consensus that, for the treatment of peri-implant infections, the mechanical removal of biofilm from the implant surface should be supplemented by chemical decontamination with surgical access (Thöne-Mühling et al. 2010).

Heitz-Mayfield and Mombelli (2014) in a systematic and meta-analysis of different treatment protocols that included mechanical, chemical, and laser detoxification concluded that due to the variety of surface decontamination treatments with limited comparative studies, no specific protocol has been shown to be more effective than the others for treatment of peri-implantitis.

Chan et al. (2014), a systematic review and meta-analysis of treatment outcomes, found that the most essential component of any treatment protocol for peri-implantitis is the decontamination of the exposed contaminated implant surface. The primary objective is to alter the microbiota in such a way so that the resident microbiota at the implant surface is compatible with the host so that the host immune system has the potential to eliminate putative pathogens effectively.

In summary, although the treatment of peri-implantitis may be challenging and the consensus on the treatment modalities is still not very well established, it is still necessary. Steps should include: infection control, non-surgical debridement, corrective/regenerative surgical procedures, and supportive therapy.

Clinical Case to Illustrate Peri-implantitis Treatment

A 35 year old male presented with purulence and discomfort on implant in position #8 that was placed 4 years earlier in an immediate placement after tooth extracted (Figure 21.1). A radiograph revealed a bone loss around the implant (Figure 21.2). A full thickness flap was elevated buccally with papilla sparing showing the inflammed tissue encapsulated with xenograft (Figure 21.3). A complete debridement using a Er,Cr:YSGG laser and hand instrumentation (Figure 21.4). This revealed the presences of a bonding cement used to cement the crown. Using high speed rotary burs consisited of very fine carbide and diamond, the cement and the contaminated rough surface

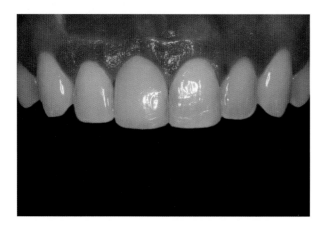

Figure 21.1 A 35 year old male presented with purulence and discomfort on implant in position #8 that was placed 4 years earlier in an immediate placement after tooth extracted.

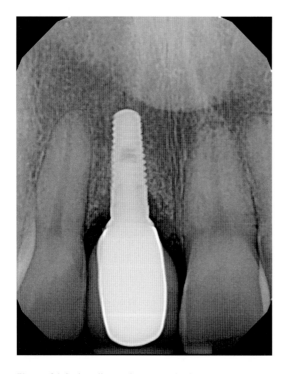

Figure 21.2 A radiograph revealed a bone loss around the implant.

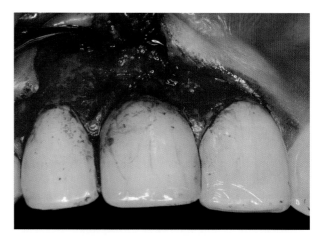

Figure 21.3 A full thickness flap was elevated buccally with papilla sparing showing the inflamed tissue encapsulated with xenograft.

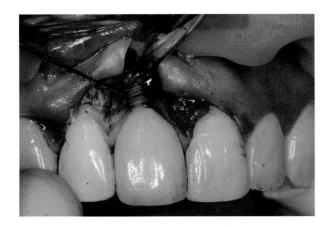

Figure 21.4 A complete debridement using a Er,Cr:YSGG laser and hand instrumentation.

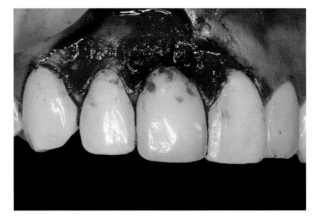

Figure 21.7 A cancellous allograft was placed.

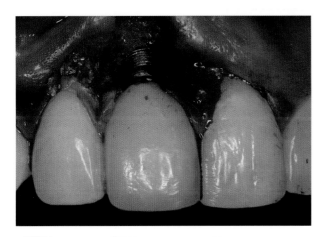

Figure 21.5 This revealed the presences of a bonding cement used to cement the crown. Using high speed rotary burs consisted of very fine carbide and diamond, the cement and the contaminated rough surface of the implant were mechanically treated under copious irrigation.

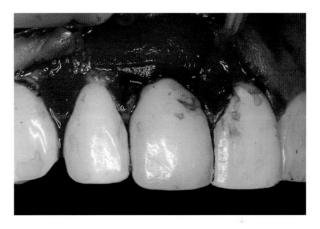

Figure 21.8 And covered by a resorbable collagen membrane.

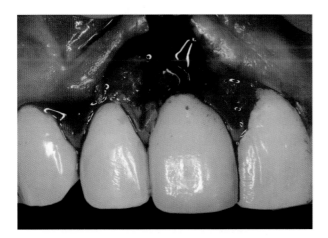

Figure 21.6 An acid etch was applied for 1 minute and thoroughly rinsed.

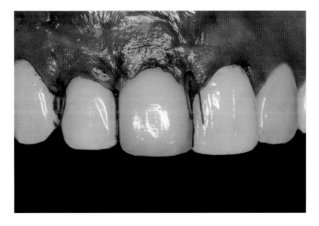

Figure 21.9 A coronally advanced flap was passivated and covered the graft.

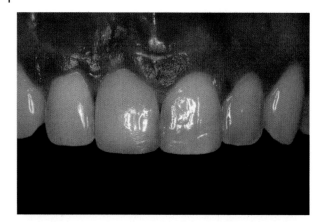

Figure 21.10 A five year follow-up clinical picture shows the healthy outcome.

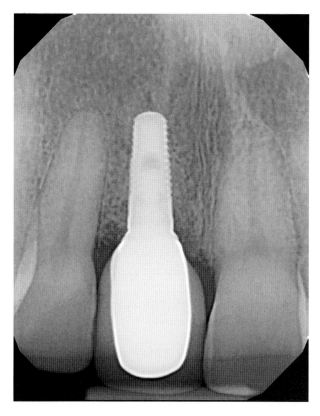

Figure 21.11 A radiograph showing the stability of the grafted site.

of the implant were implantoplastied (Figure 21.5). After an acid etch was applied for 1 minute and thoroughly rinsed (Figure 21.6). At this point a cancellous allograft was placed (Figure 21.7) and covered by a resorbable collagen membrane (Figure 21.8). A coronally advanced flap was passivated and covered the exposed implant (Figure 21.9).

A five years follow-up clinical picture shows the healthy outcome and a radiograph showing the stability of the grafted site. (Figures 21.10 and 21.11)

References

Aghazadeh, A., Persson, G.R., and Renvert, S. (2012). A single-centre randomized controlled clinical trial on the adjunct treatment of intra-bony defects with autogenous bone or a xenograft: results after 12 months. *J. Clin. Periodontol.* 39: 666–673.

Canullo, L., Tallarico, M., Radovanovic, S. et al. (2016). Distinguishing predictive profiles for patient-based risk assessment and diagnostics of plaque induced, surgically and prosthetically triggered peri-implantitis. *Clin. Oral Implants Res.* 27 (10): 1243–1250.

Chambrone, L., Wang, H.L., and Romanos, G.E. (2018). Antimicrobial photodynamic therapy for the treatment of periodontitis and peri-implantitis: an American Academy of Periodontology best evidence review. *J. Periodontol.* 89 (7): 783–803.

Chan, H.L., Lin, G.H., Suarez, F. et al. (2014). Surgical management of peri-implantitis: a systematic review and meta-analysis of treatment outcomes. *J. Periodontol.* 85 (8): 1027–1041.

Chen, H., Liu, N., Xu, X. et al. (2013). Smoking, radiotherapy, diabetes and osteoporosis as risk factors for dental implant failure: a meta-analysis. *PLoS One* 8 (8): e71955. https://doi .org/10.1371/journal.pone.0071955.

Claffey, N., Clarke, E., Polyzois, I., and Renvert, S. (2008). Surgical treatment of peri-implantitis. *J. Clin. Periodontol.* 35: 316–332.

Costa, F.O., Takenaka-Martinez, S., Cota, L.O. et al. (2012). Peri-implant disease in subjects with and without preventive maintenance: a 5-year follow-up. *J. Clin. Periodontol.* 39 (2): 173–181.

Daubert, D.M., Weinstein, B.F., Bordin, S. et al. (2015). Prevalence and predictive factors for peri-implant disease and implant failure: a cross-sectional analysis. *J. Periodontol.* 86 (3): 337–347.

Derks, J., Schaller, D., Håkansson, J. et al. (2016). Effectiveness of implant therapy analyzed in a Swedish population: prevalence of peri-implantitis. *J. Dent. Res.* 95 (1): 43–49.

DeWaal, Y.C.M., Raghoebar, G.M., Huddleston Slater, J.J.R. et al. (2013). Implant decontamination during surgical peri-implantitis treatment: a randomized, double-blind, placebo-controlled trial. *J. Clin. Periodontol.* 40: 186–195.

Hallström, H., Persson, G.R., Lindgren, S. et al. (2012). Systemic antibiotics and debridement of peri-implant mucositis. A randomized clinical trial. *J. Clin. Periodontol.* 39 (6): 574–581.

Heitz-Mayfield, L.J. and Mombelli, A. (2014). The therapy of peri-implantitis: a systematic review. *Int. J. Oral Maxillofac. Implants* (Suppl): 325–345.

Jepsen, S., Berglundh, T., Genco, R. et al. (2015). Primary prevention of periimplantitis: managing peri-implant mucositis. *J. Clin. Periodontol.* 42 (Suppl. 16): S152–S157.

Johnson, G.K. and Hill, M. (2004). Cigarette smoking and the periodontal patient. *J. Periodontol.* 75 (2): 196–209. https://doi.org/10.1902/jop.2004.75.2.196.

Karring, E.S., Stavropoulos, A., Ellegaard, B., and Karring, T. (2005). Treatment of peri-implantitis by the Vector system. A pilot study. *Clin. Oral Implants Res.* 16: 288–293.

Koldsland, O.C., Scheie, A.A., and Aass, A.M. (2011). The association between selected risk indicators and severity of peri-implantitis using mixed model analyses. *J. Clin. Periodontol.* 38 (3): 285–292.

Lang, N.P. and Berglundh, T. (2011). Working Group 4 of Seventh European Workshop on Periodontology. Periimplant diseases: where are we now? – Consensus of the Seventh European Workshop on Periodontology. *J. Clin. Periodontol.* 38 (Suppl. 11): 178–181.

Liddelow, G. and Klineberg, I. (2011). Patient-related risk factors for implant therapy. A critique of pertinent literature. *Aust. Dent. J.* 56 (4): 417–441. https://doi.org/10.1111/j.1834-7819.2011.01367.

Lindhe, J., Meyle, J., and Group DoEWoP (2008). Peri-implant diseases: consensus report of the Sixth European Workshop on Periodontology. *J. Clin. Periodontol.* 35 (Suppl. 8): 282–285.

Maximo, M.B., De Mendonça, A.C., Renata Santos, V. et al. (2009). Short-term clinical and microbiological evaluations of peri-implant diseases before and after mechanical anti-infective therapies. *Clin. Oral Implants Res.* 20 (1): 99–108.

Mellado-Valero, A., Buitrago-Vera, P., Solá-Ruiz, M.-F., and Ferrer-García, J.-C. (2013). Decontamination of dental implant surface in peri-implantitis treatment: a literature review. *Med. Oral Patol. Oral Cir. Bucal.* 18 (6): e869–e876.

Menezes, K.M., Fernandes-Costa, A.N., Silva-Neto, R.D. et al. (2016). Efficacy of 0.12% chlorhexidine gluconate for non-surgical treatment of peri-implant mucositis. *J. Periodontol.* 87 (11): 1305–1313.

Mombelli, A. and Décaillet, F. (2011). The characteristics of biofilms in peri-implant disease. *J. Clin. Periodontol.* 38: 203–213.

Mombelli, A., Van Oosten, M.A., Schürch, E. Jr., and Lang, N.P. (1987). The microbiota associated with successful or failing osseointegrated titanium implants. *Oral Microbiol. Immunol.* 2 (4): 145–151.

Mombelli, A., Feloutzis, A., Brägger, U., and Lang, N.P. (2001). Treatment of peri-implantitis by local delivery of tetracycline: clinical, microbiological and radiological results. *Clin. Oral Implants Res.* 12 (4): 287–294.

Monje, A., Alcoforado, G., Padial-Molina, M. et al. (2014). Generalized aggressive periodontitis as a risk factor for dental implant failure: a systematic review and meta-analysis. *J. Periodontol.* 85 (10): 1398–1407.

Muthukuru, M., Zainvi, A., Esplugues, E.O., and Flemmig, T.F. (2012). Non-surgical therapy for the management of peri-implantitis: a systematic review. *Clin. Oral Implants Res.* 23: 77–83.

Ogita, M., Tsuchida, S., Aoki, A. et al. (2015). Increased cell proliferation and differential protein expression induced by low-level Er: YAG laser irradiation in human gingival fibroblasts: proteomic analysis. *Lasers Med. Sci.* 30 (7): 1855–1866.

Padial-Molina, M., López-Martínez, J., O'Valle, F., and Galindo-Moreno, P. (2016). Microbial profiles and detection techniques in peri-implant diseases: a systematic review. *J. Oral Maxillofac. Res.* 7 (3): e10.

Pimentel, S.P., Shiota, R., Cirano, F.R. et al. (2018). Occurrence of peri-implant diseases and risk indicators at the patient and implant levels: a multilevel cross-sectional study. *J. Periodontol.* 89 (9): 1091–1100.

Quirynen, M. and Van Assche, N. (2011). Microbial changes after full-mouth tooth extraction, followed by 2-stage implant placement. *J. Clin. Periodontol.* 38 (6): 581–589.

Renvert, S. and Polyzois, I. (2000). Treatment of pathologic peri-implant pockets. *Periodontology* 2018 (76): 180–190.

Renvert, S., Lessem, J., Dahlén, G. et al. (2006). Topical minocycline microspheres versus topical chlorhexidine gel as an adjunct to mechanical debridement of incipient peri-implant infections: a randomized clinical trial. *J. Clin. Periodontol.* 33 (5): 362–369.

Renvert, S., Samuelsson, E., Lindahl, C., and Persson, G.R. (2009). Mechanical non-surgical treatment of peri-implantitis: a double blind randomized longitudinal clinical study. I: clinical results. *J. Clin. Periodontol.* 36: 604–609.

Renvert, S., Polyzois, I., and Maguire, R. (2009). Re-osseointegration on previously contaminated surfaces: a systematic review. *Clin. Oral Implants Res.* 20: 216–227.

Sahm, N., Becker, J., Santel, T., and Schwarz, F. (2011). Non-surgical treatment of peri-implantitis using an air-abrasive device or mechanical debridement and local application of chlorhex idine: a prospective, randomized, controlled clinical study. *J. Clin. Periodontol.* 38: 872–878.

Sanz, M. and Chapple, I.L. (2012). Working Group 4 of the VEWoP. Clinical research on peri-implant diseases:

consensus report of Working Group 4. *J. Clin. Periodontol.* 39 (Suppl 12): 202–206.

Sanz, M. and Chapple, I.L. (2012). Working Group 4 of the VIII European Workshop on Periodontology. Clinical research on peri-implant diseases: consensus report of working group 4. *J. Clin. Periodontol.* 39 (Suppl 12): 202–206.

Schenk, G., Flemmig, T.F., Betz, T. et al. (1997). Some clinical and radiographical features of submerged and non-submerged titanium implants. A 5-year follow-up study. *Clin. Oral Implants Res.* 8 (5): 427–433.

Schwarz, F., Bieling, K., Nuesry, E. et al. (2006). Clinical and histological healing pattern of peri-implantitis lesions following non-surgical treatment with an Er: YAG laser. *Lasers Surg. Med.* 38 (7): 663–671.

Schwarz, F., John, G., Mainusch, S. et al. (2012). Combined surgical therapy of peri-implantitis evaluating two methods of surface debridement and decontamination. A two-year clinical follow up report. *J. Clin. Periodontol.* 39 (8): 789–797.

Schwarz, F., Derks, J., Monje, A., and Wang, H.-L. (2018). Peri-implantitis. *J. Periodontol.* 89 (Suppl 1): S267–S290.

Shibli, J.A., Melo, L., Ferrari, D.S. et al. (2008). Composition of supra and subgingival biofilm of subjects with healthy and diseased Implants. *Clin. Oral Implants Res.* 19: 975–982.

Stein, J.M., Hammächer, C., and Michael, S.S. (2018). Combination of ultrasonic decontamination, soft tissue curettage, and submucosal air polishing with povidone-iodine application for non-surgical therapy of peri-implantitis: 12-month clinical outcomes. *J. Periodontol.* 89 (2): 139–147.

Strooker, H., Rohn, S., and Van Winkelhoff, A.J. (1998). Clinical and microbiological effects of chemical versus mechanical cleansing in professional supportive implant therapy. *Int. J. Oral Maxillofac. Implants* 13: 845–850.

Subramani, K. and Wismeijer, D. (2012). Decontamination of titanium implant surface and re-osseointegration to treat peri-implantitis: a literature review. *Int. J. Oral Maxillofac. Implants* 27: 1043–1054.

Takagi, T., Aoki, A., Ichinose, S. et al. (2018). Effective removal of calcified deposits on microstructured titanium fixture surfaces of dental implants with erbium lasers. *J. Periodontol.* 89 (6): 680–690.

Tamura, N., Ochi, M., Miyakawa, H., and Nakazawa, F. (2013). Analysis of bacterial flora associated with peri-implantitis using obligate anaerobic culture technique and 16S rDNA gene sequence. *Int. J. Oral Maxillofac. Implants* 28 (6): 1521–1529.

Tan, W.C., Ong, M.M.A., and Lang, N.P. (2017). Influence of maintenance care in periodontally susceptible and non-susceptible subjects following implant therapy. *Clin. Oral Implants Res.* 28: 491–494.

Teughels, W., Van Assche, N., Sliepen, I., and Quirynen, M. (2006). Effect of material characteristics and or surface topography on bio- film development. *Clin. Oral Implants Res.* 17 (Suppl. 2): 68–81.

Thöne-Mühling, M., Swierkot, K., Nonnenmacher, C. et al. (2010). Comparison of two full-mouth approaches in the treatment of peri-implant mucositis: a pilot study. *Clin. Oral Implants Res.* 21 (5): 504–512.

Wilson, T.G. Jr. (2009). The positive relationship between excess cement and peri-implant disease: a prospective clinical endoscopic study. *J. Periodontol.* 80 (9): 1388–1392.

Zitzmann, N.U. and Berglundh, T. (2008). Definition and prevalence of peri-implant diseases. *J. Clin. Periodontol.* 35: 286–291.

Zitzmann, N.U., Berglundh, T., Marinello, C.P., and Lindhe, J. (2001). Experimental peri-implant mucositis in man. *J. Clin. Periodontol.* 28 (6): 517–523.

Index